TUMORS OF THE KIDNEY

THIS VOLUME IS ONE OF A SERIES

International Perspectives In Urology

EDITED BY
John A. Libertino, M.D.

International Perspectives In Urology

Volume 13

John A. Libertino, M.D.
series editor

TUMORS OF
THE KIDNEY

Editors

Jean B. deKernion, M.D.

Professor of Surgery/Urology
Chief, Division of Urology
Director for Clinical Programs
University of California, Los Angeles
Jonsson Comprehensive Cancer Center
Los Angeles, California

M. Pavone-Macaluso

Professor
Institutodi Clinica Urologica
Dell' Università di Palermo
Palermo, Italy

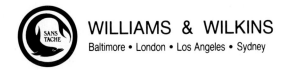

WILLIAMS & WILKINS
Baltimore • London • Los Angeles • Sydney

Editor: Kimberly Kist
Associate Editor: Victoria M. Vaughn
Copy Editor: Deborah K. Tourtlotte
Design: Bob Och
Illustration Planning: Lorraine Wrzosek
Production: Raymond E. Reter

Printed in the United States of America

Library of Congress Cataloging-in-Publication Data

Tumors of the kidney.

  (International perspectives in urology; v. 13) Includes bibliographies and index.
  1. Kidneys—Cancer. 2. Adenocarcinoma. 3. Kidneys—Tumors. I. deKernion, Jean
B., 1940–   . II. Pavone-Macaluso, Michele. III. Series. [DNLM: 1. Kidney Neo-
plasms—diagnosis. 2. Kidney Neoplasms—therapy. W1 IN827K v.13 / WJ 358
T9248] RC280.K5T86 1986   616.99′461   85-22543
ISBN 0-683-02426-4

Composed and printed at the   86 87 88 89 90
Waverly Press, Inc.   10 9 8 7 6 5 4 3 2 1

Series Editor's Foreword

Renal cell carcinoma accounts for an estimated 5,000 to 7,000 deaths yearly in the United States. These tumors occur most frequently in the 40-year to 69-year age group, but the incidence in patients in the fifth decade of life seems to be increasing. Although uncommon, renal cell carcinoma is occasionally seen in the pediatric population.

Even though considerable effort has been used to determine the cause and pathogenesis of renal cell carcinoma in humans, the cause still remains unknown. The discovery that administration of diethylstilbestrol can produce renal tumors in the Syrian hamster led to an interesting series of experiments, including the demonstration of all stages of tumor development from tubular hyperplasia to invasive carcinoma.

Dr. Jean deKernion, Professor and Chairman of the Department of Urology at the University of California School of Medicine in Los Angeles, provides us with a contemporary view of the management of patients who have renal cell carcinoma. In editing this book, Dr. deKernion has included authors who have been responsible for many of the advances made in the diagnosis and management of renal cell carcinoma.

This book provides an up-to-date summary of advances made in the field and will be of great benefit to urologists engaged in the care of patients with renal cell carcinoma.

JOHN A. LIBERTINO, MD
Series Editor

Preface

Neoplasms of the adult kidney remain a major problem in urologic oncology. Although management of advanced renal cancer has not improved significantly due to the lack of effective systemic agents, advances in the surgical management and the diagnosis of renal mass lesions have improved the care of patients with renal tumors. The paucity of known effective treatment modalities for tumors of the kidney has encouraged a profusion of experimental approaches with respect to both diagnosis and treatment. Sophisticated new diagnostic approaches—both radiographic and in vitro—have been developed at many centers and show promise for improved long-term survival rates and more timely selection of treatment modalities. Investigators at many centers throughout the world have dedicated themselves to the study of these new diagnostic and therapeutic techniques. The wide dissemination of this information to an international audience is both timely and essential. This book provides a common forum in which experts from many countries report the results from their institutions and outline their own theories and practices based on these experiences. The chapter authors' synthesis of the data and analysis of the results from the various centers place into perspective the current controversies which are of concern to urologists worldwide. Such analysis of the prospects for success and the known and projected limitations of these methods is vital to the world community of urologists.

For the first time, an international panel of experts presents their experiences under a single cover, providing a ready reference to urologists, radiologists, and oncologists. Such an assimilation of current international expertise will encourage the improved management of renal tumors and provide a foundation for identification of future research needs.

J. B. deKernion, M.D.
M. Pavone-Macaluso, M.D.

Contributors

Christian Barré, M.D.
Chapter 1
Clinique Urologique de l'Hôpital
 Cochin
Paris, France

Richard Bihrle, M.D.
Chapter 8
Assistant Professor of Urology
Indiana University Medical Cen-
 ter
Indianapolis, Indiana

M. O. Bitker
Chapter 7
Clinique Urologique
Hôpital de la Pitié
C. H. U. Pitié-Salpetrière
Paris, France

Laurent Boccon-Gibod, M.D.
Chapter 1
Clinique Urologique de l'Hôpital
 Cochin
Paris, France

Aldo V. Bono, M.D.
Chapter 14
Urological Department
Regional Hospital
Varese, Italy

Christian Chatelain
Chapter 7
Clinique Urologique
Assistance Publique
Hôpitaux de Paris
Paris, France

Jean B. deKernion, M.D.
Chapter 19
Professor of Surgery/Urology
Chief, Division of Urology
Director for Clinical Programs
University of California, Los An-
 geles
Jonsson Comprehensive Cancer
 Center
Los Angeles, California

Ricardo Delgado, M.D.
Chapter 3
Pathological Institute
University of Innsbruck
Innsbruck, Austria

Anthony Golio, M.D.
Chapter 4
Department of Urology
State University of New York at
 Buffalo
The Buffalo General Hospital
The Roswell Park Memorial Insti-
 tute
Buffalo, New York

Y. Hammoudi
Chapter 7
Clinique Urologique
Hôpital de la Pitié
C. H. U. Pitié-Salpetrière
Paris, France

Ferdinand Hofstädter, M.D.
Chapter 3
Abteilung Pathologie der
 Medizinischen Fakultätat an der
 RWTH
Aachen FRG

Gerhard Jakse, M.D.
Chapter 3
Urological Department
University of Innsbruck
Innsbruck, Austria

Alain Jardin
Chapter 7
Clinique Urologique
Hôpital de la Pitié
C. H. U. Pitié-Salpetrière
Paris, France

Saad Khoury, M.D.
Chapter 13
Professor of Urology
Clinique Urologique
Hôpital de la Pitié
Paris, France

Karl F. Klippel, M.D.
Chapter 18
Urological Clinic
General Hospital
Celle, Federal Republic of Germany

Karl Heinz Kurth, M.D.
Chapter 15
Department of Urology
Erasmus University
Rotterdam, The Netherlands

Erich K. Lang, M.D.
Chapter 2
Professor and Chairman
Department of Radiology
Louisiana State University Medical Center
Professor of Radiology
Tulane School of Medicine
Director, Department of Radiology
Charity Hospital
New Orleans, Louisiana

John A. Libertino, M.D.
Chapter 8
Department of Urology
Lahey Clinic Medical Center
Burlington, Massachusetts

Michael M. Lieber, M.D.
Chapters 15, 16, and 20
Professor of Urology
Mayo Medical School
Consultant in Urology and Cell Biology
Director, Urology Research Laboratory
Mayo Clinic
Rochester, Minnesota

Michael Marberger, M.D.
Chapter 10
Department of Urology
Rudolfstiftung
Vienna, Austria

Fray F. Marshall, M.D.
Chapter 6
Associate Professor of Urology
The James Buchanan Brady Urological Institute
The Johns Hopkins Hospital
The Johns Hopkins School of Medicine
Baltimore, Maryland

Gerald P. Murphy, M.D.
Chapter 4
Department of Urology
State University of New York at Buffalo
The Buffalo General Hospital
The Roswell Park Memorial Institute
Buffalo, New York

Giorgio Pizzocaro, M.D.
Chapter 5
Chief, Urologic Section
Department of Clinical Oncology
Istituto Nazionale per lo Studio e la Cura dei Tumori
Milan, Italy

J. Edson Pontes, M.D.
Chapter 17
Head, Section of Urologic Oncology
Cleveland Clinic Foundation
Cleveland, Ohio

Hans Rauschmeier, M.D.
Chapter 3
Urological Department
University of Innsbruck
Innsbruck, Austria

J. C. Romijn, M.D.
Chapter 15
Department of Urology
Erasmus University
Rotterdam, The Netherlands

A. Saul, M.B., B.S.
Chapter 13
Clinique Urologique
Hôpital de la Pitié
Paris, France

Fritz H. Schröder, M.D.
Chapter 15
Department of Urology
Erasmus University
Rotterdam, The Netherlands

Robert B. Smith, M.D.
Chapter 9
Professor of Surgery/Urology
University of California, Los Angeles Medical Center
Chief of Urology
Wadsworth Veterans Administration Hospital
Los Angeles, California

Adolphe Steg, M.D.
Chapter 1
Clinique Urologique de l'Hôpital Cochin
Paris, France

Urs E. Studer, M.D.
Chapter 19
Urologische Universitaets Klinik
Berne, Switzerland

Gerald Sufrin, M.D.
Chapter 4
Department of Urology
State University of New York at Buffalo
The Buffalo General Hospital
The Roswell Park Memorial Institute
Buffalo, New York

David A. Swanson, M.D.
Chapter 12
Department of Urology
The University of Texas
M. D. Anderson Hospital and Tumor Institute at Houston
Houston, Texas

Taiji Tsukamoto, M.D.
Chapter 20
Department of Urology
Mayo Clinic
Rochester, Minnesota

J. W. van Dongen, M.D.
Chapter 15
Department of Urology
Erasmus University
Rotterdam, The Netherlands

Sidney Wallace, M.D.
Chapter 12
Department of Diagnostic Radiology
The University of Texas
M. D. Anderson Hospital and Tumor Institute at Houston
Houston, Texas

Grant Williams, M.S., F.R.C.S.
Chapters 11 and 21
Consultant Urologist
Charing Cross Hospital
London, England

Contents

Section 1. Diagnosis and Staging

1
Section

Diagnosis and Staging

1

Computerized Tomography for Diagnosis and Staging of Renal Adenocarcinoma

Christian Barré, M.D.
Laurent Boccon-Gibod, M.D.
Adolphe Steg, M.D.

The dramatic developments in imaging techniques provide the urologist dealing with renal cell carcinoma (RCC) with a wide range of investigative procedures. Obviously in these days of cost containment, a choice has to be made so that all of the information relevant to the selection of the suitable therapeutic option can be gathered while keeping expenses and invasiveness at their lowest. The investigation protocol currently used at the Clinique Urologique de l'Hôpital Cochin (Paris, France) is presented here, focusing on the value of the computerized tomography (CT) scan in the evaluation of local and regional tumor spread.

Imaging techniques currently used in the management of RCC include intravenous urography (IVU), ultrasonography (USG), CT scan, and arteriography and venacavography (1).

INTRAVENOUS UROGRAPHY

IVU is usually the first procedure leading to a diagnosis of renal mass. Evans (2) has shown the great diagnostic yield of early nephrotomograms, which nevertheless can miss tumors growing out from the anterior or posterior aspect of the kidney.

ULTRASONOGRAPHY

Total noninvasive and relatively inexpensive, USG tends to replace IVU as a first-line procedure. The wide use of abdominal USG in the investigation of abdominal symptoms has led to a sharp increase in the detection of asymptomatic renal masses, which sometimes are not readily apparent on a routine IVU. USG is useful in distinguishing between cystic and solid masses seen on IVU. Its main diagnostic advantage is that modifications of the kidney contour and the presence of abnormal echogenic zones within the renal parenchyma are shown.

USG and IVU are diagnostic of a solid renal mass in the vast majority of cases (3), so the use of the CT scan as a *diagnostic* procedure, in the authors' opinion, should be limited to such specific problems as hypoechogenic tumor developed by or within the renal hilum where the diagnosis of hypertrophy of Bertin's column or sinusal lipomatosis remains questionable, or necrotic tumor with a central anechogenic zone and distortion of the renal hilum or cortex contour suggestive of renal pseudotumors.

The efficacy of USG as far as evaluation of local tumor spread is concerned remains questionable; extracapsular invasion and lymphatic extension are difficult to demonstrate at their early stages. The patency of the renal vein and of the vena cava is not always easily assessed due to technical difficulties (intestinal gas, patient compliance, and morphology). On the other hand, USG is a valuable investigation to rule out the presence of liver metastasis.

CT SCAN

CT can be useful when USG is nondiagnostic. A solid tumor appears as an irregular mass, the density of which is enhanced after contrast infusion, remaining lower than that of adjacent renal parenchyma (Fig. 1.1) (4, 5). In the vast majority of cases, however, CT only confirms the diagnosis already provided by IVU and USG and, therefore, is not mandatory as far as diagnostic problems are concerned. Nevertheless, CT has great value in the evaluation of local and regional extension of the tumor (6), as also shown in the authors' series of 40 patients (3). In 10 cases, an operation was considered unwarranted, as the CT scan showed *local/regional* extension, incompatible with radical surgery. In the 30 other cases, the results of the CT scan were compared to those of surgical exploration and pathologic examination of the specimen. Following many authors (7–9), Robson et al's (10) classification has been used to compare CT scan interpretation and pathologic patterns of invasion.

Extracapsular Invasion

PERIRENAL SPACE

Poor delineation of the tumor and trabeculated hyperdense extension into the perirenal fat are considered to be specific of perirenal fat involvement (Fig. 1.2), whereas simple thickening of Gerota's fascia is not diagnostic and can occur in inflammatory or traumatic processes. This analysis is not free from pitfalls. In lean subjects, the paucity of

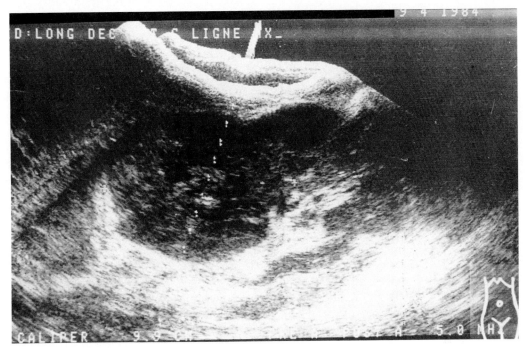

Figure 1.1 Ultrasonogram showing a hypoechogenic tumor of the upper pole of the right kidney.

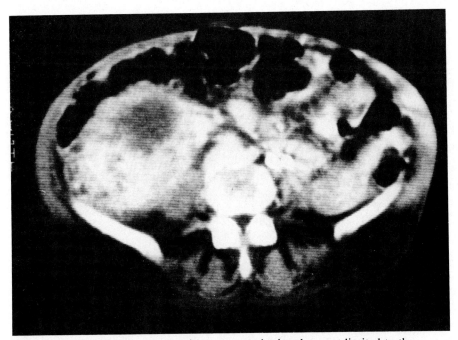

Figure 1.2 Right kidney tumor with extracapsular involvement limited to the perirenal space.

perirenal and retroperitoneal fat can mimic tumoral involvement, and a large tumor may compress perirenal fat, although it remains totally intracapsular. In the authors' series, CT misevaluated perirenal fat in

36% of the cases—four false negatives due to the microscopic invasion and seven false positives due to previously cited causes of error.

PARARENAL SPACE AND OTHER ORGANS

Although infiltration of the retroperitoneal fat associated with extension to Gerota's fascia is characteristic, direct invasion of a contiguous organ should be sought—i.e., the tumor image is prolonged by a zone of heterogeneous density extending into another organ (Fig. 1.3) or angioscannography (CT scan together with intravenous injection of contrast medium) shows a continuous zone of neovascularization—whereas different characteristics can be used to demonstrate pathologic adhesions (11). Six of the authors' patients had such lesions and were not operated. Three died of cancer within the following year; three are alive with a follow-up of 2 to 6 months, but two of them have developed pulmonary metastases. Thus, it appears that CT cannot differentiate Robson's stages I and II. However, this limitation has no surgical implication, as radical nephrectomy removes en bloc Gerota's fascia, perirenal fat, and the kidney. On the other hand, CT can demonstrate with certainty extension into a contiguous organ (7, 9), thus sparing unnecessary surgery in patients beyond the scope of radical nephrectomy.

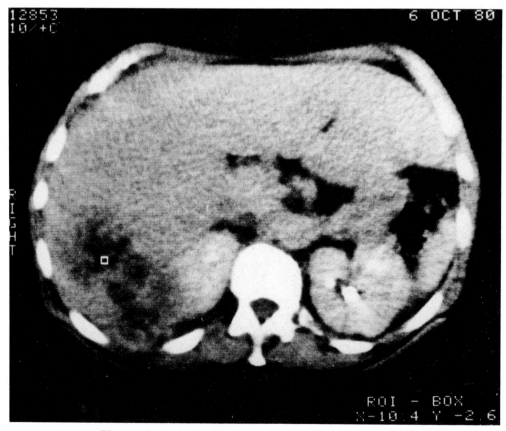

Figure 1.3 Tumor of the right kidney with involvement of the liver.

VENOUS INVOLVEMENT

Assessment of the venous status is critical in the evaluation of RCC as far as surgical technique is concerned. There is a wide range of opinions (12) concerning the value of the CT scan in this setting, due to the use of many different imaging techniques (angioscan) in the published series (13, 14). Indeed, the study of the renal veins requires a special procedure: location of the vein with a scout film and study of the densities using the angioscan technique. If the vein's obliquity precludes a complete study, the investigation should be focused on the proximal part of the vessel.

Renal vein thrombosis induces modification of morphology and densities. A diameter over 1.5 cm (15) is a good diagnostic sign when associated with modification of the densities, which appear like a heterogeneous filling defect with no or slight enhancement (10 to 20 Hounsfield units (HU)) after contrast infusion. Some aspects may be misleading; highly vascularized neoplastic thrombi can reach high densities (100 HU), thus mimicking the blood flow (Fig. 1.4). In these cases, the angioscan may be helpful by showing simultaneous enhancement in the tumor itself. The vena cava is easier to study (16); sagittal and frontal reconstructions (17) make its analysis easier. The shape and

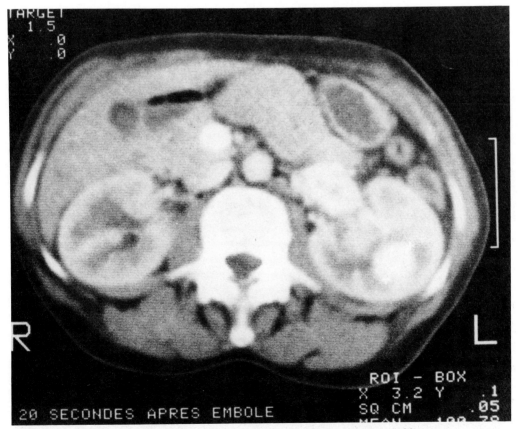

Figure 1.4 Thrombosis of the left renal vein; the density of the thrombus (100 HU) is higher than that of the tumor.

diameter of the cava vary with respiration from 1.5 to 3.7 cm (15). Whenever the angioscan cannot rule out a renal vein thrombosis, the status of the cava can be readily assessed using injection of contrast in a foot vein (18, 19).

Caval thrombosis can be suspected in the presence of a large tumor, extending into the renal hilum and associated with renal vein thrombosis. The diagnosis is confirmed by one of the following: diameter over 3.7 cm, or heterogeneous intraluminal filling defects sometimes surrounded by a ring- or crescent-like hyperdense zone.

CT can also differentiate between different types of thrombi. A heterogeneous defect is characteristic of a neoplastic thrombus, whereas a hyperdense, ring-like image is suggestive of an organizing clot with its hypervascularity. As the upper limit of the thrombus is not always easily demonstrated, cavography is often mandatory.

The authors observed three cases of venous involvement, all before the advent of the angioscan, always limited to the renal vein. There were no false negatives but two false positives in the authors' series.

LYMPH NODE ASSESSMENT

CT detects metastatic lymph nodes as round masses of more than 5 mm in diameter, with a weaker contrast uptake than surrounding vessels (Fig. 1.5). In the authors' series, there were no false negatives but four false positives. In these cases, the actual node enlargements proceeded

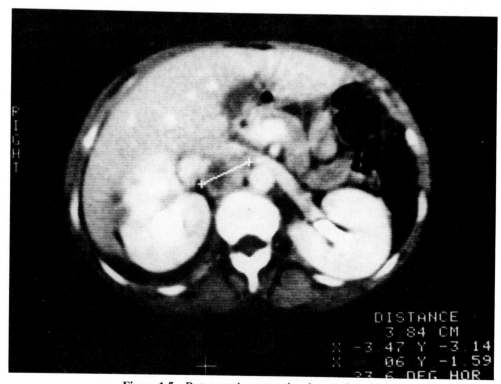

Figure 1.5 Retrocaval metastatic adenopathy with central necrosis.

Table 1.1
Performance of CT Scan in 30 Operated Patients

	Extracapsular Involvement	Venous Involvement	Nodal Involvement
True positives	5	3	2
True negatives	14	25	24
False positives	7	2	4
False negatives	4	0	0

from inflammatory processes. Thus, CT detects enlarged nodes but does not tell the nature of the nodal enlargement.

In conclusion, in the authors' hands, CT did not permit a precise preoperative staging of the tumor because of errors in evaluation of nodes and perirenal fat involvement (Table 1.1). However, CT definitely can detect venous involvement, thus helping to select the surgical approach, as well as contiguous organ involvement, thereby sparing these patients unnecessary surgery.

REFERENCES

1. Karp W, Ekelund L, Olafsson G, Losson A: Computed tomography, angiography, and ultrasound in staging of renal carcinoma. *Acta Radiol* 22:626–633, 1981.
2. Evans JA: The accuracy of diagnostic radiology: arteriography and nephrotomography. *JAMA* 204:225–226, 1968.
3. Bocon-Gibod L, Benoit G, Steg A: Diagnostic des tumeurs du rein. Le scanner est-il un luxe ou une necessite? *Nouv Presse Med* 10:3575, 1981.
4. Caron-Pointreau C, Soret JY, Lavenet F, Rieux D, Vialle M, Rognon LM: L'apport de la tomodensitometrie au diagnostic des masses renales. *Chirurgie* 105:489, 1979.
5. Sagel SS, Stanley RJ, Levitt RG, Geiss G: Computed tomography of the kidney. *Radiology* 124:359–370, 1977.
6. Love L, Churchill R, Reynes C, Schuster GA, Moncada R, Berkow M: Computed tomography staging of renal carcinoma. *Urol Radiol* 1:3–10, 1979.
7. Lemaitre G, Delambre Y: Place de la tomodensitometrie dans le diagnostic et le therapie d'extension des tumeurs malignes du rein. *J Radiol (Paris)* 64:91–98, 1983.
8. Probst P, Hoogewoud HM, Haertel M, Zingg E, Fuchs WA: Computerized tomography versus angiographie in the staging of malignant renal neoplasm. *Br J Radiol* 54:744–753, 1981.
9. Richard F, Khoury S, Kuss R: Computed tomography in the diagnosis and evaluation of renal cell carcinoma. *Prog Clin Biol Res* 100:377–397, 1982.
10. Robson CJ, Churchill BM, Anderson W: The results of radical nephrectomy for renal cell carcinoma. *J Urol* 101:297–301, 1969.
11. Robson CJ: Staging of renal cell carcinoma. *Prog Clin Biol Res* 100:439–445, 1982.
12. Kothari K, Segal AJ, Spitzer RM, Peartree RJ: Pre-operative radiographic evaluation of hypernephroma. *J Comput Assist Tomogr* 5:702–704, 1981.
13. Barre C, Caron-Pointereau C, Francois H, Rognon L: Apport de la tomodensitometrie dans la recherche de l'extension veineuse des cancere su rein. *Ann Urol*, in press.
14. Vasile N, Lacrosniere L, Abbou C, Larde D: Extension veineuse des cancers du rein. Role de la tomodensitometrie. *J Radiol (Paris)* 62:615–620, 1980.
15. Marks WM, Korobkin M, Callen PW, Kaiser JA: CT diagnosis of tumour thrombosis of the renal vein and inferior vena cava. *AJR* 131:843–845, 1978.
16. Steel JR, Sones PJ, Heffner LT: The detection of inferior vena canal thrombosis with computed tomography. *Radiology* 128:385–386, 1978.
17. Smith WP, Levine E: Sagittal and coronal CT image reconstruction: application in assessing the inferior vena cava in renal cancer. *J Comput Assist Tomogr* 4:531–535, 1980.

18. Pillari G, Kumari S, Phillips G, Cruz V, Pochaczevsky R, Marc J: Computed tomography in ileo femoral venous thrombosis extension to inferior vena cava defined with foot vein infusion. *J Comput Assist Tomogr* 5:375–377, 1981.
19. Vujic I, Stanley J, Tyminski LJ: Computed tomography of suspected caval thrombosis secondary to proximal extension of phlebitis from the leg. *Radiology* 140:437–441, 1981.

2

Current Cost-Effective Diagnosis of Asymptomatic Renal Mass Lesions

Erich K. Lang, M.D.

The introduction of new imaging modalities, particularly the computed tomogram, has swelled the number of patients known to harbor asymptomatic mass lesions of the kidney. Once considered rare, renal mass lesions are discovered now in 20% of older age group patients (1–4). While exploration of upper urinary tract mass lesions was once held obligatory, this large patient population begs for a cost-effective and minimally invasive diagnostic approach (5).

The ever increasing number of asymptomatic space-occupying lesions of the kidney discovered on computed tomograms has also greatly altered need and approach to further diagnostic workup. The much higher specificity and accuracy of diagnosis by computed tomogram often obviates the need for further or additional diagnostic investigation (4–6).

The inherent disparity of the confidence level of diagnosis of such lesions by the discovering examinations, the intravenous urogram and computed tomogram, calls for significantly different diagnostic pathways for definitive workup (3).

CURRENT APPROACH TO THE ASSESSMENT OF ASYMPTOMATIC SPACE-OCCUPYING LESIONS OF THE KIDNEY

The increased use of computed tomography for the study of a wide variety of abdominal conditions has resulted in recognition of a substantial number of unsuspected and asymptomatic space-occupying lesions of the kidney (3, 6).

In the past, the intravenous urogram was largely responsible for discovery of asymptomatic space-occupying lesions of the kidney. Today, more than 50% of all asymptomatic renal mass lesions are discovered by computed tomograms (3). The vastly different ability of these two examinations toward establishing a definitive diagnosis has resulted in different algorithmic approaches to finalize the diagnosis (3).

If computed tomograms are the discovering examination, the majority of the lesions can be diagnosed by the computed tomogram with acceptable confidence (3, 4, 6).

Lesions with cystic characteristics that cannot be definitively diagnosed on the computed tomogram are then examined by either guided percutaneous aspiration biopsy or the ultrasonogram (Table 2.1).

For lesions with solid tumor characteristics, guided percutaneous aspiration biopsy is advocated as next examination (Table 2.1).

However, solid masses suspected to be pseudotumors should be examined by radionuclide studies to establish a definitive diagnosis. Only rarely will guided percutaneous aspiration biopsy become necessary to affirm this diagnosis (7) (Table 2.1).

Only suspected vascular abnormalities are slated for arteriography. Most recently, arteriography may be replaced by magnetic resonance imaging when attempting to establish a definitive diagnosis of such vascular lesions (H. Hricak, personal communication).

The much lower rate of definitive diagnosis of such lesions by the intravenous urogram necessitates confirmatory diagnostic studies for the vast majority of asymptomatic space-occupying lesions discovered on intravenous urograms.

Ultrasonography is recommended as a second examination, principally to identify and diagnose definitely all lesions suspected to be cystic in nature (Table 2.2). If the diagnosis cannot be established with acceptable confidence by the ultrasonogram in a lesion presumed to be cystic, guided percutaneous aspiration biopsy is recommended as the next step (3, 4, 6).

Conversely, if the ultrasonogram suggests a solid rather than cystic lesion, computed tomograms are advocated for the next study to be complimented by guided percutaneous aspiration biopsy if the computed tomogram alone cannot establish the diagnosis (3, 4) (Table 2.2). Lesions thought to be solid on the basis of the intravenous urogram are handled in a like fashion (Table 2.2).

Masses suspected to be caused by a "column of Bertin" are most easily diagnosed on radionuclide studies; computed tomograms are recommended as the third study if the nature of the lesion remains indeterminate. Guided percutaneous aspiration biopsy remains the last resort. Lesions suspected to be of vascular etiology are best examined by arteriogram or magnetic resonance imaging. Computed tomograms and guided percutaneous aspiration biopsy are deployed for those lesions remaining refractory to diagnosis after the previous studies (3; H. Hricak, personal communication) (Table 2.2).

CONFIDENCE LEVEL OF DIAGNOSIS

Sensitivity, specificity, and accuracy of diagnosis vary for different entities and diagnostic studies. The vastly different rate of occurrence

Table 2.1
Diagnostic Pathway Proposed for the Assessment of Asymptomatic Space-Occupying Lesions of the Kidney Discovered on Computed Tomograms[a]

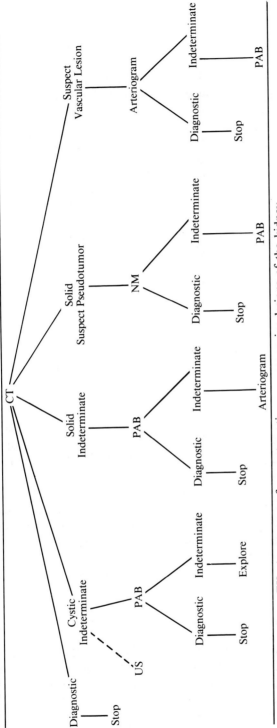

[a] Adapted from Lang EK: Assessment of asymptomatic space-occupying lesions of the kidney, 1984. Presented at the Radiological Society of North America, Washington, DC, 1984. US, ultrasonography; PAB, percutaneous aspiration biopsy; NM, nuclear medicine.

Table 2.2
Diagnostic Pathway Proposed for the Assessment of Asymptomatic Space-Occupying Lesions of the Kidney Discovered on the Intravenous Urogram[a]

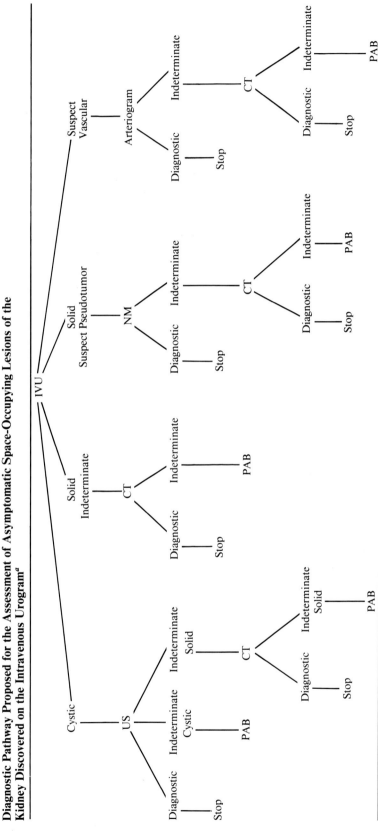

[a] Adapted from Lang EK: Assessment of asymptomatic space occupying lesions of the kidney, 1984. Presented at the Radiological Society of North America, Washington, DC, 1984. IVU, intravenous urogram; US, ultrasonography; PAB, percutaneous aspiration biopsy; NM, nuclear medicine.

14

of various etiologic entities, however, emphasizes the need for weighing the diagnostic approach in favor of the most common lesions (Table 2.3).

Benign renal cysts account for 66 to 89% of all asymptomatic space-occupying lesions of the kidney (1, 3, 4, 6, 8, 9). If the computed tomogram is the discovering examination, it establishes the definitive diagnosis of benign renal cyst in 96% of the patients harboring this lesion (3, 6, 9) (Table 2.4). Ultrasonograms can be used to confirm the diagnosis of benign renal cyst in patients failing to meet all four computed tomography criteria (sharply delineated, eliptical or round mass with smooth borders, attenuation coefficients of -10 to $+10$, and lack of enhancement during dynamic phase or on postenhancement computed tomograms) (Fig. 2.1).

The combination of computed tomograms and ultrasonograms can be expected to establish the definitive diagnosis of benign renal cyst in another 2% of these patients. Guided cyst puncture and aspiration and biochemical, cytologic, and radiographic assessment may be necessary to establish the diagnosis in the remaining 2% of patients with benign renal cysts (1, 3, 4, 6, 9).

If, however, the intravenous urogram was the discovering examination, only about 6% of benign renal cysts are diagnosed definitively by this study (Table 2.4). The vast majority of benign renal cysts, more

Table 2.3
The Etiologic Composition of 1594 Asymptomatic Space-Occupying Lesions of the Kidney[a]

Benign cysts	1055	66%
Benign cystic lesions	228	14%
Malignant neoplasms	72	5%
Benign neoplasms	13	<1%
Inflammatory mass lesions	125	8%
Pseudotumors	93	6%
Vascular lesions	8	0%

[a] Adapted from Lang EK: Assessment of asymptomatic space occupying lesions of the kidney, 1984. Presented at the Radiological Society of North America, Washington, DC, 1984.

Table 2.4
Percentile Diagnostic Contribution of Different Investigations in Benign Renal Cysts Discovered on Either Computed Tomogram or Intravenous Urogram[a]

Computed Tomogram		Intravenous Urogram	
Computed tomogram	96%	Intravenous urogram	6%
Percutaneous aspiration biopsy	2%	Ultrasonogram	77%
Ultrasonogram	2%	Computed tomogram	8%
		Percutaneous aspiration biopsy	8%
		Arteriogram	<1%

[a] Adapted from Lang EK: Assessment of asymptomatic space occupying lesions of the kidney, 1984. Presented at the Radiological Society of North America, Washington, DC, 1984.

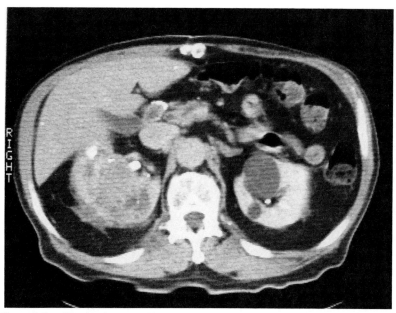

Figure 2.1. The early parenchymal phase of a computed tomogram demonstrates a characteristic parapelvic and cortical cyst in the left kidney. Note the sharp delineation, smooth borders, and lack of enhancement of the lesions. An ill defined mass enhancing less than normal renal parenchyma has replaced most of the right kidney. This appearance is characteristic of an infiltrating renal cell carcinoma.

than 77%, can be diagnosed on ultrasonograms, generally performed as the second examination (Table 2.2).

For a small group of lesions that fail to meet all of the ultrasonographic criteria (sharp definition against adjacent parenchyma, more or less spherical mass lesion, absence of internal echoes, and enhanced transmission through the cystic lesion as compared to adjacent renal parenchyma), guided percutaneous aspiration or computed tomograms must be performed to establish the diagnosis (Table 2.4). Failure to establish the diagnosis of benign renal cyst on ultrasonogram is most often attributable to an incompatibility of transducer frequency and depth of the lesion, thus erroneously producing echogenicity (1). Benign cystic lesions tend to be more refractory to diagnosis than simple cysts because of their composite mode of presentation. Septated benign cysts, multilocular benign cysts, benign cysts with calcifications in the wall, hemorrhagic cysts, parapelvic cysts, cystic dysplastic elements, and polycystic disease present with a multitude of criteria which often make diagnosis with an acceptable confidence level impossible (Figs. 2.2–2.4).

Computed tomograms establish the definitive diagnosis of these entities in about 42% of such patients (Table 2.5). Ultrasonograms and arteriograms can confirm the diagnosis in another 10% and 7% of the patients, respectively. Guided percutaneous aspiration, histochemical and cytologic examination of the aspirate, and double contrast studies, however, are necessary to complement the diagnostic criteria provided by the discovering computed tomograms and to establish a definitive diagnosis of such benign cystic disease entities in the remaining 41% of such patients. Cytologic and histochemical criteria are often necessary to differentiate composite benign cystic lesions, particularly if they contain hemorrhagic debris, from similar lesions that are associated with malignant neoplasms (10–14) (Fig. 2.2C).

Intravenous urograms, as the discovering examination, provide reliable criteria for the diagnosis of polycystic disease and some parapelvic and peripelvic cysts. The diagnosis of subsepted cysts, hemorrhagic cysts, cystic dysplastic kidney, multilocular cysts and calcified benign cysts, however, rests in essence on second and sometimes third examinations. Ultrasonograms are usually capable of establishing the diagnosis of septated cysts. Benign calcified cysts, multilocular cysts and cystic dysplastic elements are easiest diagnosed on computed tomograms (Table 2.4) (Fig. 2.5).

Guided cyst puncture and aspiration, cytologic and histochemical assessment of the aspirate and double contrast studies, however, are often necessary to affirm the diagnosis of hemorrhagic cysts, benign calcified cysts as well as some multilocular or cystic dysplastic elements (10, 12, 14) (Fig. 2.6). Arteriograms were favored in the past to exclude neoplastic disease but are replaced today by the less expensive and more definitive guided percutaneous aspiration biopsy procedure.

Malignant neoplasms represent only 5% of all asymptomatic space-occupying lesions of the kidney but are the principal reason for diagnostic efforts (Table 2.3).

Forty-seven percent of malignant neoplasms are diagnosed by the computed tomogram if it is the initial examination. The arteriogram and radionuclide studies diagnose another 14% and 3%, respectively. Thirty-six percent of these lesions are diagnosed by guided percutaneous aspiration biopsy (Table 2.6).

If the lesion is discovered on the intravenous urogram, the choice of subsequent investigations is influenced by the presumptive diagnosis of the intravenous urogram. Most often, the ultrasonogram is performed as the second examination. It tends to be inconclusive for malignant tumors. Depending on whether it suggests a solid or composite cystic lesion, a computed tomogram and an arteriogram or a guided percutaneous aspiration biopsy would be advocated for the next examination. For these reasons, the largest number of malignant neoplasms are diagnosed by guided percutaneous aspiration biopsy in patients in whom the lesion was discovered on intravenous urograms (55.5%). Computed tomograms and arteriograms account for 14% and 25% of the diagnoses, respectively. A relatively large number of refractory cases (5.5%) attests to the difficulty of making this diagnosis (15, 16) (Table 2.6).

Benign tumors are a relatively rare cause for renal mass lesions. If CT is the discovering examination, 66% were also definitively diagnosed by the computed tomogram, although the confidence level of the diagnosis can be improved by added criteria constellations from the ultrasonogram. This combined diagnostic approach is particularly appropriate for the assessment of angiomyolipomas (17, 18) (Fig. 2.7, Table 2.7). The diagnoses of benign renal adenoma, fibroma, and hamartoma, however, prove more difficult and, at times, refractory even to guided percutaneous aspiration biopsy (Table 2.8). The intravenous urogram provides no specific criteria for the diagnosis of benign renal tumors. Marked radiolucency of the mass may raise suspicion of an angiomyolipoma, but confirmation of the diagnosis by other examinations, such as the computed tomogram or ultrasonogram, is necessary.

About 60% of all inflammatory mass lesions first suggested on computed tomograms are also diagnosed with acceptable confidence by this examination (Table 2.9). The criteria constellation of heterogeneous enhancement during the phase of capillary transit of contrast medium and on the subsequent postenhancement computed tomograms is considered quite characteristic for areas of localized infection, such as lobar nephronia (Fig. 2.8). Conversely, abscess formation is characterized by a heterogeneous but low density mass reflecting debris. Lack of enhancement during the phase of capillary transit or on the postenhancement phase is due to liquefaction necrosis of the afflicted tissue. Rim enhancement of the abscess, particularly during the phase of capillary transit of contrast medium, is a reflection of the age of the process and maturation of the abscess wall (19, 20) (Fig. 2.9).

Scintiscanograms assessing accumulation of gallium 67 offer another noninvasive and reliable method to confirm this diagnosis. Arteriography and guided percutaneous aspiration biopsy establish the diagnosis

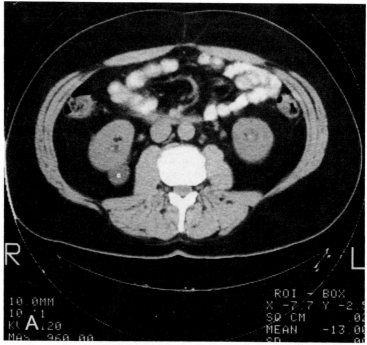

Figure 2.2. *A,* A spherical low density mass is seen to project from the posterior circumference of the right kidney into the perirenal space. *B,* The postenhancement CT shows a set-up of attenuation coefficients from −13 to +27, raising the question of a parenchymal tumor rather than a cyst. *C,* Under CT guidance, cyst puncture and aspiration are carried out. Cytologic and histochemical criteria confirmed the diagnosis of the benign cyst.

18   TUMORS OF THE KIDNEY

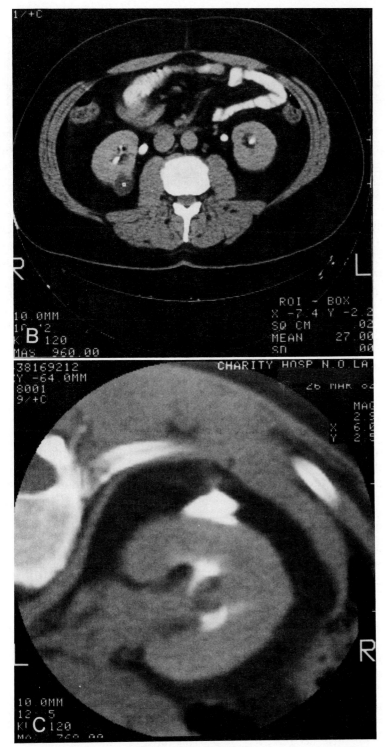

Figure 2.2. *B* and *C*

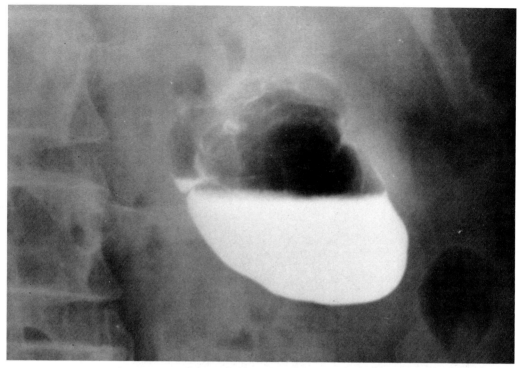

Figure 2.3. Guided puncture and aspiration yielded crystal yellowish aspirate. Cytologic and histochemical examination of the fluid confirmed the diagnosis of a benign cyst. The subsequent double contrast study demonstrates multiple septae within the cyst, suggesting a septated benign cyst or possibly a communicating multilocular benign cyst.

in most of the remaining patients with inflammatory mass lesions (Tables 2.7 and 2.9).

The intravenous urogram as the discovering examination establishes a definitive diagnosis of an inflammatory mass lesion only rarely. The computed tomogram or radionuclide study deploying gallium 67 scintiscanograms as well as the arteriogram and guided percutaneous aspiration biopsy must be utilized to confirm the diagnosis. A small number of such lesions will remain refractory to these diagnostic investigations, attesting to the inherent difficulty of this diagnosis.

The diagnosis of pseudotumor or column of Bertin causing a renal mass is established in about two-thirds of such patients by the discovering computed tomogram. Radionuclide scintiscanograms can confirm the diagnosis in the remainder of the patients by demonstrating normal or slightly increased uptake of technetium glucoheptonate in the area of concern (7) (Fig. 2.10).

Conversely, if this type of mass lesion is suggested by the intravenous urogram, the radionuclide scintiscanogram advocated as the second study renders a definitive diagnosis in about 94% of the patients. Only rarely is there need to revert to arteriography to differentiate this lesion from a true neoplasm. However, there remain a small number of lesions refractory to this diagnostic approach (Table 2.10).

The diagnosis of vascular lesions, such as arteriovenous fistulae or

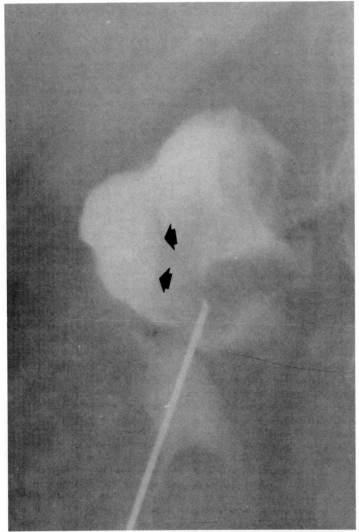

Figure 2.4. Guided aspiration of a cystic lesion yields aspirate of crank oil consistency. This is characteristic for cystic dysplastic elements. The contrast study demonstrates the dysplastic element of the upper moiety of the right kidney (*arrows*). (From Lang EK: Assessment of asymptomatic space occupying lesions of the kidney. *Radiology*, in press.)

arteriovenous malformation, rests on the dynamic computed tomogram, the arteriogram, or magnetic resonance imaging. A correct diagnosis tends to evolve if the computed tomogram augmented by dynamic series recording was the discovering examination.

If, however, the mass lesion was first discovered on the intravenous urogram, the normal algorithmic progression suggests the ultrasonogram for the second examination, which in turn would tend to make the erroneous diagnosis of a cystic lesion. Guided percutaneous aspiration biopsy may well be opted as the third examination and result in deleterious effects.

Table 2.5
Percentile Diagnostic Contribution of Different Investigations in Benign Cystic Entities Discovered on Computed Tomogram or Intravenous Urogram[a]

Computed Tomogram		Intravenous Urogram	
Computed tomogram	42%	Intravenous urogram	23%
Percutaneous aspiration biopsy	41%	Ultrasonogram	18%
Ultrasonogram	10%	Computed tomogram	12%
Arteriogram	7%	Percutaneous aspiration biopsy	43%
		Arteriogram	4%

[a] Adapted from Lang EK: Assessment of asymptomatic space occupying lesions of the kidney, 1984. Presented at the Radiological Society of North America, Washington, DC, 1984.

COST-EFFECTIVE APPROACH TO THE ASSESSMENT OF ASYMPTOMATIC SPACE-OCCUPYING LESIONS OF THE KIDNEY

The impact of setting remuneration according to diagnosis related groups mandates careful reassessment of one's approach to the management of all medical problems (21). Almost by definition asymptomatic space-occupying lesions of the kidney tend not to be related to the presenting problem for which the patient sought medical care. Ninety percent of the lesions discovered have little or no impact on the future well-being of the patient (1, 3, 6, 21–23) (Table 2.5). The 10% of patients discovered to harbor a malignant or inflammatory mass lesion, however, mandate and benefit from appropriate therapy.

Although concern has been expressed about the rising costs of health care related to the introduction of new technology, this does not appear applicable to the evaluation of renal mass lesions (21). In fact, recent statistical analysis by Zimmer et al has shown conclusively that the average cost of evaluating such patients has declined by 30% over the last 7 years (21). Zimmer et al, in their study, attributed this decline in cost largely to the significant decrease in the use of angiography.

The cost of a diagnostic workup can be broken down into several major groups: (*a*) direct cost for the diagnostic test, (*b*) hospitalization costs for diagnostic procedures mandating inpatient status, and (*c*) loss of income attributable to time committed for the test procedure and recuperation thereof.

The advent of noninvasive diagnostic studies—such as the computed

Figure 2.5. *A*, The capillary phase of the dynamic computed tomogram demonstrates multiple rounded, low density mass lesions, originating from the anterior circumference of the midpole of the left kidney (*arrows*). *B*, The attenuation coefficients of the lesions located along the anterolateral circumference are in the range of benign renal cysts. The attenuation coefficient of the anterior cystic lesion, however, is clearly in the range of a parenchymal mass or hyperdense cyst. Moreover, shell-like calcifications (*arrow*) limited to the wall are noted. A hemorrhagic cyst was proven by CT guided puncture, aspiration, and cytologic and histochemical assessment of the aspirate.

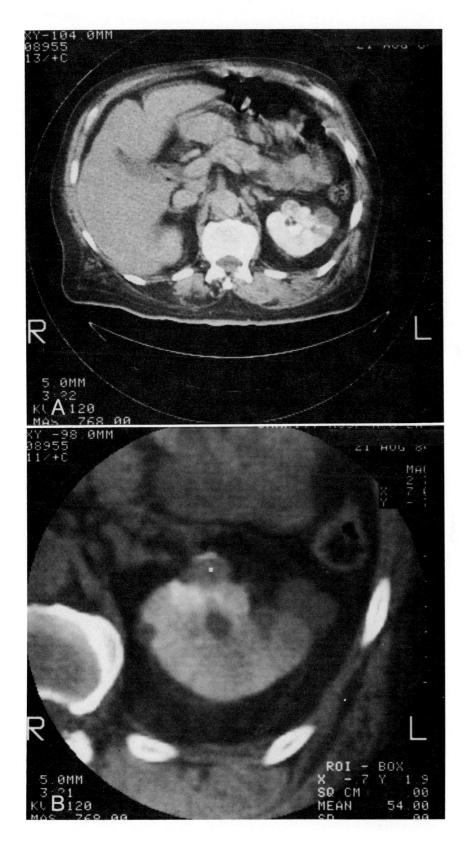

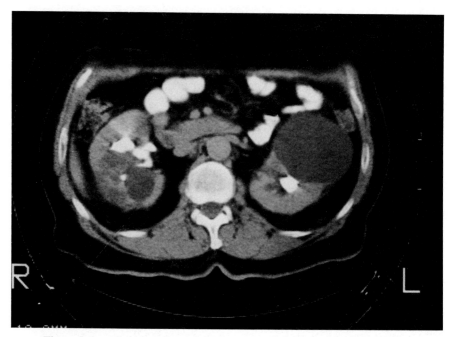

Figure 2.6. The parenchymal phase computed tomogram demonstrates a typical benign cyst replacing the anterior half of the midpole of the left kidney. On the right side there are multiple low density masses that appear to intercommunicate and compress and displace the pelvis; the appearance is characteristic of a cystic dysplastic element involving a portion or moiety of the kidney.

Table 2.6
Number of Patients Diagnosed as Malignant Neoplasms by Various Techniques in a Group of Asymptomatic Space-Occupying Lesions of the Kidney Discovered on Computed Tomogram or Intravenous Urogram[a]

Computed Tomogram		Intravenous Urogram	
Computed tomogram	17	Computed tomogram	5
Percutaneous aspiration biopsy	13	Percutaneous aspiration biopsy	20
Arteriogram	5	Arteriogram	9
Radionuclide Scintiscanogram	1	Undiagnosed	2

[a] Adapted from Lang EK: Assessment of asymptomatic space occupying lesions of the kidney, 1984. Presented at the Radiological Society of North America, Washington, DC, 1984.

tomogram, the ultrasonogram, magnetic resonance imaging, and radionuclide scanning—has greatly impacted on the overall cost of diagnostic assessment of renal masses. These noninvasive procedures can be carried out on an outpatient basis. This eliminates costs for hospitalization but also reduces the indirect cost associated with loss of income incurred by the patient during hospitalization and aggravated by work time lost to recuperation.

The present trend to complete screening procedures on an outpatient basis prior to admission of the patient for intended definitive therapy has, therefore, greatly reduced the "hotel component" of medical costs.

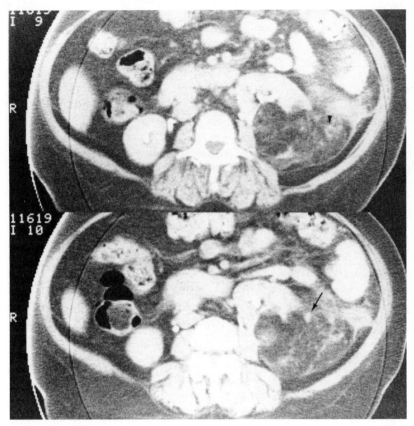

Figure 2.7. Dynamic computed tomograms obtained during the phase of capillary transit of contrast medium demonstrate a low density multilobulated mass replacing the posterior and lateral circumference of the mid and lower pole of the left kidney. Isolated high density structures identified within the fat are opacified vessels (*arrows*). The diagnosis of angiomyolipoma is established by these findings. (From Lang EK: Assessment of asymptomatic space occupying lesions of the kidney. *Radiology*, in press.)

Table 2.7
Asymptomatic Space-Occupying Lesions of the Kidney—Study Period July 1, 1977 to June 30, 1984[a]

Asymptomatic space-occupying lesions of the kidney	1594
Number of patients	1578
Age range	8 to 91 years
Mean age	60.4 years
Male	991
Female	587

[a] Adapted from Lang EK: Assessment of asymptomatic space occupying lesions of the kidney, 1984. Presented at the Radiological Society of North America, Washington, DC, 1984.

The high specificity of the computed tomogram and ultrasonogram, which establish the definitive diagnosis in about 85% of all asymptomatic space-occupying lesions of the kidney, makes complete workup on an outpatient basis possible, and "hotel component" costs, loss of

Table 2.8
Number of Patients Diagnosed as Benign Neoplasms by Various Techniques in a Group of Asymptomatic Space-Occupying Lesions of the Kidney Discovered on Computed Tomogram or Intravenous Urogram[a]

Computed Tomogram		Intravenous Urogram	
Computed tomogram	4		
Percutaneous aspiration biopsy	2	Ultrasonogram	2
		Arteriogram	1
Undiagnosed	3	Undiagnosed	1

[a] Adapted from Lang EK: Assessment of asymptomatic space occupying lesions of the kidney, 1984. Presented at the Radiological Society of North America, Washington, DC, 1984.

Table 2.9
Number of Patients Diagnosed with Inflammatory Mass Lesions by Various Examinations in a Group Found to Harbor a Space-Occupying Lesion of the Kidney on Initial Computed Tomogram or Intravenous Urogram[a]

Computed Tomogram		Intravenous Urogram	
Computed tomogram	47	Intravenous urogram	1
Percutaneous aspiration biopsy	36	Computed tomogram	16
Radionuclide scintiscano-gram	10	Percutaneous aspiration biopsy	29
Arteriogram	2	Arteriogram	10
Undiagnosed	1	Radionuclide scintiscano-gram	12
		Undiagnosed	2

[a] Adapted from Lang EK: Assessment of asymptomatic space occupying lesions of the kidney, 1984. Presented at the Radiological Society of North America, Washington, DC, 1984.

income-producing time, and direct procedural costs are thus kept to a minimum.

The mode of discovery of asymptomatic space-occupying lesions of the kidney also has a major impact on the ultimate cost of establishing a diagnosis with acceptable confidence.

The computed tomogram, a highly specific and accurate test, renders the definitive diagnosis in 79% of all such patients (Table 2.11). The intravenous urogram can establish a definitive diagnosis in only 7% of the patients.

In conjunction with a second noninvasive examination, the ultrasonogram or radionuclide scintiscanogram, computed tomograms then establish the definitive diagnosis in another 6% of the patients (Table 2.12). Thus, better than 85% of all patients are definitively diagnosed by means of noninvasive tests easily performed on an outpatient basis. Only 14% of the patients require an invasive study to establish the diagnosis (Table 2.12). However, even among the invasive studies, guided percutaneous aspiration biopsy can be carried out safely on an outpatient basis. Only 1% of the patients need to be hospitalized to perform diagnostic studies—namely, the group assessed by arteriograms (Table 2.13).

Even in the group of patients in whom the mass lesion was discovered

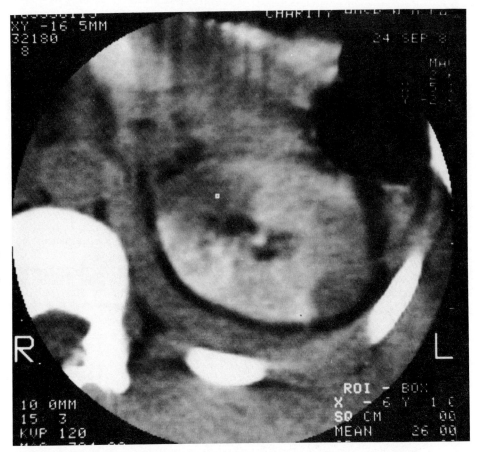

Figure 2.8. The dynamic phase computed tomogram demonstrates several areas of decreased, yet heterogeneous enhancement of parenchyma in the left kidney. The appearance is quite characteristic of a lobar nephroma. Cloudy swelling and edema result in suppressed perfusion causing the decreased and heterogeneous enhancement. Lack of a wedge-shaped appearance and dense enhancement of the appropriate cortical segments serve to differentiate it from a parenchymal infarct.

on the intravenous urogram, 82% can be definitively diagnosed by noninvasive procedures easily performed on an outpatient basis—7% by the discovering intravenous urogram and another 75% by a combination of two examinations, the intravenous urogram with either the ultrasonogram, the computed tomogram, or a radionuclide scintiscanogram (Table 2.14). In approximately 17% of these patients, invasive procedures become necessary (Table 2.12). The higher use of arteriograms in this group is probably attributable to the sometimes contradictory criteria provided by preliminary intravenous urogram and ultrasonogram, particularly in patients with inflammatory mass lesions. The current trend to deploy the computed tomogram preferentially as the third examination in such patients will undoubtedly reduce the use of arteriography.

Regardless of the discovering examination, there remains a group of approximately 0.5% of the patients who prove refractory to diagnostic

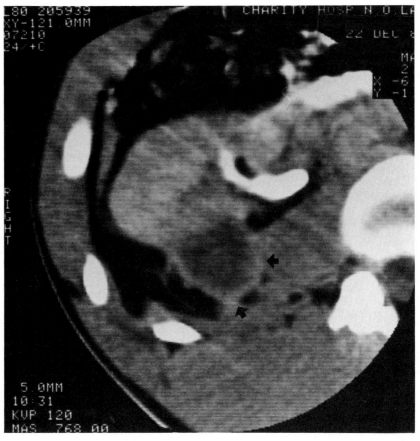

Figure 2.9. A low density mass with a thick wall projects into the posterior perirenal space (*arrows*). Enhancement of the wall during the phase of late capillary transit of contrast medium is characteristic for a vascularized abscess wall. Conversely, the center of the abscess (an area of liquefection necrosis) does not show enhancement.

investigation. Exploration is the most cost-effective method to deal with this group of patients since a plethora of conflicting diagnostic criteria has usually been assembled at this point that will preclude diagnosis with acceptable confidence.

The level of confidence demanded to accept diagnosis has a major economic implication. A prudent approach individualizes for each patient and takes into consideration his age, his general medical condition, and the need to address the principal complaint that brought the patient to medical attention.

In this group of asymptomatic space-occupying lesions of the kidney, there are a number of lesions that test the capability of the diagnostic armamentarium. Multilocular cysts; cystic and dysplastic renal elements; septated cysts; inflammatory and hemorrhagic cysts; such benign tumors as adenoma, fibroma, and hamartoma; and such malignant tumors as lymphoma, capsular sarcoma, cystic and necrotic hypernephroma, and metastatic carcinoma tend to present diagnostic problems (3, 4, 10–12, 15, 24–26). However, "soft criteria" provided by imaging

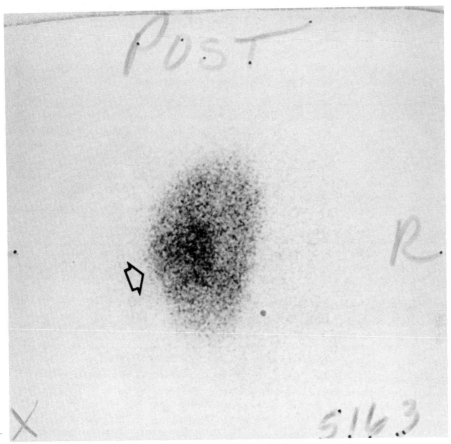

Figure 2.10. A technetium 99m glucoheptonate scintiscanogram demonstrates increased accumulation of radiotracer (*arrow*) in a segment of the right kidney previously implicated as possible pseudotumor (column of Bertin). Normal or slightly increased accumulation of technetium glucopheptonate is characteristic for a column of Bertin.

studies can be "hardened" if complemented by guided percutaneous aspiration biopsy. This approach is particularly useful to establish a diagnosis—though with admittedly a somewhat lower but yet acceptable confidence level—for conditions such as inflammatory or hemorrhagic (hyperdense) cysts, calcified benign cysts, cystic and dysplastic elements, and multilocular cysts as well as some of the malignant lesions (3, 9, 10, 15, 22, 24, 25) (Figs. 2.3 and 2.4).

Cost-effective management of asymptomatic space-occupying lesions of the kidney is based on maximal but judicious use of such noninvasive imaging examinations as the ultrasonogram, the computed tomogram complemented by dynamic phase recording, the radionuclide scintiscanogram, and, as of late, magnetic resonance imaging. The high sensitivity and specificity of criteria generated by these examinations will allow diagnosis with acceptable confidence for about 85% of all lesions.

Appropriate deployment of guided percutaneous aspiration biopsy procedures should bring the rate of diagnosis to about 98%. Since guided percutaneous aspiration biopsy is likewise a relatively noninvasive pro-

Table 2.10
Number of Patients Diagnosed as Pseudotumors by Various Techniques in a Group of Asymptomatic Space-Occupying Lesions of the Kidney Discovered on Computed Tomogram or Intravenous Urogram[a]

Computed Tomogram		Intravenous Urogram	
Computed tomogram	8	Radionuclide scintiscanogram	67
Radionuclide scintiscano-gram	14	Arteriogram	3
		Undiagnosed	1

[a] Adapted from Lang EK: Assessment of asymptomatic space occupying lesions of the kidney, 1984. Presented at the Radiological Society of North America, Washington, DC, 1984.

Table 2.11
Percentage of Asymptomatic Space-Occupying Lesions of the Kidney Diagnosed by the Discovering Examination[a]

Computed tomogram	79%
Intravenous urogram	7%

[a] Adapted from Lang EK: Assessment of asymtomatic space occupying lesions of the kidney, 1984. Presented at the Radiological Society of North America, Washington, DC, 1984.

Table 2.12
Invasiveness of Diagnostic Studies Deployed in Assessment of Asymptomatic Space-Occupying Lesions of the Kidney[a]

	Discovering Examination	
	Computed Tomogram	Intravenous Urogram
Noninvasive	Less than 86%	82%
Invasive	14%	17%
Undiagnosed	Less than 1%	Less than 1%

[a] Adapted from Lang EK: Assessment of asymptomatic space occupying lesions of the kidney, 1984. Presented at the Radiological Society of North America, Washington, DC, 1984.

Table 2.13
Percentage of Asymptomatic Space-Occupying Lesions of the Kidney Diagnosed by Two Examinations (the Computed Tomogram Discovering the Lesion)[a]

Computed tomogram and guided percutaneous aspiration biopsy	13%
Computed tomogram and ultrasonogram	3%
Computed tomogram and arteriogram	less than 1%
Computed tomogram and radionuclide scintiscanogram	3%

[a] Adapted from Lang EK: Assessment of asymptomatic space occupying lesions of the kidney, 1984. Presented at the Radiological Society of North America, Washington, DC, 1984.

Table 2.14
Percentage of Asymptomatic Space-Occupying Lesions of the Kidney Diagnosed by Two Examinations (the Intravenous Urogram (IVU) Discovering the Lesion)[a]

IVU and ultrasonogram	56%
IVU and computed tomogram	9%
IVU and radionuclide scintiscanogram	10%
IVU and guided percutaneous aspiration biopsy	5%
IVU and arteriogram	1%

[a] Adapted from Lang EK: Assessment of asymptomatic space occupying lesions of the kidney. 1984. Presented at the Radiological Society of North America, Washington, DC, 1984.

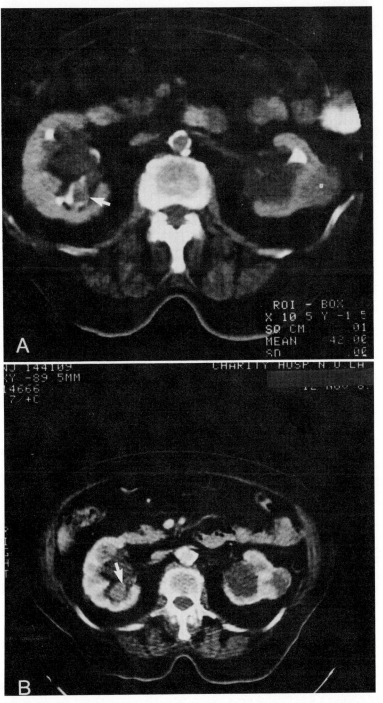

Figure 2.11. *A*, A postenhancement computed tomogram demonstrates a heterogeneously enhancing mass projecting into the left perirenal space. A filling defect is demonstrated in a posterior calyx of the right kidney (*arrow*). *B*, During the phase of capillary transit a dynamic CT demonstrates characteristic enhancement of the rim of this left renal mass. The area lacking enhancement in the center suggests necrosis of the renal cell carcinoma. A homogeneously enhancing mass corresponds to the previously seen filling defect in the posterior calyx on the right side (*arrow*). The staining quality is characteristic for a transitional cell carcinoma. The dynamic computed tomogram establishes the diagnosis of two histologically different, asymptomatic neoplasms involving the right and left kidneys, respectively. (From Chisholm GD (ed): *Percutaneous and Interventional Urology and Radiology.* London, Springer-Verlag, 1986.)

31

cedure, the entire diagnostic workup of such lesions can be performed on an outpatient basis.

The remaining 2% of patients require hospital admission for further clarification. Either arteriography or exploration may be deemed necessary to establish the diagnosis.

Despite the initial higher cost of new technology procedures, the much higher diagnostic yield of these procedures has more than offset their cost and has resulted in the reduction of cost per diagnosis as compared to the past era, which depended heavily on invasive diagnostic procedures.

REFERENCES

1. Pollack HM, Banner MP, Arger PH, Goldberg BB, Mulhern CB Jr: Comparison of computed tomography in ultrasound in diagnosis of renal masses. *Clin Diagn Ultrasound* 2:25–72, 1979.
2. Lang EK: Asymptomatic space occupying lesions of the kidney. *Minn Med* 63:773–778, 1980.
3. Lang EK: Assessment of asymptomatic space occupying lesions of the kidney. Presented as Paper 1 at 70th Scientific Assembly and Annual Meeting of the Radiological Society of North America, Washington, DC, November 25–30, 1984.
4. Balfe DM, McClennan BL, Stanley RJ, Weyman PJ, Sagel SS: Evaluation of renal masses considered indeterminate on computed tomography. *Radiology* 142:421–428, 1982.
5. Lang EK: Asymptomatic space occupying lesions of the kidney: a programmed sequential approach and its impact on quality and cost of health care. *South Med J* 70:277–286, 1977.
6. McClennan BL, Stanley RJ, Melson GL, Levitt RG, Sagel SS: CT of the renal cyst: is cyst aspiration necessary? *AJR* 133:671–675, 1979.
7. Pollack HM, Edell S, Morales JO: Radionuclide imaging in renal pseudotumors. *Radiology* 111:639–676, 1974.
8. Kissane JM: The morphology of renal cystic disease. *Persp Nephrol Hypertension* 4:31–63, 1976.
9. Lang EK: Roentgenologic approach to diagnosis in management of cystic lesions of the kidney: is cyst exploration mandatory? *Urol Clin North Am* 7:677–688, 1980.
10. Saxton HM, Golding SJ, Chantler C, Haycock GD: Diagnostic puncture in renal cystic dysplasia (multicystic kidney): evidence on the etiology of the cyst. *Br J Radiol* 54:555–561, 1981.
11. Segal AJ, Spitzer RM: Pseudo thick walled renal cysts by CT. *AJR* 132:827–828, 1979.
12. Banner MP, Pollack HM, Chatten J, Witzleben C: Multilocular renal cysts, radiologic pathologic correlation. *AJR* 136:239–247, 1981.
13. Mayer DP, Baron RL, Pollack HM: Increase in CT attenuation values of parapelvic renal cysts after retrograde pyelography. *AJR* 139:991–993, 1982.
14. Lang EK: Coexistence of cyst and tumor in the same kidney. *Radiology* 101:7–14, 1971.
15. Sussman S, Cochran ST, Pagani JJ, McArdle C, Wong W, Austin R, Curry N, Kelly KM: Hyperdense renal masses: a CT manifestation of hemorrhagic renal cysts. *Radiology* 150:207–211, 1984.
16. Hilton S, Bosniak MA, Megibow AJ, Ambos MA: Computed tomographic demonstration of spontaneous subcapsular hematoma due to a small renal cell carcinoma. *Radiology* 141:743–744, 1981.
17. Sherman JL, Hartman DS, Friedman AC, Madewell JE, Davis CJ, Goldman SM: Angiomyolipoma: computed tomographic pathologic correlation of 17 cases. *AJR* 137:1221–1226, 1981.
18. Totty WG, McClennan BL, Melson GL, Patel R: Relative value of computed tomography and ultrasonography in the assessment of renal angiomyolipoma. *J Comput Assist Tomogr* 5:173–178, 1981.

19. Lee JKT, McClennan BL, Melson GL, Stanley RJ: Acute focal bacterial nephritis: emphasis on gray scale sonography and computed tomography. *AJR* 135:87–92, 1980.
20. Mendez G, Isikoff MB, Morillo G: The role of computed tomography in the diagnosis of renal and perirenal abscess. *J Urol* 122:582–586, 1979.
21. Zimmer WD, Williamson BE Jr, Hartman GW, Hattery RR, O'Brien TC: Changing patterns in the evaluation of renal masses: economic implications. *AJR* 143:285–289, 1984.
22. Lang EK: Diagnosis and management of renal cysts. In *Interventional Uroradiology*. Heidelberg, Springer-Verlag, 1985.
23. Clayman RV, Williams RD, Fraley EE: The pursuit of the renal mass. *N Engl J Med* 300:72–74, 1979.
24. Parienty RA, Pradel J, Imbert M, Picard JD, Savart P: Computed tomography of multilocular cystic nephroma. *Radiology* 140:135–139, 1981.
25. Kim WS, Goldman SM, Gatewood OMB, Marshall FF, Siegelman SS: Computed tomography in calcified renal masses. *J Comput Assist Tomogr* 5:555–560, 1981.
26. Weyman PJ, McClennan BL, Lee JKT, Stanley RJ: CT of calcified renal masses. *AJR* 138:1095–1099, 1982.

3

The Value of DNA Cytophotometry for the Prognostic Evaluation of Renal Adenocarcinoma

Ferdinand Hofstädter, M.D.
Gerhard Jakse, M.D.
Hans Rauschmeier, M.D.
Ricardo Delgado, M.D.

THE GRADING OF RENAL CELL CARCINOMA: THE PROBLEM

Human renal cell carcinoma (RCC) has kept histopathologists busy since its first description by Grawitz (1). Even the diagnostic term "RCC" indicates insecurity concerning histogenesis. The histopathologic grading and classification should be relevant for the treatment and prognosis. The morphologic criteria should be simple and transferable from one pathologist to the other. Numerous attempts have been made.

There have been two principal approaches. The first was to find out one predominant prognostic criterion. The most frequently discussed phenomenon is the prognostic value of the discrimination of clear cells and granular (dark) or plasma-rich cells (2). A large series of clinico-pathological studies suggest that granular tumor cells indicate worse prognosis (3–15). Fuhrman et al (16) and Selli et al (17) principally agreed, but they showed that the prognostic value of the cell type is in part a function of the nuclear grade. Angervall and Wahlquist (18) found a partial correlation of cell type with elevation of erythrocyte sedimentation rate. Interestingly, Sarosdy and Lamm (19) have found a noticeable trend of a higher percentage of blood group isoantigen-positive tumors among clear cell carcinomas when compared with mixed or granular cell type tumors. This finding, too, indicates a higher malignancy of granular cell type tumors and of granular cell type RCC. On the other hand, a series of studies has been published strictly denying correlations between cell type and prognosis (20–25).

In most studies, histologic structure alone—with the exception of the sarcoma-like tumors—does not seem to bear a major influence on the clinical prognosis. But papillary carcinoma has been suggested to indicate a better prognosis than other types of cellular structure (26, 27).

The second principal approach to the prognostic classification of RCC is the combination of different histologic and cytologic parameters (65). The original grading of Hand and Broders (28) included both histologic and cytologic criteria. They used a semiquantitative technique in order to evaluate the proportional percentages of differentiated cells. Foot and Humphreys (7) have combined the size of the type cell, the nature of its cytoplasm (clear or granular), the size and regularity of the nuclei, and the architecture of the growth (cords, tubules, papillae, etc). This combination of histostructural and cytologic parameters enabled the authors to distinguish between RCC with good prognosis (5-year survival: 87.5%) and fair or poor prognosis (5-year survival: 31.7%) (29). Riches et al (30) used a combination based upon histostructural and nuclear criteria with three grades of malignancy (5-year survival: 71, 39, and 25%) (31). Mathisen et al (32) and McNichols et al (24) used other combinations of histostructural and cytologic criteria.

Arner et al (33) added the relationship of the tumor to the circumjacent tissue to the criteria of cellular differentiation and nuclear grading. They subdivided the group of moderately differentiated RCC into clearly circumscribed tumors and into not clearly circumscribed ones. The predictive value of this grading system was shown to be very exact (5-year survival: 93, 63, and 41.7%). But the reproducibility of the grading system was criticized to be as low as 50% (34). Syrjanen and Hjelt (34) therefore combined the criterion of the demarcation of the carcinoma with a more detailed nuclear grading (grades 1 to 3), thus obtaining six grades of malignancy. Hermanek et al (35) introduced a grading system based upon histoarchitecture and cytomorphology which fulfills three important criteria: (a) it correlates with the histopathologic stage, (b) tumors of different grades of malignancy show different prognosis, and (c) it is simple.

Skinner et al (14) proposed to record all of the microscopic features mentioned above, but concentrated their grading technique upon the nuclear morphology (grades 1 to 4). They found nuclear morphology to be of definite predictive value. This finding was corroborated by the work of Fuhrman et al (16). Comparing such different variables as cell arrangement, tumor size, and cell type, they found that the nuclear grading was the most significant prognostic criterion for the outcome of patients with stage I RCC.

The critical comparison of the different grading systems reveals that each of them shows close correlation with the biologic behavior of the respective tumors. Their practicability, however, is diminished by two facts: (a) The cellular heterogeneity of RCC, stressed by several authors (3, 34, 36), leads to confusion in the application of the respective morphologic criterion. (b) Most criteria used are based upon the subjective interpretation of the histopathologist. This point crucially diminishes the intra- and especially the interobserver reproducibility. Therefore, from that critical point of view, there is rather little progress in the grading of RCC since the statement of Melicow (9) that "grading, especially in the clear cell group, is not possible."

DNA CYTOPHOTOMETRY AS A METHOD FOR THE ANALYTICAL INVESTIGATION AND STANDARDIZED CLASSIFICATION OF HUMAN TUMORS

Malignant transformation in most human tumors is accompanied by changes of the content of nuclear DNA (37). These alterations can be measured by DNA cytophotometry (38, 39). Two main systems of measurement are widely used: single cell cytophotometry, and DNA flow cytometry (FCM).

Single cell cytophotometry is based upon the work of Caspersson (40). The preferred staining technique used was the Feulgen reaction. Freshly prepared cells (imprint preparations from tumor cut surface, cytologic specimens, etc) are fixed according to Bohm (37). Recently, Delgado et al (41) developed a technique for the DNA cytophotometric analysis of paraffin-embedded tissues. After Feulgen staining, the relative DNA content of tumor cell nuclei is determined by a microdensitometer (either an integrating system or, more recently, a scanning table directed by a connected computer). Measurements are done at a defined wavelength (570 nm). The extinction values are expressed as arbitrary units (AU). The number of cell nuclei measured varies between 50 and 1000. The extinction values of normal, non-neoplastic cells (diploid extinction value: 2c) are determined by means of the analysis of the nuclei of small lymphocytes or polymorphonuclear leukocytes in each of the specimens.

Several statistical modes are used for analyzing the measurements: (*a*) The determination of the *DNA tumor stem line* (37). The stem line is defined as the first distinguishable peak of relative DNA values confirmed by a respective doubled value. The latter represents nuclei in the G_2 and M phases of the cell cycle. The position of the DNA stem line is expressed graphically as a histogram (Fig. 3.1). This allows the simple differentiation into tumors with a diploid (2c) stem line and those with a nondiploid stem line (tetraploid: 4c, hypotetraploid, or all other variations up to 32c). This method does not reflect the proliferative activity of the measured cell population. The statistical analysis of a large number of tumors or the comparison of different tumor types is difficult using this mode. For the analysis of large series of specimens, Hofstädter et al (42) have introduced the *stem line quotient* (SQ), which

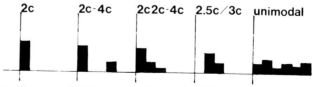

Figure 3.1 Some typical histogram figures in DNA Feulgen cytophotometry. From left: diploid, near diploid, diploid-tetraploid, triploid, without stem line (unimodal).

defines the stem line mathematically by division by the normal DNA value (2c standard).

(b) Another parameter used is the mean value of the measured relative DNA content. This value, however, is dependent upon the staining intensity of the individual specimen. Although using standardized procedures, staining intensity shows variations between the different preparations. Therefore, Fossa (43) introduced the *diploid deviation quotient* (DDQ), which is the mean value of all measured nuclei divided by the normal extinction value (2c standard.) Therefore, DDQ is independent of individual staining intensity and, contrary to SQ, includes the proliferative activity of the respective cell population. It includes the dispersion pattern of the relative DNA contents of tumor cell nuclei. Of course, DDQ is not identical with the true proliferation rate as can be determined by autoradiography (44). It must be considered that not all nuclei at the tetraploid doubling peak are indeed proliferating cells. Indeed Ogino (45) has shown that in a cultured cell line of RCC of Syrian hamster (HKC-400), 9% of the cells in the G_2 DNA region are in a quiescent state.

(c) Other parameters analyzed by single cell photometry (using scanning techniques) are nuclear area, chromatin density (46), chromatin arrangement (47), nuclear form, and atypism. The latter leads to sophisticated methods of cellular and nuclear image analysis and mathematical morphology.

The second main technique for analyzing the DNA content of tumor cells is *DNA flow cytometry* (48). The staining technique mostly uses fluorochromes (ethidium, bromide-mithramycin). The relative content of nuclear DNA per cell is quantitated by measuring the intensity of fluorescent light emitted when the cell passes through the sensing region of a fluorometer. The major advance of this technique against the single cell technique is the high speed of measurement, exceeding 10^3 cells/second (49). Therefore, large numbers of nuclei may be analyzed. Furthermore, cytometers have been developed that are equipped with high power laser light sources, allowing multiparameter analyses and cell-sorting procedures. The large number of cells enables better statistical resolution. The quantitative distribution of the different populations is documented much more precisely. Paraffin-embedded material, too, may be used for FCM (50).

In cases of heterogeneously composed solid tumors, in the authors' opinion, it seems possible that a small group of cells with excessively high DNA values may be suppressed by the overall majority of uniform tumor cell nuclei. However, in general, the results of single cell cytophotometry and FCM are surprisingly uniform concerning the analysis of DNA distribution in human solid tumor specimens. Both principal techniques have been widely used to study the ploidy and the proliferative state of human tumors.

Some of the main purposes of these investigations are: (a) objectification and standardization of the histologic diagnosis and especially the histopathologic grading (42); in particular, nuclear grading is a very subjective technique, even in the hands of experienced histopathologists (51); (b) early detection and classification of preneoplastic states (52);

(*c*) control of therapy; (*d*) more detailed and objective information about prognosis, independent from subjective influences of histopathology (53, 54); (*e*) specific decision base for the choice of therapy (55).

CONVENTIONAL IMPRINT DNA CYTOPHOTOMETRY AS A BASE FOR THE GRADING OF RCC

Hermanek et al (35) introduced a simple, morphologically well defined classification system for RCC. It combines both histologic and cytopathologic criteria and is deduced from the biologic behavior. There are three grades of malignancy. Grade 1—solid tumors with clear cells and tumors of doubtful malignancy, and questionable benign Grawitz tumors after the definition of Largiader (56) and Zollinger (57). Grade 3—tumors which are exclusively of glandular or glandular-papillary pattern, or tumors exhibiting sarcoma-like features in some areas, or tumors which show at least in one low power field (64×) exclusively dark cells. Grade 2—all tumors not fulfilling the criteria of grade 1 or grade 3. The first goal of quantitative cell analysis should be to find correlations between the subjective grading and the objective cytometric data.

The present authors have investigated 101 freshly prepared imprint specimens from 36 RCC (20 males; 16 females; mean age 65.6 ± 10.9, range 44 to 81). Tumor size was 7.4 ± 3.0 cm (range 2.5 to 15.0 cm). The distribution of malignancy grades was as follows: grade 1 = 7; grade 2 = 38; grade 3 = 56. Figure 3.2 shows DDQ at different malignancy grades. There is a clear correlation between the increase of histologically stated malignancy grade and the proliferation of tumor cell nuclei. Very similar results give the analysis of the stem lines at different grades (Table 3.1). Grade 1 tumors show diploid or nearly diploid stem lines with some tetraploid nuclei. Grade 3 tumors show nondiploid stem lines in most cases. Grade 2 RCC seem to take an intermediate position, with about 45% nondiploid cases. The analysis of the areas of the tumor cell nuclei (Fig. 3.3) shows results strictly differing from the features given

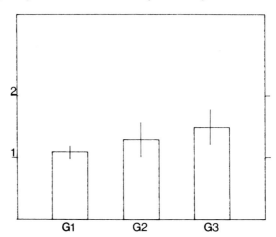

Figure 3.2 Imprint DNA cytophotometry. DDQ at different grades of malignancy (35): grade 1 (*n* = 7), grade 2 (*n* = 38), grade 3 (*n* = 56). Differences of mean values between grade 1 (*G1*) and grade 2 (*G2*) ($\alpha < 0.01$) and grade 2 and grade 3 (*G3*) ($\alpha < 0.002$) are significant.

Table 3.1
DNA Distribution Pattern in RCC (Histograms)—Freshly Prepared Imprint Specimens

	2c	2c/4c	2c2c/4c	2.5c–3c	4c, 4c
Grade 1[a]	2	2	3		
Grade 2	4	17	5	11	1
Grade 3	4	11	14	21	6

[a] Grading according to Hermanek et al (35).

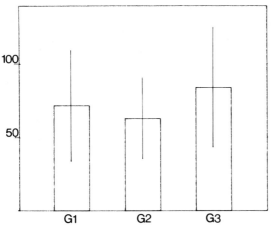

Figure 3.3 Imprint DNA cytophotometry. Nuclear area (μm^2) at different grades of malignancy. Difference between grade 2 (*G2*) and grade 3 (*G3*) is significant ($\alpha < 0.001$).

above. Again, grade 3 nuclei represent the highest values of nuclear area; but, interestingly, grade 1 tumors show considerable increase in nuclear area. Thus, in contrast with DDQ and stem line analysis (histograms), there is no stepwise increase of cytometric values according to the grade of malignancy in nuclear area.

FCM gives more precise information, especially about proliferative activity. FCM produces very similar results concerning ploidy of RCCs (55, 58). These authors found a close correlation between cytologic grading (according to Arner et al (33)) and ploidy: 19 of 22 high grade tumors (grades 3 and 4) were found to be aneuploid, whereas 29 of 44 low grade tumors were diploid. It is of interest to note that 15 low grade tumors contained nondiploid nuclei. This finding agrees well with the authors' results that even in small, strictly histologically defined specimens, cytometrically high malignant tumors may be hidden under the cytologic features of grades 1 or 2 RCC.

Based upon the large number of cells measured by FCM, it is possible to give more detailed results concerning the proliferative activity of the tumor. Interestingly, Baisch et al (58) found that the proliferative activity of diploid and nondiploid tumors is nearly the same. The proliferative activity of RCC, surprisingly, is rather low (diploid: $5 \pm 3\%$; nondiploid: $12 \pm 9\%$). This finding is substantiated by autoradiographic studies done by Rabes (44), who reported labeling indices of RCC of 1 to 5.8%.

In general, both single cell cytophotometry and FCM show significant correlations with histopathologic grading. DNA cytometry, therefore, can serve as a base for the objectification and standardization of histopathology in RCC. However, current results do not completely explain (*a*) the direct correlations between cytometric data and the actual histopathologic substrate because of the morphologic heterogeneity of most RCCs; (*b*) the lack of congruence between DNA data and nuclear area in grades 1 and 2 tumors; and (*c*) the possibilities of cytometry to serve as a base for the cytologic investigation of RCC, e.g., preoperative grading by means of fine needle puncture biopsy.

CAN DNA CYTOMETRY SUPPORT THE PREOPERATIVE CYTOLOGIC GRADING OF RCC?

The fine needle biopsy of RCC—guided by either computerized tomography or ultrasound—has been proven to be a relevant diagnostic technique (59). Preoperative grading of cytologic specimens could be of some importance for the choice of treatment. For example, in cases of metastasizing RCC it could be shown that nephrectomy is of no mean benefit to patients with high grade tumors. In cases of low grade RCC, on the other hand, nephrectomy increases survival rates (60).

The present authors have investigated a series of 27 RCCs (grade 1 = 3; grade 2 = 11; grade 3 = 13). Intraoperatively, we have prepared four fine needle biopsy specimens from different tumor areas. The specimens have been Feulgen stained and investigated by means of single cell cytophotometry as discussed above. When taking into account the position of stem lines, there is a clear correlation between cytometry and histologic grade of malignancy (35) (Fig. 3.4). This finding is in good agreement with the results of von Schreeb et al (61), who found concordance between cytology and histopathology in 36 of 47 cases. However, the predictive value of cytometry in the authors' study is diminished by two facts: (*a*) The number of tumor areas investigated

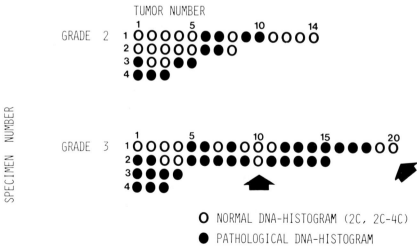

Figure 3.4 DNA cytophotometry from intraoperative fine needle biopsies. Diploid and nondiploid stem lines in different regions of each tumor.

must be at least three in order to detect a nondiploid tumor stem line indicating a high grade of malignancy (62). (*b*) Although the percentage of specimens exhibiting nondiploid stem lines is significantly higher in grade 3 tumors than in grade 2, the safe distinction between grades 2 and 3 RCC is not possible by means of cytometry in individual cases.

The cytometric results of the cytologic biopsy specimens reflect the histopathologic features of the respective tumor areas; but as in conventional imprint cytophotometry, it is difficult to obtain close correlations between cytometric data and histopathology because of the heterogeneity of RCC even in small tumor areas. The authors tried to mark the tumor regions after biopsy and to reinvestigate them histopathologically, but did not get correlations exceeding the findings mentioned above.

POSTEMBEDDING DNA CYTOPHOTOMETRY LEADS TO DISTINCT CORRELATIONS BETWEEN THE ACTUAL HISTOPATHOLOGIC FEATURE AND THE OBJECTIVE CYTOMETRIC DATA

DNA cytometry can be performed not only on freshly prepared cells, but also on fixed and routinely embedded tissues (50, 63, 64). Recently, Delgado et al (41) developed a technique for single cell cytophotometry using paraffin-embedded specimens. This method enables the investigation of histologically defined ("pure") tumor areas in order to find out the cytometric characteristics of the respective features of the tumor. The authors' series of RCCs now includes 106 specimens obtained from 21 tumors. For this part of the studies, the authors chose nuclear grading according to Skinner et al (14) as well as the cell type (clear, dark, mixed) and the histostructural pattern (solid, cystic, adenomatous, papillary, undifferentiated). The main cytometric parameters used in this section are DDQ, SQ, and nuclear area (μm^2). A number of conclusions can be drawn.

First, the stem line values (SQ) clearly reflect the pathohistologic features of the tumor. The nuclear grading according to the criteria of Skinner et al (14) correlates well with the mean values of SQ (Fig. 3.5). As could be supposed by the earlier studies mentioned above, all grade 1 specimens exhibit diploid tumor stem lines expressed as SQ = 1. Additionally, most grade 3 specimens show nondiploid tumor stem lines (SQ < 1.2). Interestingly, there is no difference between the SQ of grade 3 specimens and that of grade 4—i.e., with the exception of the grade 3:grade 4 ratio, the nuclear grading accurately reflects the ploidy of RCC.

Also, the small specimens taken for pepsin extraction and DNA measurement in this study are not completely homogeneous, as can be seen from Figure 3.6. In about a third of the cases investigated, the tumor cells are of mixed type, i.e., they are composed of clear cells intermingled with granular cells. The stem lines of clear cells are positioned near the diploid value, whereas granular cells (and mixed) show considerable variation of their SQ. The mean values of the SQ of clear cells and of granular and mixed cells differ significantly.

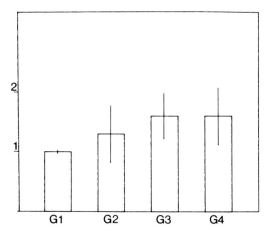

Figure 3.5 Single cell DNA cytophotometry from paraffin-embedded, histo-logically defined tumor specimens—nuclear grading (14): grade 1 ($n = 16$), grade 2 ($n = 37$), grade 3 ($n = 38$), grade 4 ($n = 6$). Stem line quotient (SQ). Differences of mean values of SQ are significant between grade 1 (*G1*) and grade 2 (*G2*) ($\alpha < 0.001$) and grade 2 and grade 3 (*G3*) ($\alpha < 0.01$). No difference between grade 3 and grade 4 (*G4*).

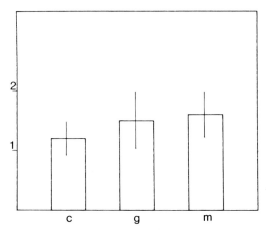

Figure 3.6 Single cell DNA cytophotometry from paraffin-embedded, histo-logically defined tumor specimens: Cell type is clear (*c*), granular (*g*), or mixed (*m*). Stem line quotient (mean values). The difference between clear cells and granular/mixed cells is significant ($\alpha < 0.001$).

The third histopathologic feature to be taken into account is the histopathologic structure (Fig. 3.7). As could be supposed, undifferen-tiated areas show a high SQ, reflecting the high malignant potential of the respective tumor areas. Adenomatous tumor areas are situated between solid and undifferentiated tumor types. Papillary structure, interestingly, reveals a low SQ, similar to solid tumors.

Topographic position within the tumor was another parameter of cytometric analysis (Fig. 3.8). By use of a simple description mode (tumor center, medium position, periphery) the ploidy of the tumor stem line remains equal over the different tumor areas in most cases (28:32). In contrast, malignancy increases when comparing the central

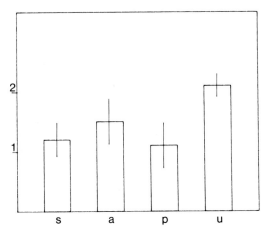

Figure 3.7 Single cell DNA cytophotometry from paraffin-embedded, histologically defined tumor specimens. Histopathologic structure is solid (*s*), adenomatous (*a*), papillary (*p*), or undifferentiated (*u*). $N = 41, 7, 15,$ and 13, respectively). Stem line quotient (SQ), mean values. Difference between solid structure and undifferentiated RCC is significant ($\alpha < 0.01$). Solid, adenomatous and papillary show no differences.

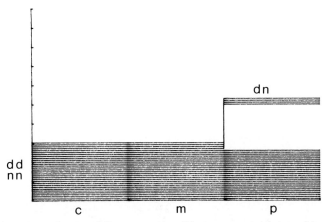

Figure 3.8 Stem lines at different topographic tumor areas (center (*c*), medium (*m*), periphery (*p*)). Same quality of SQ in 28 cases (diploid/diploid (*dd*) or nondiploid/nondiploid (*nn*)); qualitative change (diploid/nondiploid (*dn*)) in 4 cases against the periphery.

tumor mass with infiltrating parts of the tumor within the renal vein in two of four cases.

Second, DDQ values (including the proliferative potential) in general show consistency with histopathology but differ with respect to the topographic position of the investigated specimen within the tumor. The nuclear grading, according to Skinner et al (14), is confirmed by cytophotometry (Fig. 3.9). In contrast to the SQ, there is no significant difference between groups 2, 3, and 4. In general, RCC can be subdivided into two groups: a low proliferating group (grade 1) and a high proliferating group (grades 1 to 3). This finding reflects the fact that diploid tumors commonly show low proliferation, whereas nondiploid tumors reveal a high proliferation rate, as already suggested by Baisch et al (58).

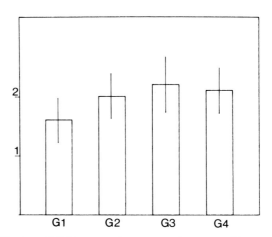

Figure 3.9 Single cell DNA cytophotometry from paraffin-embedded, histologically defined tumor specimens. Nuclear grading (14): grade 1 (*G1*) (*n* = 16), grade 2 (*G2*) (*n* = 27), grade 3 (*G3*) (*n* = 39), grade 4 (*G4*) (*n* = 6). Diploid deviation quotient (DDQ), mean values. Difference between grade 1 and grade 2 is significant ($\alpha < 0.002$). Grade 2 to grade 3 and grade 3 to grade 4 show no differences.

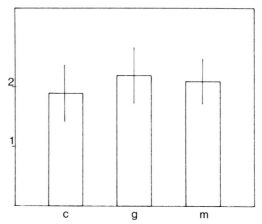

Figure 3.10 Paraffin-embedded specimens. Single cell cytophotometry. Cell type is clear (*c*) (*n* = 49), granular (*g*) (*n* = 24), or mixed (*m*) (*n* = 30). DDQ (mean values). Difference between clear and granular/mixed is significant ($\alpha < 0.001$). Granular and mixed show no difference.

At DDQ, there is a clear distinction between clear cells and granular/mixed cells (Fig. 3.10). The histopathologic structure (Fig. 3.11), too, is reflected by the DDQ values. Again, there is no detectable difference between solid and papillary tumor areas, whereas adenomatous and especially undifferentiated areas reveal a marked increase of DDQ. In contrast to the findings of SQ, there is considerable increase of DDQ at the periphery of the tumor mass (Fig. 3.12). The proliferative activity increases within the renal vein infiltrations, too, whereas, interestingly, the proliferation in lymph node metastases seems to be very low. However, the number of specimens investigated is rather small.

Third, the analysis of nuclear area givens further information concerning especially adenomatous and papillary differentiation and undif-

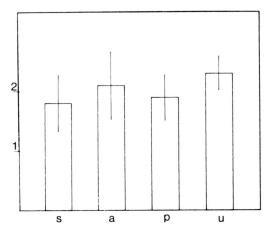

Figure 3.11 Paraffin-embedded specimens. Single cell cytophotometry. Histopathologic structure is solid (*s*) (*n* = 41), adenomatous (*a*) (*n* = 7), papillary (*p*) (*n* = 16), or undifferentiated (*u*) (*n* = 13). Difference between solid and undifferentiated is significant ($\alpha < 0.01$). Adenomatous shows little increase against solid, but the difference is not significant. Solid and papillary show very similar DDQ values.

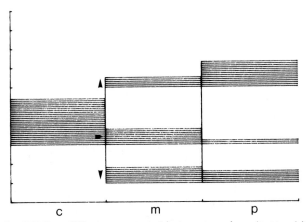

Figure 3.12 DDQ at different topographic tumor regions (center (*c*), medium (*m*), periphery (*p*)). Fourteen cases show increase of DDQ at the peripheral tumor regions.

ferentiated cancer areas. Nuclear area (μm^2) shows an increase from grade 1 to grade 3 (Fig. 3.13), as could be expected from the definition criteria of the grading system (14). Very interestingly, nuclear area sharply decreases in grade 4 specimens, almost down to the area of grade 1. This surprising finding may be explained by the hypothesis that there is a certain percentage of giant nuclei in grade 4, leading to the cytopathologic diagnosis; but, in general, the nuclei of these anaplastic carcinomas are rather small. The nuclei of clear cells are smaller than those of granular/mixed ones (Fig. 3.14). Nuclear area shows similar correlations to histopathologic structure as to nuclear grading (Fig. 3.15). Again, undifferentiated RCC shows small nuclei not significantly differing from solid tumor areas. Papillary regions are even smaller than solid tumor parts. Interestingly, adenomatous tumor areas show the highest

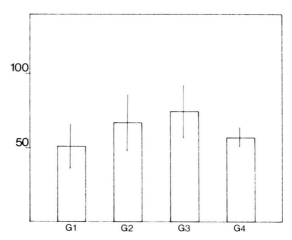

Figure 3.13 Paraffin-embedded specimens. Single cell cytophotometry. Nuclear grading (14): grade 1 (*G1*) (*n* = 16), grade 2 (*G2*) (*n* = 37), grade 3 (*G3*) (*n* = 39), grade 4 (*G4*) (*n* = 6). Nuclear area (μm^2). Difference between grade 1 and grade 2 is significant (α < 0.01).

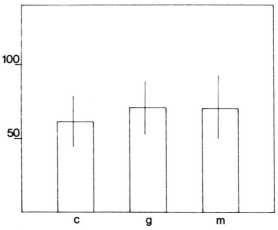

Figure 3.14 Paraffin-embedded specimens. Single cell cytophotometry. Cell type is clear (*c*) (*n* = 49), granular (*g*) (*n* = 24), or mixed (*m*) (*n* = 30). Nuclear area (μm^2) mean values. Difference between clear and granular/mixed is significant (α < 0.02).

values extending beyond all other histopathologic structures. The finding that papillary structure shows the smallest nuclear areas (and low values in DDQ and SQ) supports the view that the papillary type should be separated from adenomatous carcinoma in histopathologic classification (26, 27).

DOES DNA CYTOPHOTOMETRY HAVE ANY INFLUENCE ON PROGNOSIS OF RCC?

Baisch et al (58) and Otto et al (55) published the first results of RCC measurements with clinical follow-up from 1 to 4 years. Beyond the correlations between cytometry and grading, the results of DNA cytom-

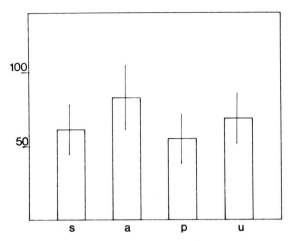

Figure 3.15 Paraffin-embedded specimens. Single cell cytophotometry. Histopathologic structure is solid (*s*) (*n* = 41), adenomatous (*a*) (*n* = 7), papillary (*p*) (*n* = 16), or undifferentiated (*u*) (*n* = 13). Nuclear area (μm^2) mean values. Difference between solid and adenomatous is significant ($\alpha < 0.01$). Undifferentiated and papillary show no differences.

etry clearly influence the prediction of prognosis: 31 of 35 patients with aneuploid RCC developed metastases, as did only 7 of 35 with diploid tumors. The proliferative activity of aneuploid tumors from patients without metastases was lower than the proliferation rate of all aneuploid tumors. It is of special interest that 87% of nondiploid tumors with high malignancy in cytophotometry developed metastases. Therefore, it seems reasonable to suggest that DNA values and nuclear grading are, in part, independent prognostic parameters (55).

CONCLUSIONS

1. Histopathologic grading of RCC represents an important prognostic factor. A review of previous attempts at an exact grading system shows, however, that the different histopathologic systems are hardly comparable and that each system is substantially influenced by subjective factors.
2. Cytometry (both FCM and single cytophotometry) may be useful for standardization and objectification of histopathologic grading and classification.
3. Cytometry gives new information about histopathologic criteria not detectable by conventional microscopy (papillary RCC, undifferentiated RCC).
4. Cytometry is of greater prognostic value than classical histopathologic grading.

REFERENCES

1. Grawitz P: Die sogenannten Lipome der Niere. *Virchow's Arch* 93:39–63, 1883.
2. Apitz K: Geschwülste und Gewebsmißbildungen der Nierenrinde. *Virchow's Arch (Pathol Anat)* 311:285–431, 1943.
3. Amtrup F, Bech Hausen J, Thybo E: Prognosis in renal cell carcinoma evaluated from histological criteria. *Scand J Urol Nephrol* 8:198–202, 1974.

4. Angervall L, Carlström E, Wahlquist L, Åhrén C: Effects of clinical and morphological variables on spread of renal cell carcinoma in an operative series. *Scand J Urol Nephrol* 3:134–140, 1969.
5. Claes G: Concerning the relationship between the morphology and the symptomatology of hypernephroma. *Urol Int* 15:265–279, 1963.
6. Cahill GF: Cancer of the kidney. *JAMA* 138:357–362, 1948.
7. Foot NC, Humphreys GA: The importance of accurate pathologic classification in the prognosis of renal tumors. *Surgery* 23:369–376, 1948.
8. Kay S: Renal cell carcinoma. A 10-year study. *Am J Clin Pathol* 50:428–432, 1968.
9. Melicow MM: Classification of renal neoplasms: a clinical and pathological study based on 199 cases. *J Urol* 51:333–385, 1944.
10. Murphy GP, Fishbein RH: Clinical manifestations and cytology of hypernephromas. *J Urol* 85:483–487, 1961.
11. Murphy GP, Schirmer HK: The diagnosis and treatment of hypernephroma. *Geriatrics* 18:354–360, 1963.
12. Murphy GP, Mostofi FK: The significance of cytoplasmic granularity in the prognosis of renal cell carcinoma. *J Urol* 94:48–54, 1965.
13. Ochsner MG, Brannan W, Pond HS, Goodier EH: Renal cell carcinoma: review of 26 years of experience at the Ochsner Clinic. *J Urol* 110:643–646, 1973.
14. Skinner DG, Colvin RB, Vermillion CD, Pfister RC, Leadbetter WF: Diagnosis and management of renal cell carcinoma. A clinical and pathological study of 309 cases. *Cancer* 28:1165–1177, 1971.
15. Deleted in proof.
16. Fuhrman SA, Lasky LC, Limas C: Prognostic significance of morphologic parameters in renal cell carcinoma. *Am J Surg Pathol* 6:655–663, 1982.
17. Selli C, Hinshaw WM, Woodard BH, Paulson DF: Stratification of risk factors in renal cell carcinoma. *Cancer* 52:899–903, 1983.
18. Angervall L, Wahlquist L: Follow-up and prognosis of renal carcinoma in a series operated by perifascial nephrectomy combined with adrenalectomy and retroperitoneal lymphadenectomy. *Eur Urol* 4:13–17, 1978.
19. Sarosdy MF, Lamm DL: Application of the mixed cell agglutination test for cell surface antigens to renal cell carcinoma. *J Urol* 128:693–696, 1982.
20. Fryfogle J, Dockerty M, Clagett O: Dark-cell adenocarcinomas of the kidney. *J Urol* 60:221–234, 1948.
21. Fuselier HA, Guice SL, Brannan W, Ochsner MG, Sangisetty KV, Beckman EN: Renal cell carcinoma: the Ochsner Medical Institution experience (1945–1978). *J Urol* 130:445–448, 1983.
22. Kofler K, Reichl ER, Zischka-Konorsa W: Statistische Untersuchungen zur Frage der Beziehungen zwischen Morphologie und Prognose bei Nierenparenchymkarzinomen. *Virchow's Arch* (*Pathol Anat*) 368:347–359, 1975.
23. Lieber MM, Tomera FM, Taylor WF, Farrow GM: Renal adenocarcinoma in young adults: survival and variables affecting prognosis. *J Urol* 125:164–168, 1981.
24. McNichols DW, Segura JW, DeWeerd JH: Renal cell carcinoma: long term survival and late recurrence. *J Urol* 126:17–23, 1981.
25. Patel NP, Lavengood RW: Renal cell carcinoma: natural history and results of treatment. *J Urol* 119:722–726, 1978.
26. Boczko S, Fromowitz FB, Bard RH: Papillary adenocarcinoma of the kidney. A new perspective. *Urology* 14:491–495, 1979.
27. Mancilla-Jiminez R, Stanley RJ, Blath RA: Papillary renal carcinoma. A clinical, radiologic and pathologic study of 34 cases. *Cancer* 38:2469–2480, 1976.
28. Hand JR, Broders AC: Carcinoma of the kidney: the degree of malignancy in relation to factors bearing on prognosis. *J Urol* 28:199–216, 1932.
29. Foot NC, Humphreys GA, Whitmore WF: Renal tumors: pathology and prognosis in 295 cases. *J Urol* 66:190–197, 1951.
30. Riches EW, Griffiths IH, Thackray AC: New growths of the kidney and ureter. *Br J Urol* 23:297, 1951.
31. Riches EW: Factors in the prognosis of carcinoma of the kidney. *J Urol* 79:190–195, 1958.
32. Mathisen W, Muri O, Myhre E: Pathology and prognosis in renal tumors. *Acta Chir Scand* 130:303–313, 1965.

33. Arner O, Blanck C, van Schreeb T: Renal adenocarcinoma. Morphology, grading of malignancy, prognosis. A study of 197 cases. *Acta Chir Scand* 346, suppl, 1965.
34. Syrjänen K, Hjelt L: Grading of human renal adenocarcinoma. *Scand J Urol Nephrol* 12:49–55, 1978.
35. Hermanek P, Sigel A, Chlepas S: Histological grading of renal cell carcinoma. *Eur Urol* 2:189–191, 1976.
36. Matsuda M, Osafume M, Nakano E, Asano S, Arima M, Hada T, Watanabe S, Higashino K: Renal cell carcinoma having heterogeneous histological appearance and homogeneous enzymatic property. *Cancer* 45:528–533, 1980.
37. Böhm N, Sandritter W: DNA in human tumors: a cytophotometric study. *Curr Top Pathol* 60:151–219, 1975.
38. Atkin NB, Kay R: Prognostic significance of modal DNA value and other factors in malignant tumors, based on 1465 cases. *Br J Cancer* 40:210–221, 1979.
39. Sandritter W, Kleinhaus D: Über das Trockengewicht, den DNS- und Histonprotein-gehalt von menschlichen Tumoren. *Z Krebsforsch* 66:333–348, 1964.
40. Caspersson T, Lomakka G: Recent progress in quantitative cytochemistry: instru-mentation and results. In Bahr G, Wied G (eds): *Introduction to Quantitative Cyto-chemistry.* New York, Academic Press, 1970, pp. 27–56.
41. Delgado R, Mikuz G, Hofstädter F: DNA-Feulgen-cytophotometric analysis of single cells isolated from paraffin embedded tissue. *Pathol Res Pract* 179:92–94, 1984.
42. Hofstädter F, Jakse G, Lederer B, Mikuz G: Cytophotometric investigations of DNA content in transitional cell tumors of the bladder. Comparison of results with clinical follow up. *Pathol Res Pract* 167:254–264, 1980.
43. Fosså SD: Feulgen DNA-values in transitional cell carcinoma of the human bladder. *Beitr Pathol* 155:44–55, 1975.
44. Rabes MM: Growth kinetics of human renal adenocarcinoma. *UICC Tech Rep Ser* 49:78–81, 1980.
45. Ogino T: Cell kinetic analysis of the quiescent cell compartment in cultured renal carcinoma of syrian hamster. *Gan* 71:381–386, 1980.
46. Fosså SD, Kaalhus O: Nuclear size and chromatin concentration in transitional carcinoma of the human urinary bladder. *Beitr Pathol* 157:109–125, 1976.
47. Mittermayer C, Madreiter H, Lederer B, Sandritter W: Differential acid hydrolysis of euchromatin and heterochromatin (biochemical, histochemical and morphological studies). *Beitr Pathol* 143:157–161, 1971.
48. Braylan RC: Flow cytometry. *Arch Pathol Lab Med* 107:1–6, 1983.
49. Lindmo T, Steen HB: Characteristics of a simple, high-resolution flow cytometer based on a new flow configuration. *Biophys J* 28:33–44, 1979.
50. Hedley DW, Friedlander ML, Taylor IW, Rugg CA, Musgrove EA: Method for analysis of cellular DNA content of paraffin-embedded pathological material using flow cytometry. *J Histochem Cytochem* 31:1333–1335, 1983.
51. Ooms ECM, Anderson WAD, Alons CL, Boon ME, Veldhuizen RW: Analysis of the performance of pathologists in the grading of bladder tumors. *Hum Pathol* 14:140–143, 1983.
52. Klein FA, Herr HW, Whitmore WF, Sogani PC, Melamed MR: An evaluation of automated flow cytometry (FCM) in detection of carcinoma in situ of the urinary bladder. *Cancer* 50:1003–1008, 1982.
53. Hofstädter F, Jakse G, Lederer B, Mikuz G, Delgado R: DNA-Feulgen-cytopho-tometry and biological behavior of urothelial bladder carcinoma. *Br J Urol* 56:289–295, 1984.
54. Kreicbergs A, Boquist L, Borssén B, Larsson SE: Prognostic factors in chondrosar-coma. A comparative study of cellular DNA content and clinicopathological features. *Cancer* 50:577–583, 1982.
55. Otto U, Baisch H, Huland H, Klöppel G: Tumor-cell deoxyribonucleic acid content and prognosis in human renal adenocarcinoma. *J Urol* 132:237–239, 1984.
56. Largiader F: Morphologie, Histogenese und Klassifikation der Nierentumoren. *Urol Int* 6:273–367, 1958.
57. Zollinger HU: *Niere und ableitende Harnwege.* Berlin, Springer, 1966.
58. Baisch M, Otto U, König K, Klöppel G, Köllermann M, Linden WA: DNA content of human kidney carcinoma cells in relation to histological grading. *Br J Cancer* 45:878–886, 1982.

59. Zaijzek J: *Aspiration Biopsy Cytology. II: Cytology of Infradiaphragmatic Organs.* Basel, Karger, 1979.
60. Pauer W, Mikuz G, Jakse G: Ist die Nephrektomie beim metastasierenden Nierenzellkarzinom sinnvoll? *Aktuel Urol* 12:146–149, 1981.
61. von Schreeb T, Franzén E, Ljungquist A: Renal adenocarcinoma. Evaluation of malignancy on a cytologic basis: a comparative cytologic and histologic study. *Scand J Urol Nephrol* 1:265–269, 1967.
62. Rauschmeier H, Hofstädter F, Jakse G: Prognostic relevance of cytologic grading in metastatic renal cell carcinoma. In Pavone-Macaluso M, Smith PH (eds): *Cancer of the Prostate and Kidney.* New York, Plenum, 1983, pp 587–593.
63. Inokuchi K, Kodama Y, Sasaki O, Kamegawa T, Okamura T: Differentiation of growth patterns of early gastric carcinoma determined by cytophotometric DNA analysis. *Cancer* 52:1138–1141, 1983.
64. Kreicbergs A, Zetterberg A: Cytophotometric DNA measurements of chondrosarcoma. Methodological aspects on measurements in tissue sections from old paraffin embedded specimens. *Anal Quant Cytol* 2:84–92, 1980.
65. Griffiths IH, Thackray AC: Parenchymal carcinoma of the kidney. *Br J Urol* 21:128–135, 1949.

4

Serologic Markers, Paraneoplastic Syndromes, and Ectopic Hormone Production in Renal Adenocarcinoma

Gerald Sufrin, M.D.
Anthony Golio, M.D.
Gerald P. Murphy, M.D.

INTRODUCTION

Since the present authors' previous review of the hormonal syndromes and serologic manifestations of renal adenocarcinoma, important advances in the paraneoplastic syndrome associated with malignancy in general and with hypernephroma in particular have been reported (1–4). Indeed, a wider recognition of the serologic markers associated with renal carcinoma, both eutopic and ectopic, has immediate clinical relevance since these may facilitate earlier diagnosis, may allow timely therapy of metabolic abnormalities associated with ectopic hormone production, and may serve as a means to assess response to therapy (3). In view of this and in view of expanding diagnostic capabilities, including monoclonal antibodies, recognition of serologic factors may provide new insights into the management of renal adenocarcinoma.

The presenting manifestations of renal adenocarcinoma in man may be ubiquitous—may be nonurologic—and it is of interest that in about 30% of patients specific genitourinary symptoms are absent, and systemic effects often are the initial mode of presentation (5–7). In addition, since the kidney has well recognized endocrine functions, it is not unexpected that hormonal syndromes and serologic markers should be associated with hypernephroma (8). Thus, the kidney is normally involved in the production of renin, erythropoietin, prostaglandins, and

1,25-dihydroxycholecalciferol, and the inappropriate production of at least the first three have been described in association with renal adenocarcinoma (7). In addition and possibly of greater significance is the fact that renal carcinomas are capable of elaborating ectopic factors, including parathormone, insulin, glucagon, enteroglucagon, chorionic gonadotropin, and ferritin (6, 9, 10).

The classification of ectopic hormonal syndromes, of paraneoplastic syndromes, and of serologic markers associated with renal carcinoma may be based on the specific factors in question, such as parathormone, renin, or erythropoietin; on the clinical syndromes which occur as a result of the inappropriate elaboration of these factors, e.g., hypercalcemia, erythropoietosis, or hypertension; or on whether the factors or syndromes produced are eutopic (that is, customarily associated with the kidney) or ectopic (that is, not typically associated with the kidney). While such classifications may be relevant to providing new biologic insights, it should be noted that diverse systemic effects have been associated with renal carcinoma, including amyloidosis, cachexia, anemia, thrombocytosis, and alterations in plasma protein levels, that evidence for a humoral mechanism in the etiology of these abnormalities is unconvincing, and that immunologic factors may possibly be of significance (7). This review will address only the paraneoplastic syndromes, syndromes of inappropriate hormonal secretion, and serologic markers whose production has been related to renal adenocarcinoma.

PARANEOPLASTIC SYNDROMES

Hypertension

Hypertension has been noted in up to 40% of patients with renal adenocarcinoma, although this association is not surprising in view of the kidney's role in the regulation of blood pressure (11, 12). While this figure may require modification since renal carcinoma occurs in a population with an expected 20% incidence of hypertension, mechanisms for this association are diverse (13). Thus, hypernephromas may produce hypertension through a variety of mechanisms, including hyperreninemia, renal arteriovenous fistulae, polycythemia, hypercalcemia, ureteral obstruction, or elevated intracranial pressure secondary to cerebral metastases (7, 14, 15).

The hyperreninemia found in some cases of renal carcinoma may be due to a variety of etiologies, including secretion of renin by the tumor itself, secretion of renin by adjacent non-neoplastic renal tissue, and iatrogenic factors (15–17). The secretion of renin by renal carcinoma has been reported in both clear and granular cell tumors and usually in lesions of low histologic grade (11, 15, 17, 18). In these cases a decline in elevated blood pressure and in plasma renin levels was noted to occur following nephrectomy, and tumor tissue renin determinations further confirmed renin production by the tumors (15, 17). Renal tumors may also elicit hyperreninemia and hypertension by renal artery encasement and production of a Goldblatt effect; in these cases, hypertension improved and plasma renin levels declined following nephrectomy (16). Subcapsular or perirenal hemorrhage, a well documented complication of renal carcinoma, may also produce extrinsic renal parenchymal compression, renal ischemia, hyperreninemia, and hypertension that is relieved by nephrectomy (19).

Yet another source of hyperreninemia in patients with renal neoplasia occurs in those whose tumors arise from the juxtaglomerular cell and who exhibit elevated tumor and plasma renin levels (20–22). Finally, iatrogenic factors may relate to the hyperreninemia and hypertension seen in patients with renal carcinoma, and in this regard the use of renal artery embolization prior to nephrectomy is of interest (23). Thus, following palliative renal artery embolization in a patient with metastatic renal carcinoma, severe hypertension developed and angiography showed only partial vascular occlusion (23). Plasma renin levels lateralized to the side of embolization, and hypertension persisted despite efforts to embolize the collateral vessels (23).

While approximately 90% of renal carcinomas are roentgenographically hypervascular, hemodynamically significant arteriovenous fistulae are uncommon, and only when extensive arteriovenous communications exist do such clinical manifestations as bruits, arterial hypertension, and cardiac failure occur (24–26). These fistulous communications are located within the substance of the tumor or its metastases and may cause elevation of cardiac output with systemic hypertension (24, 27). Diastolic hypertension, however, is less common and results from "renovascular steal"—that is, ischemia and hyperreninemia arising in renal parenchyma distal to the fistula (26). It is of interest that over 70% of patients with hypernephroma and symptomatic arteriovenous fistulae are females, in contrast to the general male preponderance of this tumor, and that in patients manifesting the cardiovascular effects of fistulae, nephrectomy may ameliorate those symptoms (26,28).

Paradoxically, renal carcinoma has been related to an antihypertensive effect, and a vasodilator, prostaglandin A, has been isolated from a hypernephroma (29). Thus, a patient with a history of severe refractory hypertension was noted spontaneously to become normotensive (29). Following nephrectomy, however, the patient once again became hypertensive. In this patient, tumor tissue and preoperative plasma prostaglandin A levels were elevated, and postoperatively plasma prostaglandin levels fell in association with a rise in blood pressure (29).

While arterial hypertension and renal carcinoma may be causally unrelated, a 10-fold higher incidence of renal carcinoma has been described in asymptomatic patients being screened for hypertension (13). Hypertension in association with renal carcinoma is usually seen in low stage, low grade, clear cell lesions and does not appear to relate to prognosis; although nephrectomy may alleviate hypertension, the reappearance of hypertension may be a harbinger of tumor recurrence (11, 15, 24). Moreover, reduction in levels of hypertension has correlated with reductions in plasma renin levels or with the obliteration of arteriovenous fistulae, and these observations serve to confirm a causal relation between hypernephroma and hypertension (17, 26).

Nonmetastatic Hepatic Dysfunction

Hepatic dysfunction in the absence of liver metastases occurring in patients with renal carcinoma—that is, nonmetastatic hepatic dysfunction or the so-called "Stauffer syndrome"—has been reported in 15 to 33% of patients with this tumor (5, 30–32). Classically, those liver function studies, listed in order of frequency, which have been reported to be abnormal are as follows: prolonged sulfobromophthalein (BSP) retention (91%), hypoprothrombinemia (73%), elevated α_2-globulin (71%), elevated indirect bilirubin (70%), and increased alkaline phosphatase (60%) (33). Indeed, subsequent studies have confirmed this syndrome, and a recent study revealed an elevated alkaline phosphatase level in 100% of patients, prolonged prothrombin time or an increased α_2-globulin level or hypoalbuminemia in 63%, hypergammaglobulinemia in 54%, increased hepatic alkaline phosphatase in 36%, increased bilirubin in 27%, and increased glutamyl transpeptidase in 18% (31, 32). By agreement, the diagnosis of nonmetastatic hepatic dysfunction requires abnormalities in at least three of these parameters of hepatic function (32, 34). Moreover, while about one-half of patients with this syndrome exhibit a diffuse, nontender hepatomegaly, this syndrome has also been reported in patients with xanthogranulomatous pyelonephritis (34, 35).

The specific pathogenesis of this disorder is unclear, although two theories have been suggested (32, 36, 37). One hypothesis suggests that hypernephromas may secrete either hepatotoxins or lysosomal enzymes, either of which may enhance hepatic lysosomal enzyme activity, including cathepsins, acid phosphatase, and β-glucuronidase (36). The precise mechanism whereby increased hepatic lysosomal enzyme activity leads to disordered liver functions, however, remains obscure, and attempts to reproduce this syndrome were experimentally unsuccessful (32). On the other hand, the immunologic theory suggests that secretion of a hepatotoxin by renal adenocarcinoma may result in recruitment of helper T cells, with stimulation of a β cell response and production of autoantibodies to putative neoantigens on the hepatocyte (37). In any event, reversal of hepatic dysfunction and normalization of the abnormal liver function tests following nephrectomy have been observed in 62% of reported cases, clearly implicating a hepatotoxic factor elaborated by the tumor or produced by the host in response to this neoplasm (33, 38, 39).

Hepatic morphology in nonmetastatic hepatopathy shows a reactive hepatitis with Kupffer cell proliferation, sinusoidal dilation, varying degrees of hepatocellular degeneration, focal necrosis, and portal triaditis (32, 34). Although these changes are somewhat nonspecific, clinical resolution of hepatic dysfunction is associated with histologic evidence of healing and would seem to correlate with the nonmetastatic hepatopathy of renal carcinoma (32, 38).

In 86 to 100% of reports a clear cell renal carcinoma, and in about 70% a high grade lesion was found in patients with this syndrome (31–33, 39). Moreover, while the occurrence of this syndrome was unrelated to tumor stage, its reversibility, as, for example, following nephrectomy, was related to the extent of the disease and to the presence of metastases (32). It is also of interest that, despite these biochemical abnormalities, clinical symptoms of the syndrome are nonspecific and jaundice is uncommon (33).

Nonmetastatic hepatic dysfunction in association with renal carcinoma is not of prognostic significance and should not be a contraindication to aggressive surgical management (34). However, when this syndrome is the presenting manifestation of renal carcinoma, recognition of the tumor may be delayed because of nonlocalizing, nonurologic symptoms. Hence, diagnosis may be delayed, accounting in some reports for a high incidence of advanced lesions (32). Indeed, the effect of nephrectomy on these abnormal liver function tests may be of prognostic value since of those patients whose hepatic abnormalities returned to normal following nephrectomy, 88% were alive and well after 1 year in contrast to patients whose hepatic function was unchanged after nephrectomy, in whom a 26% 1-year survival rate was reported (35, 38). Similarly, of those patients whose abnormal liver functions tests persisted postnephrectomy, about 90% had evidence of metastases, whereas such involvement was absent in patients whose postnephrectomy studies returned to normal (34).

It would appear that serial liver function studies are of value in monitoring patients with nonmetastatic hepatopathy and that a persistence of abnormalities indicates residual disease and thus a poor prognosis (33). Moreover, patients in whom postnephrectomy liver function studies become normal and who then show a recrudescence of abnormal values have been shown to have recurrent disease (34). Indeed, even delayed recurrences in the absence of hepatic metastases may be associated with this syndrome, and in one report recurrence of renal carcinoma 22 years after nephrectomy was associated with the appearance of this syndrome (40).

Pyrexia

Recurrent fever in the absence of other identifiable causes is a common manifestation of certain neoplasms, including lymphomas, acute leukemia, and hypernephromas (41, 42). Indeed, an unexplained fever coinciding with tumor growth may remit with excision but then reappear with tumor recurrence. Mechanisms which have been suggested for such fevers include tumor-produced toxins, tumor necrosis with release of tissue pyrogens, abnormal hepatic metabolism of steroids, particularly etiocholanolone, and the elaboration of a specific tumor pyrogen (41–43). Moreover, investigators have demonstrated the presence of an endogenous pyrogen in extracts prepared from renal carcinoma tissue but not from adjacent normal renal tissue (43).

The incidence of fever in association with hypernephroma is about 20%, and temperature levels in over 90% of patients are generally below 39°C (42). Fever, however, is the sole presenting manifestation of hypernephroma in 2% of cases, although it is an initial symptom among others in 12% and occurs sometime during the course of the disease in up to 41% of patients (6).

Fever associated with renal carcinoma does not correlate with several important clinical aspects of this tumor, including patient age, tumor stage, tumor size, degree of tumor necrosis, prognosis, or duration of survival (4, 42, 44, 45). Fever, however, has been reported to be more common in tumors with a granular cell pattern, in females with renal carcinoma as compared to males, in patients exhibiting weight loss, and in patients with an elevated erythrocyte sedimentation rate (7, 46). Nephrectomy in the absence of metastases has been associated with defervescence, although growth of residual tumor or appearance of metastases has caused a reappearance of febrile episodes (45). The presence of fever is not an adverse prognostic sign among patients with hypernephroma, and no difference in survival could be detected between patients whose fever resolved postnephrectomy and patients who remained febrile (7).

Cushing's Syndrome

Ectopic adrenocorticotropic hormone (ACTH) production and Cushing's syndrome are well recognized in association with a variety of neoplasms, although renal adenocarcinoma accounts for less than 2% of reported ectopic ACTH-secreting neoplasms (47). Indeed, the availability of sensitive assay procedures has suggested that ectopic ACTH production is a widespread concomitant of certain neoplasms, although corresponding clinical and biochemical abnormalities are uncommon (48). In the ectopic production of ACTH, serum ACTH and cortisol levels and urinary 17-hydroxycorticosteroids and 17-ketosteroids are often profoundly elevated despite a paucity of the clinical stigmata of Cushing's disease, such as moon facies, hirsutism, striae, and truncal obesity, which occur in less than 50% of patients (49, 50). In patients with ectopic ACTH production, manifestations most commonly include hypokalemia, alkalosis, myopathy, and mental confusion, and usually result in adrenal cortical hyperplasia and failure of large doses of dexamethasone (8 mg) to suppress corticosteroid levels (49, 51).

Although ectopic ACTH production and Cushing's syndrome have only rarely been reported in association with renal carcinoma, a discordance between biologic activity and immunoreactivity of ectopic ACTH may exist, and hence the true incidence of ectopic ACTH production may be higher than reports would indicate (52–54).

Consistent with the occasionally prolonged clinical course of patients with renal carcinoma are well documented illustrations of Cushing's syndrome in association with hypernephroma (52, 53). Thus, in contrast to other ectopic ACTH-producing tumors, e.g., bronchogenic carcinoma, where a rapid clinical course may preclude development of cushingoid manifestations, in patients with renal carcinoma, clinical stigmata of Cushing's syndrome have been noted (48). The associated renal carcinomas were low stage, low grade, and of the clear cell pattern, and the adrenal glands showed diffuse hyperplasia (52). Nephrectomy and subtotal adrenalectomy were associated with remission of Cushing's syndrome, although recrudescence of Cushing's syndrome was noted in association with tumor recurrence, suggesting that serial ACTH measurement may be of value in early detection of recurrences (51). Similarly, in a patient with a long history of Cushing's syndrome in association with hypernephroma, refractory hypotension occurred following nephrectomy, suggesting that in the absence of metastatic replacement, ectopic ACTH suppressed the pituitary, thereby preventing endogenous ACTH production following excision of the tumor. Despite this, Cushing's syndrome in association with renal carcinoma is not an unfavorable sign, and resection of the tumor may result in reversal of the symptoms noted (52).

Galactorrhea

Non-puerperal galactorrhea has been noted in association with hypothalamic disorders, various drug therapies, and pituitary neoplasms; in view of the role of prolactin in lactation, it is of interest that ectopic production of this hormone has been documented in patients with renal adenocarcinoma (55–57). Thus, a 49-year-old female was found to have nonpuerperal galactorrhea, renal adenocarcinoma, and elevated serum prolactin levels (57). That the hyperprolactinemia was causally related to the renal tumor was suggested by the fall in prolactin levels following nephrectomy, although whether the galactorrhea remitted was not mentioned. Further evidence that this tumor did indeed elaborate prolactin was the demonstration of prolactin synthesis by these renal carcinoma cells when they were grown in tissue culture (57).

Moreover, galactorrhea has been reported in other cases of hypernephroma, although serum prolactin determinations were unavailable at the time these patients were studied (58, 59). In addition, it is possible that hyperprolactinemia may occur in the absence of galactorrhea and that the true incidence of hyperprolactinemia may be higher than the frequency of galactorrhea would suggest (57). Thus, since renal carcinoma is 2 to 3 times more common in males than it is in females, and since the male breast is not appropriately primed for lactation with hormones such as estrogens, hyperprolactinemia may be present but may fail to elicit galactorrhea (60). Furthermore, the sensitivity of immunoassay techniques along with the heterogeneity of peptide hormones associated with neoplasia may result in immunoassay activity but not in biologic activity (61).

SEROLOGIC MARKERS

Hypercalcemia

Hypercalcemia, perhaps the commonest systemic metabolic aberration associated with malignancies in general, has been reported in from 3 to 13% of patients with renal carcinoma (62–65). The etiology of the hypercalcemia of malignancy, however, is varied, and multiple factors, including osteoclast activating factor, 1,25-dihydroxyvitamin D, prostaglandins, direct erosion of bone by tumor cells, parathyroid hormone, transforming growth factors, factors that interact with parathormone receptors, and colony stimulating factor, have all been implicated (65).

In some cases, however, the etiology of hypercalcemia remains obscure, although urinary nephrogenous cyclic adenosine monophosphate may be an important marker of humorally mediated, cancer-related hypercalcemia (66, 67).

The skeletal metastases of renal carcinoma are typically osteolytic and bone destruction due either to direct mechanical pressure exerted by an expanding tumor mass or to tumor-induced stimulation of osteoclastic bone resorption (65, 68). In any case, the accelerated skeletal resorption and release of calcium in excess of renal excretory capabilities may result in hypercalcemia.

Pseudohyperparathyroidism, that is, the syndrome of hypercalcemia, in the presence of malignancy without osseous metastases but with normal parathyroid glands has been noted in patients with renal carcinoma (69, 70). Indeed, pseudohyperparathyroidism is often found in association with hypernephroma, and documentation that parathormone or a parathormone-like peptide is responsible for the hypercalcemia of pseudohyperparathyroidism has been provided by immunoassay of tumor extracts and of serum (71, 72). In addition, secretion of a factor which is recognized by cellular parathormone receptors and which was isolated for the media in which human renal carcinoma cells were grown has been reported (67). Moreover, when the cells were grown in nude mice, hypercalcemia was noted, and resection of the tumors was associated with a fall in blood calcium levels in these animals (67).

Prostaglandins, particularly those of the E series, have also been shown both clinically and experimentally to have a causal role in the hypercalcemia of malignancy, and prostaglandins have been identified in human renal carcinoma tissue (73, 74). Additional confirmation that prostaglandins are capable of mediating the hypercalcemia of renal carcinoma in the absence of osseous metastases is found in the reports of patients with hypernephroma, hypercalcemia, and elevated plasma prostaglandin levels but without osseous metastases (74). In these patients, nephrectomy was followed by a fall in elevated calcium and in prostaglandin levels.

The coexistence of primary hyperparathyroidism and renal carcinoma has been described, and in such patients the etiology of hypercalcemia is an important diagnostic challenge since the therapy of primary hyperparathyroidism differs from the treatment of pseudohyperparathyroidism (75–77). Differentiation between these levels may be difficult, but a history of hypercalcemia which antedates recognition of the cancer, and the effect of anticancer therapy on the hypercalcemia are relevant diagnostic considerations (76). In addition, and for a given level of serum calcium, parathormone levels are generally higher in ectopic hyperparathyroidism than they are in primary hyperparathyroidism (71). In contrast to primary hyperparathyroidism where the symptoms of hypercalcemia may be subtle, the symptoms of hypercalcemia secondary to ectopic hormone production in renal carcinoma may be more florid and of shorter duration, and such symptoms reflect the higher serum calcium levels seen in patients with the ectopic hyperparathyroidism of hypernephroma (71, 78). Symptoms of hypercalcemia may be nonspecific—e.g., weakness, anorexia, and mental changes—and despite elevated urinary calcium levels, there is only an 8% incidence of renal calculi in association with the hypercalcemia, in contrast to a 40% incidence of urolithiasis in primary hyperparathyroidism (78, 79).

In evaluating available reports the present authors noted that 75% of patients with hypernephroma and hypercalcemia tended to exhibit high stage lesions of the clear cell type (80–85). Histologic grade, however, had no apparent relation to serum calcium levels, although ultrastructural and immunohistochemical studies may provide insight into the etiology of hypercalcemia in hypernephroma (86). Thus, ultrastructural studies of carcinomatous renal tissue in patients with hypercalcemia without osseous metastases showed cytoplasmic membrane-bound, electron-dense granules identified as parathormone granules, and this was confirmed by immunohistochemistry (86).

Therapeutic strategies in the management of the hypercalcemia associated with renal carcinoma include saline infusion, a furosemide-induced diuresis, corticosteroids, and mithramycin (87). In addition to these general measures, however, specific therapy, such as nephrectomy, and the extirpation or other treatment of metastases may normalize serum calcium levels and should be pursued aggressively (69, 80, 84, 88). Additionally, serum calcium levels have served as an effective tumor marker since recrudescence of disease was heralded by elevation of a previously normalized calcium level. Moreover, when hypercalcemia has been related to elevated prostaglandin levels, indomethacin has effectively lowered serum calcium and prostaglandin levels (89). Finally, the treatment of hypercalcemia due to hyperparathyroidism in patients with renal carcinoma is parathyroidectomy (76).

Erythropoietin

Erythropoietin (EP), a glycoprotein produced by the renal cortex in response to hypoxia, is a principal factor regulating erythropoiesis and is believed to act by inducing erythrocyte differentiation (90). In view of the kidney's role in EP production, it is understandable that elevated EP levels have been detected in association with a variety of renal lesions, including cysts, Wilms' tumor, hydronephrosis, and renal adenocarcinoma (91–93). The mechanisms which have been proposed to account for the increased EP levels that have been reported to occur in over 40% of patients with renal adenocarcinoma include synthesis of EP by the neoplastic cells themselves or enhanced EP production by the nonmalignant portion of the kidney in response to tumor-induced hypoxia (94, 95).

Recently, evidence that renal carcinoma cells themselves can synthesize biologically active EP has been presented, and potent EP extracts from the primary tumor and from pulmonary metastases were demonstrated (93). In addition, when pulmonary metastases from a patient with renal adenocarcinoma and elevated EP levels were transplanted into nude mice, 50% of the animals developed erythrocytosis, and elevated EP levels and extracts of the tumor grown in nude mice demonstrated elevated EP levels (93). Similarly, mechanisms whereby renal tumors may reduce renal perfusion and produce renal hypoxemia have been outlined: (*a*) elevated intrarenal pressure due to extracapsular or intracapsular tumors; (*b*) tumor impairment of renal arterial supply or venous drainage; (*c*) ureteral obstruction with hydronephrosis and elevated intrarenal pressure (96). Further mechanisms proposed for elevated EP levels in renal carcinoma include tumor-induced systemic hypoxia, tumor impairment of EP metabolism, and extrarenal production of EP (96).

Elevated EP levels have been reported in up to 47% of patients with metastatic renal carcinoma and in up to 37% of patients with nonmetastatic disease (94). However, since erythrocytosis has been noted in no more than 10% of patients with renal carcinoma, a discordance between the production of EP and hemoglobin levels might be due to failure of end organ, that is, bone marrow response, or to the elaboration of a biologically inactive tumor EP (96). It is of interest that opposing trends, namely, a polycythemic propensity tending to produce erythrocytosis and dyshematopoietic trend tending to produce anemia, occur in renal carcinoma and that the relative rarity of the former suggests predominence of the latter mechanism (97).

A relation between tumor stage and serum EP levels was documented by studies showing that elevated EP levels were more common in high stage (47%) than in low stage (37%) lesions and that EP levels were 3½ times higher in patients with high stage lesions than in patients with low stage lesions (98). Erythrocytosis, however, was found with equal frequency irrespective of stage (98). While previous reports suggest that erythrocytosis tends to occur in association with clear cell carcinoma, other investigators have been unable to confirm this association (99).

Additional evidence regarding EP levels and and renal adenocarcinoma relates to the effect of nephrectomy on EP levels. Thus, in patients with renal carcinoma and elevated EP levels, nephrectomy reduced serum EP in both high and low stage lesions (94, 98). Moreover, while postnephrectomy EP levels fell to normal in patients with nonmetastatic disease, patients with metastases merely exhibited a lowering of EP. However, a constant relationship between EP and clinical prognosis in patients with renal carcinoma may, in individual cases, be uncertain, although a significant correlation between elevated hemoglobin values and survival 1 year following nephrectomy has been reported (99).

Prostaglandins

The prostaglandins are ubiquitous substances with diverse biologic properties which regulate a variety of physiologic processes. It is of interest, therefore, that their inappropriate production has been reported in association with renal adenocarcinoma, and in this regard their association with hypercalcemia and the amelioration of arterial hypertension is noteworthy (20, 29, 100). While these latter syndromes are described elsewhere in this review, recently a carcinoid-like syndrome in association with renal adenocarcinoma and elevated prostaglandin levels was reported (101). Thus, in a patient who had previously undergone nephrectomy for renal carcinoma and who subsequently developed pulmonary metastases, recurrent episodes of flushing, facial congestion, sweating, palpitations, and abdominal pain were noted (101). During one of these episodes systolic blood pressure was noted to be 60 mm Hg and urinary excretion of 5-hydroxyindoleacetic acid and catecholamines was normal. However, plasma prostaglandin E and 13,14-dehydro-15-ketoprostaglandin $F_{2}\alpha$ levels were elevated during these attacks and normal when the patient was asymptomatic (101). While incontrovertible evidence of prostaglandin synthesis by the tumor itself was not provided, it is of particular importance that the attacks of flushing and of other carcinoid-like symptoms were eliminated by administration of aspirin and that cessation of aspirin resulted in reappearance of symptoms (101). Moreover, antihistamines, phenothiazines, and prednisone were ineffective in preventing flushing, and this report, therefore, would appear to document a causal association between a carcinoid-like syndrome in a patient with metastatic renal carcinoma and elevated prostaglandin levels (101).

Chorionic Gonadotropin

Chorionic gonadotropin is a glycoprotein produced by the placental syntrophoblast and is, therefore, normally found in the plasma of pregnant females (102, 103). Indeed, its presence in the serum of an adult male or nonpregnant female may suggest its ectopic production and neoplasia (103). Since chorionic gonadotropin and luteinizing hormone have similar biologic activity and since luteinizing hormone is secreted by the pituitary, the development of a radioimmunoassay to distinguish these hormones was an important advance (104). Indeed, ectopic chorionic gonadotropin production by nontrophoblastic tumors, including renal carcinoma, has been discussed (103, 105).

In males with renal carcinoma producing ectopic chorionic gonadotropin, signs and symptoms have included feminization and loss of libido which were most likely due to elevated estradiol levels (6). Proposed mechanisms whereby ectopic chorionic gonadotropin results in elevated estradiol levels in males include enhanced Leydig cell production of testosterone with subsequent peripheral conversion to estradiol, or a direct increase in testicular estrogen production itself (106). In females, virilization and amenorrhea due to elevated androgen levels have been noted (107). The mechanism of this relates to stimulation of the ovarian granulosa-theca cells and/or ovarian hilar cells, with resulting overproduction of androgens (6, 108).

The frequency of ectopic chorionic gonadotropin (hCG) production by renal adenocarcinoma may be higher than the number of reported cases would indicate owing to a disparity between the biologic potency and the serologic reactivity of hCG. Thus, the development of sensitive assays may result in detection of ectopic gonadotropin production in the absence of overt clinical manifestations (106). Ectopic hCG production has been reported in association with clear, granular, and mixed renal cell carcinoma (6, 106, 109). However, no relation between chorionic gonadotropin production and tumor stage or grade or between hCG production and patient survival has been reported (6, 109). Despite this, the clinical relevance of serial hCG monitoring in patients with renal adenocarcinoma is acknowledged, and both nephrectomy and successful chemotherapy have been associated with a reduction in hCG levels, while tumor recrudescence was accompanied by a rise in gonadotropin titer (6, 102, 106).

Alkaline Phosphatase

Alkaline phosphatase, a ubiquitous enzyme found in the serum and in association with membranes in a variety of tissues, can be classified into three main forms: intestinal, liver/bone/kidney, and placental (101). In patients with renal carcinoma, elevated serum alkaline phosphatase levels may be associated with hepatic or osseous metastases or with nonmetastatic hepatopathy, or it may be the result of the production and release of alkaline phosphatase by the tumor itself (110, 111). In view of this, it is of note that a recent study demonstrated histochemically detectable alkaline phosphatase activity in both the stromal cells and tumor cells in three of four patients with renal adenocarcinoma (112). This further confirms the belief that the elevated alkaline phosphatase levels found in the sera of patients with renal carcinoma may, in the absence of hepatic or osseous disease, originate from the tumor itself owing to release of the enzyme from tumor cells. Indeed, it is of note that in patients with localized renal carcinoma without evidence of nonmetastatic hepatopathy, elevated serum alkaline phosphatase activity has been observed; and following nephrectomy, alkaline phosphatase activity returned to normal, further suggesting a tumor-related source for this enzyme (10).

Despite these provocative findings, evidence for unique placental-like alkaline phosphatase activity was found in only one of the four patients studied with renal carcinoma (112). Although tumor tissue of the other three patients showed alkaline phosphatase activity, the enzyme did not react with polyclonal antisera or monoclonal antibodies to placental alkaline phosphatase (112). Thus, while alkaline phosphatase may indeed be a legitimate marker for the study of renal carcinoma, further study will be required to ascertain whether the alkaline phosphatase found in this tumor is the product of different genes or represents differences due to post-translational modification of the same enzyme molecule or differences due to post-transcriptional RNA processing (112).

Insulin, Glucagon, and Enteroglucagon

The ectopic production and secretion of insulin, glucagon, and enteroglucagon have been described only rarely in association with renal carcinoma, although associated clinical symptoms are of interest (9, 111). A patient with renal carcinoma exhibited extreme fluctuations in serum glucose levels, and subsequent investigation showed that elevated levels of blood glucose were accompanied by an elevated serum glucagon:insulin ratio. Similarly, subnormal blood glucose levels also seen in this patient were associated with a low glucagon:insulin ratio, and following nephrectomy all three parameters, namely, blood glucose, insulin, and glucagon levels, stabilized at near normal values (9). That ectopic production of either insulin or glucagon by renal carcinoma has been reported only rarely is of interest, and this case, therefore, is of further note since both hormones were shown to be present in tumor tissue extracts (9).

Following nephrectomy, an extract of the tumor tissue was prepared. The immunoreactive insulin level in renal carcinoma tissue was found to be 100 times that in control renal tissue, and the immunoreactive glucagon level in malignant renal tissue was 25 times that of control nonmalignant renal tissue (9). Production of multiple ectopic hormones or serologic markers by renal adenocarcinoma is a distinctly rare event, and in addition to this report of the concomitant production of insulin and glucagon by a renal carcinoma, attention is called to the report describing elevated serum ferritin levels and hypercalcemia in a patient with renal carcinoma (9, 10).

The ectopic production of enteroglucagon, a polypeptide normally secreted by the jejunal and ileal mucosa, has also been reported in association with renal carcinoma (113). Both pancreatic and intestinal enteroglucagon-secreting cells are believed to originate from the neural crest and thus to belong to the amine precursor uptake decarboxylation (APUD) system (111). Ectopic production of enteroglucagon by a renal carcinoma was associated with constipation, decreased intestinal transit time, thickening of the intestinal mucosa, a diabetic glucose tolerance test, and an elevated preoperative plasma enteroglucagon level (114). Following nephrectomy, constipation resolved, intestinal transit time increased, and the abnormal glucose tolerance test and plasma enteroglucagon level returned to normal (115). Biochemical and immunologic studies of the tumor revealed the presence of large amounts of enteroglucagon (115).

Symptoms, biochemical and histologic studies, and the response to nephrectomy all implicated ectopic enteroglucagon production by a renal tumor (114). Thus, this represents a significant link between the APUD series of endocrine polypeptide cells and the kidney; such an association has only rarely been described (111).

Other Serologic Markers and Syndromes

Although various other systemic syndromes and serologic perturbations have been reported in association with renal adenocarcinoma, this discussion will pay particular attention to the carcinomatous neuromyopathy and elevated serum ferritin levels that have recently been described in patients with hypernephroma.

Neurologic symptoms in the absence of metastatic involvement of the nervous system have been reported infrequently in patients with renal carcinoma (116–120). Indeed, while neuromyopathies have been noted in patients with this tumor, unequivocal evidence that this might be due to a systemic possibly serologically mediated factor has been unconvincing in some cases (117, 118) but more persuasive in others (116, 119, 120). Thus, the presence of a neuromyopathy or of a neuropsychiatric disorder may precede recognition of a renal carcinoma, and extirpation of the tumor may be associated with resolution of symptoms

(116, 119). Moreover, despite the inability to identify a neurotoxic factor in patients with these manifestations of renal carcinoma, axonal degeneration has been described and is considered an important pathologic finding (120).

Disorders of iron metabolism and of iron transport have been noted in patients with renal carcinoma, and the report of a patient with an elevated serum ferritin concentration and hypernephroma is of interest (10). Thus, a patient with localized nonmetastatic renal carcinoma was found to be anemic and to have reduced serum iron levels but with a paradoxically elevated serum ferritin concentration, which was 4-fold higher than normal (10). Following nephrectomy, the ferritin concentration fell markedly, thereby suggesting that the tumor was the source of the elevated ferritin levels or was a proximate stimulus to endogenous ferritin production (10).

DISCUSSION

Renal adenocarcinoma may result in elevated levels of such hormones as renin, erythropoietin, or prostaglandins—that is, hormones normally produced by the kidney which may, therefore, be considered to be eutopic (7). However, renal adenocarcinoma has also been associated with elevated levels of ectopic hormones—that is, substances not normally elaborated by the kidney, such as ACTH, parathormone, gonadotropin, and prolactin (7, 57). Indeed, the production of ectopic hormones by hypernephromas may be a reflection of the more general phenomenon of aberrant protein and polypeptide production by neoplastic cells; in addition to hormones, products include enzymes such as alkaline phosphatase and oncofetal substances such as carcinoembryonic antigen and α-fetoprotein (121–124).

Recent studies indicate that the incidence of clinically apparent paraneoplastic syndromes underestimates the true incidence of inappropriate production of peptides by tumors and that clinically overt syndromes call attention to only a small fraction of the neoplasms synthesizing aberrant peptides (47). Since such synthesis may represent a widespread concomitant of neoplasia, several factors have been proposed to account for the discordance between clinically recognized syndromes and the true frequency of hormone production by hypernephromas. Thus, renal tumors may elaborate substances detectable by immunoassay but which are biologically inert owing to an inability to bind to cellular receptors (3, 54). Antisera may not necessarily distinguish between the biologically active hormone, partially degraded fragments, prohormones, or materials with similar but not identical amino acid sequences. Another explanation for a dissociation between biologic and immunologic activity may be end organ failure—that is, an inability of the target organ to respond to the hormone. Additionally, since the signs of hormone excess may require a finite period of time to become clinically evident, rapid tumor growth might preclude this (125).

In patients with hypernephroma, recognition of paraneoplastic syndromes and of serologic factors, whether ectopic or eutopic, is of clinical importance. Thus, tumor-induced humoral syndromes may precede localizing symptoms of renal carcinoma and may, therefore, provide a clue to earlier diagnosis (51). In addition, localization of a tumor or of its metastases and the assessment of response to therapy may be facilitated by identification of tumor-associated humoral products (126). Moreover, such products also provide a functional label for neoplastic cells and may identify whether a tumor recurrence represents a new cell line or regrowth of the original clone. Secretion of humoral factors by renal adenocarcinomas may also add the burden of metabolic aberrations to the underlying neoplastic process, thereby adversely affecting the quality of life and possibly of survival. Furthermore, patients with renal adenocarcinoma may exhibit unexplained, bizarre, or unusual signs, and their appearance should prompt a search for humoral derangements as well as for metastatic progression.

Criteria for implicating inappropriate secretion of humoral factors to hypernephromas include: (a) demonstration of elevated plasma levels of a given substance or clinical evidence of hypersecretion in association with renal carcioma, (b) a fall in hormone levels and/or a regression in the clinical manifestations of hormone excess following successful therapy, (c) demonstration of an arteriovenous gradient across the tumor, (d) identification of the hormone in tumor tissue, (e) in vitro evidence that the tumor can synthesize and secrete the hormone, (f) failure of elevated hormone levels to respond to normal control mechanisms, and (g) persistence of elevated hormone levels and of clinical symptoms following removal of the normal gland of origin of the hormone (127, 128). While all of these criteria may not be satisfied in a given case, the unequivocal demonstration of two or three of these may be sufficient to ascribe an etiologic role in ectopic peptide production to the hypernephroma.

Various mechanisms for the ectopic production of hormones or peptides by tumors have been suggested, and several theories have been proposed (3, 123, 127). The abnormal genome hypothesis suggests that base substitutions or tumor genomic alterations result in the synthesis of abnormal products, and their release could then result in paraneoplastic syndromes. Another proposal is that nonendocrine tumors, such as renal carcinomas, do not synthesize hormones but selectively absorb them from the circulation and then on cell death release them systemically—the so-called "sponge" hypothesis (129). The concept of gene derepression, a widely held theory, argues that the genetic information necessary for the synthesis of all proteins is present on the genes of all nucleated cells, but that most genes are inactive or repressed in differentiated tissue (127). During malignant transformation, portions of DNA previously unavailable for transcription become transcribed as a result of ablation of the control mechanisms which occur with malignancy (3). An additional theory based on the view that the secretion of hormones by neoplastic cells represents the persistence of capabilities present in primitive cells which have been arrested during the process of differentiation has also been suggested (130).

Yet another mechanism for ectopic hormone production which has been proposed has been that of tumor cell hybridization (131). It is postulated that hybridized neoplastic cells arise by fusion of malignant cells with normal neuroectodermal cells which themselves have the capacity to elaborate polypeptide hormones. Finally, the endocrine cell hypothesis states that ectopic production of peptides or hormones derives from cells of the APUD system, which ultimately originates from neural crest ectoderm (111).

It is of interest that ectopic hormones associated with the paraneoplastic syndromes of renal cell carcinoma have been proteins or polypeptides and in general that ectopic catecholamine or steroid production has been not described (127, 132). Thus, a relatively less complicated mechanism is required for peptide hormone biosynthesis—that is, translation of a limited genomic region—than for steroid or catecholamine synthesis, which requires several enzymes and transport between cellular compartments (3).

SUMMARY

Paraneoplastic syndromes and ectopic hormone production in association with renal adenocarcinoma are important manifestations of this tumor. Thus, hypernephromas are associated with the inappropriate elaboration of factors normally secreted by the kidney, such as renin, erythropoietin, and prostaglandins, as well as with ectopic factors, such as parathormone, ferritin, pyrogens, hepatotoxins, glucagon, and prolactin. While syndromes caused by inappropriate production of hormones, primarily peptides, in association with renal carcinoma have been discussed, it is likely that ectopic hormone production is clinically unrecognized in many patients owing to the secretion of biologically inactive hormones or of hormones whose overproduction is unassociated with clinical sequelae (3). Wider recognition of this phenomenon and timely detection of these substances may allow earlier detection of renal carcinoma and more precise monitoring of therapy.

Acknowledgment. This investigation was supported in part by the Margaret Duffy and Robert Cameron Troup Fund of the Buffalo General Hospital, Buffalo, NY.

REFERENCES

1. Sufrin G, Murphy GP: Humoral syndromes of renal adenocarcinoma in man. *Rev Surg* 34:149, 1977.
2. Altaffer LF, Chenault OW Jr: Paraneoplastic endocrinopathies associated with renal tumors. *J Urol* 122:573, 1979.
3. Frohman LA: Ectopic hormone production. *Am J Med* 78:995, 1981.
4. Chisholm GD: Paraneoplastic syndromes: introduction. In Kuss R, Khoury S, Murphy GP, Karr JP (eds): *Renal Tumors: Proceedings of the First International Symposium on Kidney Tumors.* New York, Alan R Liss, 1982, p 277.
5. Creevy CD: Confusing clinical manifestations of malignant renal neoplasms. *Arch Intern Med* 55:895, 1935.
6. Holland JM: Cancer of the kidney—natural history and staging. *Cancer* 32 (part 2):1030, 1973.
7. Chisholm, GD: Nephrogenic ridge tumors and their syndromes. *Ann NY Acad Sci* 240:403, 1974.

8. Rubin AL, Creigh JS, Stenzel KH: Symposium on endocrine functions of the kidney. *Am J Med* 58:1, 1975.

9. Pavelic K, Popovic M: Insulin and glucagon secretion by renal adenocarcinoma. *Cancer* 48:98, 1981.

10. Mufti GJ, Hamblin TJ, Stevens J: Basic Isoferritin and hypercalcemia in renal cell carcinoma. *J Clin Pathol* 35:1008, 1982.

11. Ram MD, Chisholm GD: Hypertension due to hypernephroma. *Br Med J* 4:87, 1969.

12. Cox CE, Lacy SS, Montgomery WG, Boyce WH: Renal adenocarcinoma: 28-year review, with emphasis on rationale and feasibility of preoperative radiotherapy. *J Urol* 104:53, 1970.

13. Kirchner FK Jr, Barren V, Smith C, Wilson JP, Foster JH, Hollifield JW, Rhamy RK: Renal carcinoma discovered incidentally by arteriography during evaluation for hypertension. *J Urol* 115:643, 1976.

14. Fichman M, Bethune J: Effects of neoplasm on renal electrolyte function. *Ann NY Acad Sci* 230:448, 1974.

15. Dahl T, Eide I, Fryjordet A: Hypernephroma and hypertension. *Acta Med Scand* 209:121, 1981.

16. Lampe WTH, Crovatto AC: Renal adenocarcinoma producing hypertension: diagnosis by radioactive renogram and aortography. *J Urol* 93:673, 1965.

17. Hollifield JW, Page DL, Smith C, Michelakis AM, Staab E, Rhamy R: Renin-secreting clear cell carcinoma of the kidney. *Arch Intern Med* 135:859, 1975.

18. Editorial: renal tumours and hypertension. *Br J Med* 3:327, 1968.

19. Pollack HM, Popky GL: Roentgenographic manifestations of spontaneous renal hemorrhage. *Radiology* 110:1, 1974.

20. Robertson PW, Klidjian A, Harding LK, Walters G, Lee MR, Robb-Smith AHT: Hypertension due to renin-secreting renal tumor. *Am J Med* 43:963, 1967.

21. Kihara I, Kitamura S, Hoshino T, Seida H, Watanabe T: A hitherto unreported vascular tumor of the kidney: a proposal of "juxtaglomerular cell tumor." *Acta Pathol Jpn* 18:197, 1968.

22. Lee MR: Renin-secreting kidney tumors. *Lancet* 2:254, 1971.

23. Alavi JB, McLean GK: Hypertension with renal carcinoma. *Cancer* 52:169, 1983.

24. Howlett SA, Caranasos GJ: Metastatic renal cell carcinoma producing arteriovenous shunt. *Arch Intern Med* 125:493, 1970.

25. Sondag TJ, Patel SK, Petasnick JP, Chambliss J: Hypernephromas with massive arteriovenous fistulas. *AJR* 117:97, 1973.

26. Rodgers MW, Moss AJ, Hoffman M, Lipchik EO: Arteriovenous fistulae secondary to renal cell carcinoma. *Circulation* 52:345, 1975.

27. Malonado JE, Sheps SG, Bernatz PE, DeWeerd JH, Harrison EG: Renal arteriovenous fistula. A reversible cause of hypertension and heart failure. *Am J Med* 37:499, 1964.

28. Lopez-Majano V, Danckers U, Sullivan JD, Rajagopal T, Koven A: Renal cell carcinoma presenting as systemic hypertension of sudden onset. *Int Surg* 60:491, 1975.

29. Zusman RM, Snider JJ, Cline A, Caldwell BV, Speroff L: Antihypertensive function of a renal-cell carcinoma. *N Engl J Med* 290:843, 1974.

30. Stauffer MH: Nephrogenic hepatosplenomegaly (abstract). *Gastroenterology* 40:694, 1961.

31. Boxer RJ, Waisman J, Lieber MM, Mamfraso FM, Skinner DG: Nonmetastatic hepatic dysfunction associated with renal cell carcinoma. *J Urol* 119:468, 1978.

32. Hanash KA: The nonmetastatic hepatic dysfunction syndrome associated with renal cell carcinoma (hypernephroma). In Kuss R, Khoury S, Murphy GP, Karr JP (eds): *Renal Tumors: Proceedings of the First International Symposium on Kidney Tumors.* New York, Alan R Liss, 1982, p 301.

33. Warren MM, Kelalis PP, Utz DC: The changing concept of hypernephroma. *J Urol* 104:376, 1970.

34. Utz DC, Warren MM, Gregg JA, Ludwig J, Kelalis PP: Reversible hepatic dysfunction associated with hypernephroma. *Mayo Clin Proc* 45:161, 1970.

35. Vermillion SE, Morlock CG, Bartholomew LG, Kelalis PP: Nephrogenic hepatic

dysfunction: secondary to tumefactive xanthogranulomatous pyelonephritis. *Ann Surg* 171:130, 1970.

36. Schersten T, Wahlqvist L, Jilderos B: Lysosomal enzyme activity in liver tissue, kidney tissue, and tumor tissue from patients with renal carcinoma. *Cancer* 27:278, 1971.

37. Eddleston ALWF: Immunology and the liver. In Parker CW (ed): *Clinical Immunology.* Philadelphia, WB Saunders, 1980, p 1009.

38. Lemmon WT Jr, Holland PV, Holland JM: The hepatopathy of hypernephroma. *Am J Surg* 110:487, 1965.

39. Walsh PN, Kissane JM: Nonmetastatic hypernephroma with reversible hepatic dysfunction. *Arch Intern Med* 122:214, 1968.

40. Strum WB: Remote recurrence of renal cell carcinoma. *Urology* 23:68, 1984.

41. Bodel P: Part 1. Generalized perturbations in host physiology caused by localized tumors. Tumors and fever. *Ann NY Acad Sci* 230:6, 1974.

42. Fricourt L, Jouquan J, Khourhy S, Richard R, Chomette G, Godeau P: Fever in adult renal cancer. In Kuss R, Khoury S, Murphy GP, Karr JP (eds): *Renal Tumors: Proceedings of the First International Symposium on Kidney Tumors.* New York, Alan R Liss, 1982, p 283.

43. Rawlins MD, Luff RH, Cranston WI: Pyrexia in renal carcinoma. *Lancet* 1:1371, 1970.

44. Bottiger LE: Fever of unknown origin. IV. Fever in carcinoma of the kidney. *Acta Med Scand* 156:477, 1957.

45. Bennington JL, Kradjian RM: Presenting signs and symptoms. In *Renal Carcinoma.* Philadelphia, WB Saunders, 1967.

46. Murphy GP, Fisbein RH: Clinical manifestations and cytology of hypernephromas. *J Urol* 85:483, 1961.

47. Odell WE, Wolfsen A: Ectopic hormone secretion by tumors. In Becker FF (ed): *Cancer.* New York, Plenum Press, 1975, vol 3.

48. Imura H, Matsukura S, Nakai Y, Nakau K, Oki S, Tanaka I, Tsukada T, Yoshimasa T: Clinical and biochemical features of ectopic hormone producing tumors: possible mechanism of hormone production. In Ede F, Bresciani R, King JB, Lippman ME, Naner M, Raynaud JP (eds): *Progress in Cancer Research and Therapy: Hormones in Cancer II.* New York, Raven Press, 1984, p 569.

49. Bhattacharya SK, Sealy WC: Paraneoplastic syndromes. Resulting from elaboration of ectopic hormones, antigens and bizarre toxins. *Curr Probl Surg*, pp 3–49, May 1972.

50. Smith LH: Ectopic hormone production. *Surg Gynecol Obstet* 141:443, 1975.

51. Bartuska DC: Humoral manifestations of neoplasms. *Semin Oncol* 2:405, 1975.

52. Riggs BL, Sprague RG: Association of Cushing's syndrome and neoplastic disease. *Arch Intern Med* 108:841, 1961.

53. Maurer von H-J, Jensen T, Mauer B: Heterotoper nebennierrenrindentumor (echtes hypernephrom?) mit Cushing-syndrome. *Fortschr Rontgenstr* 118:273, 1973.

54. Yalow RS: Radioimmunoassay methodology: application to problem of heterogeneity of peptide hormones. *Pharmacol Rev* 25:161, 1973.

55. Fraser WM, Blackard WG: Medical conditions that affect the breast and laceration. *Clin Obstet Gynecol* 18:51, 1975.

56. Malarkey WB: Nonpuerperal lactation and normal prolactin regulation. *J Clin Endocrinol Metab* 40:198, 1975.

57. Turkington RW: Ectopic production of prolactin. *N Engl J Med* 285:1455, 1975.

58. Bittorf A: Nebennierentumor und Geschlectsdru senausfall beim manne. *Berl Klin Wochenschr* 56:776, 1919.

59. zum Busch JP: Gynakomastie bei hypernephrom. *Dtsch Med Wochenschr* 53:323, 1927.

60. Finn JE, Mount LA: Galactorrhea in males with tumors in the region of the pituitary gland. *J Neurosurg* 35:723, 1971.

61. Vaitukaitis JL: Peptide hormones as tumor markers. *Cancer* 37:567, 1976.

62. Warren MM, Utz DC, Kelalis PP: Concurrence of hypernephroma and hypercalcemia. *Ann Surg* 174:863, 1971.

63. Skinner DG, Colvin RB, Vermillion CD, Pfister RC, Leadbetter WF: Diagnosis and

management of renal cell carcinoma. A clinical and pathologic study of 309 cases. *Cancer* 28:1165, 1971.

64. Lokich JJ, Harrison JH: Renal cell carcinoma: natural history and chemotherapeutic experience. *J Urol* 114:371, 1975.

65. Mundy GR, Ibbotson KJ, D'Souza SM, Simpson EL, Jacobs JW, Martin TJ: The hypercalcemia of cancer. *N Engl J Med* 310:1718, 1984.

66. Gottlieb S, Rude PK, Sharp CF Jr, Singer FR: Humoral hypercalemia of malignancy: a syndrome in search of a hormone. *Am J Med* 73:751, 1982.

67. Strewler GJ, Williams RD, Nissenson RA: Human renal carcinoma cells produce hypercalcemia in the nude mouse and a novel protein recognized by parathyroid hormone receptors. *J Clin Invest* 71:769, 1983.

68. Cook SA, Tarar RA, Lalli AF: Bony metastasis in renal cell carcinoma. *Cleve Clin Q* 42:263, 1975.

69. Case records of the Massachusetts General Hospital. *N Engl J Med* 255:789, 1941.

70. Skrabanek P, McPartlin J, Powell D: Tumor hypercalcemia and "ectopic hyperparathroidism." *Medicine* 59:262, 1980.

71. Riggs BL, Arnaud CD, Reynolds JC, Smith LH: Immunologic differentiation of primary hyperparathyroidism from hyperparathroidism due to nonparathyroid cancer. *J Clin Invest* 50:2079, 1971.

72. Palmieri GMA, Nordquist RE, Omenn GS: Immunochemical localization of parathyroid hormone in cancer tissue from patients with ectopic hyperparathyroidism. *J Clin Invest* 53:1726, 1974.

73. Seyberth HW, Segre GV, Morgan JL, Sweetman BJ, Potts JT Jr, Oates JA: Prostaglandins as mediators of hypercalcemia associated with certain types of cancer. *N Engl J Med* 293:1278, 1975.

74. Robertston RP, Baylink DJ, Marini JJ, Adkison HW: Elevated prostaglandins and suppressed parathyroid hormone associated with hypercalcemia and renal cell carcinoma. *J Clin Endocrinol Metab* 41:164, 1975.

75. Farr HW, Fahey TJ, Nash AG, Farr CM: Primary hyperparathyroidism and cancer. *Am J Surg* 126:539, 1973.

76. Ackerman NB, Winer N: The differentiation of primary hyperparathyroidism from the hypercalcemia of malignancy. *Ann Surg* 181:226, 1975.

77. Purnell DC, Scholz DA, vanHeerden JA: Primary hyperparathroidism associated with hypernephroma. *Mayo Clinic Proc* 57:694, 1982.

78. Lafferty FW: Pseudohyperparathyroidism. *Medicine* 45:247, 1966.

79. Mallette LE, Bilezikian JP, Heath DA, Aurbach GD: Primary hyperparathyroidism: clinical and biochemical features. *Medicine* 53:127, 1974.

80. Plimpton CH, Gellhorn A: Hypercalcemia in malignant disease without evidence of bone destruction. *Am J Med* 21:750, 1956.

81. Goldberg MF, Tashjian AH Jr, Order SE, Dammin GJ: Renal adenocarcinoma containing a parathyroid hormone like substance and associated with marked hypercalcemia. *Am J Med* 36:805, 1964.

82. Lytton B, Rosof B, Evans JS: Parathyroid horomone-like activity in a renal carcinoma producing hypercalcemia. *J Urol* 93:127, 1965.

83. O'Grady AS, Morse LJ, Lee JB: Parathyroid hormone secreting renal carcinoma associated with hypercalcemia metabolic alkalosis. *Ann Intern Med* 63:858, 1965.

84. Buckle RM, McMillan M, Mallinson C: Ectopic secretion of parathyroid hormone by a renal adenocarcinoma in a patient with hypercalcemia. *Br Med J* 4:724, 1970.

85. Salama F, Luke RG, Hellebusch AA: Carcinoma of the kidney producing multiple hormones. *J Urol* 106:820, 1971.

86. Herrera GA, Reimann BEF, Turbat EA, Ho K-J: Hormone-producing capabilities of renal cell carcinoma. *Urology* 22:421, 1983.

87. Buescu A, Dimich AB, Myers WPL: Cancer hypercalcemia—a pragmatic approach. *Clin Bull (Mem Sloan-Kettering Cancer Cent)* 5:91, 1975.

88. Goldberg RS, Pilcher DB, Yates JW: The aggressive surgical management of hypercalcemia due to ectopic parathormone production. *Cancer* 45:2652, 1980.

89. Tahjian AH Jr: Prostaglandins, hypercalcemia and cancer. *N Engl J Med* 293:1317, 1975.

90. Goldwasser E: Erythropoietin and the differentiation of red blood cells. *Fed Proc* 34:2285, 1975.

SEROLOGIC MARKERS AND PARANEOPLASTIC SYNDROMES 69

91. Sperber MA: Malignant renal lesions and erythrocytosis (letter to the editor). *Br Med J* 1:51, 1969.
92. Kazol LA, Erslev AJ: Erythropoietin production in renal tumors. *Ann Clin Lab Sci* 5:98, 1975.
93. Toyama K, Fujiyama N, Suzuki H, Chen TP, Tamaoki N, Veyama Y: Erythropoietin levels in the course of a patient with erythropoietin-producing renal cell carcinoma and transplantation of this tumor in nude mice. *Blood* 54:245, 1979.
94. Murphy GP, Mirand EA, Johnston GS, Gibbons RP, Schirmer HKA, Scott WW: Erythropoietin alterations in human genitourinary disease states: correlation with experimental observations. *J Urol* 99:802, 1968.
95. Erslev AJ: Renal biogenesis of erythropoietin. *Am J Med* 58:25, 1975.
96. Hammond DD, Winnick S: Paraneoplastic erythrocytosis and ectopic erythropoietins. *Ann NY Acad Sci* 230:219, 1974.
97. Mohamed SD: Reversible nonmetastatic liver cell dysfunction and thrombocytosis from hypernephroma. *Lancet* 2:621, 1965.
98. Murphy GP, Kenny GM, Mirand EA: Erythropoietin levels in patients with renal tumors or cysts. *Cancer* 26:191, 1970.
99. Chisholm GD, Roy RR: The systemic effects of malignant renal tumours. *Br J Urol* 43:687, 1971.
100. Cummings KB, Robertson RP: Prostaglandin: increased production by renal cell carcinoma. *J Urol* 118:720, 1977.
101. Plaksin J, Landau Z, Coslonsky R: A carcinoid-like syndrome caused by a prostaglandin secreting renal cell carcinoma. *Arch Intern Med* 140:1095, 1980.
102. Braunstein GD, Vaitukaitis JL, Carbone PP, Ross GT: Ectopic production of human chorionic gonadotrophin by neoplasms. *Ann Intern Med* 78:39, 1973.
103. Rosen SW, Weintraub BD, Vaitukaitis JL, Sussman HH, Hershman JM, Muggia FM: Placental proteins and their subunits as tumor markers. *Ann Intern Med* 82:71, 1975.
104. Vaitukaitis JL, Braunstein GD, Ross GT: A radioimmunoassay which specifically measures human chorionic gonadotropin in the presence of human luteinizing hormone. *Am J Obstet Gynecol* 113:751, 1972.
105. Muggis FM, Rosen SW, Weintraub BD, Hansen HH: Ectopic placental proteins in nontrophoblastic tumors. *Cancer* 36:1327, 1975.
106. Case records of the Massachusetts General Hospital: weekly clinicopathological exercise (case 13). *N Engl J Med* 286:713, 1972.
107. Hanash KA, Utz DC, Ludwig J, Wakim KG, Ellefson RD, Kelalis PP: Syndrome of reversible hepatic dysfunction associated with hypernephroma. An experimental study. *Invest Urol* 8:399, 1971.
108. Jones KL: Feminization, virilization, and precocious sexual development that results from neoplastic processes. *Ann NY Acad Sci* 230:195, 1974.
109. Golde DW, Schambelan M, Weintraub BD, Rosen SW: Gonadotropin-secreting renal carcinoma. *Cancer* 33:1048, 1974.
110. Loose JH, Damjanov I, Harris H: Identity of the neoplastic alkaline phosphatase as revealed with monoclonal antibodies to the placental form of the enzyme. *Am J Clin Pathol* 82:173, 1984.
111. Pearse AG: The APUD cell concept and its implications in pathology. In Sommers SC (ed): *Pathology Annual.* New York, Appleton-Century-Crofts, 1974, Vol 9.
112. Benham FJ, Fogh J, Harris H: Alkaline phosphatase expression in human cell lines derived from various malignancies. *Int J Cancer* 27:673, 1981.
113. Pearse AGE, Polak JM: Neural crest origin of the endocrine polypeptide (APID) cells of the gastrointestinal tract and pancreas. *Gut* 12:783, 1971.
114. Gleeson MH, Bloom SR, Polak JM, Henry K, Dowling RH: Endocrine tumor in kidney affecting small bowel structure, motility and absorptive function. *Gut* 12:773, 1971.
115. Bloom SR: An enteroglucagon tumor. *Gut* 13:520, 1972.
116. Swan CHJ, Wharton BA: Polyneuritis and renal carcinoma. *Lancet* 2:383, 1963.
117. Madanagopalan N, Saratchandra R: Renal carcinoma with myopathy-like features. *Lancet* 1:1351, 1966.
118. Thrush DC: Neuropathy, IGM paraproteinemia and autoantibodies in hypernephroma. *Br Med J* 4:474, 1970.

119. Hughes GS, Turner RC: Hypernephroma presenting as acute delirium. *J Urol* 130:539, 1983.
120. Thomas NE, Passamonte PM, Sunderrajan EV, Andelin JB, Ansbacher LE: Bilateral diaphragmatic paralysis as a possible paraneoplastic syndrome from renal cell carcinoma. *Am Rev Respir Dis* 129:507, 1984.
121. Howlett SA, Caranasos GJ: Metastatic renal cell carcinoma producing arteriovenous shunt. *Arch Intern Med* 125:493, 1970.
122. Neville AM: Ectopic production of hormones by tumours. *Proc R Soc Med* 65:55, 1972.
123. Hall TC: Ectopic synthesis and paraneoplastic syndromes. *Cancer Res* 34:2088, 1974.
124. Imura H: Ectopic hormone syndromes. *Clin Endocrinol Metab* 9:235, 1980.
125. Gomez-Uria A, Pazianos AG: Syndromes resulting from ectopic hormone producing tumors. *Med Clin North Am* 59:431, 1975.
126. Liddle GW, Ball JH: Manifestations of cancer mediated by ectopic hormones. In Holland JF, Frei E III (eds): *Cancer Medicine.* Philadelphia, Lea & Febiger, 1973.
127. Landon J, Ratcliffe JG, Rees LH, Scott AP: Tumor-associated hormonal products. *J Clin Pathol* 27 (suppl R Coll Pathol 7):127, 1973.
128. Rees LH, Ratcliffe JG: Ectopic hormone production by non-endocrine tumours. *Clin Endocrinol* 3:263, 1974.
129. Unger RH, Lochner J de V, Eisentraut AM: Identification of insulin and glucagon in a bronchogenic metastasis. *J Clin Endocrinol Metab* 24:823, 1964.
130. Baylin SB, Mendelsohn G: Ectopic (inappropriate) hormone production by tumors: mechanisms involved and the biological and clinical implications. *Endocr Rev* 1:45, 1980.
131. Warner TFCS: Cell hybridisation in the genesis of ectopic hormone-secreting tumours. *Lancet* 1:1259, 1974.
132. Ellison ML, Neville AM: Neoplasia and ectopic hormone production. In Raven RW (ed): *Modern Trends in Oncology-1.* London, Butterworths, 1973.

2
Section

Surgical Treatment

5

Lymphadenectomy in Renal Adenocarcinoma

Giorgio Pizzocaro, M.D.

The value of lymphadenectomy at the time of radical nephrectomy for renal cell carcinoma remains controversial. In North Europe, and in the United Kingdom in particular, it is not performed, and even enlarged lymph nodes are left behind, because it is believed that lymphadenectomy is of no curative value in the management of renal cell carcinoma. On the other hand, several urologists from other countries have endorsed the use of lymphadenectomy as an integral part of radical nephrectomy.

As no effective adjuvant therapy has become available for renal cell carcinoma, the full pursuit of surgical therapy is indicated. However, it is important to know whether lymphadenectomy improves the surgical cure rate of renal cell carcinoma, because lymphadenectomy as a staging procedure does not offer anything of significance to the patient, due to the lack of adjuvant therapy. Virtually all reports describing lymphadenectomy for renal cell carcinoma contain flaws. Precise information on patients with positive lymph nodes is frequently unavailable. In most series the surgery varied, many patients having no lymphadenectomy or lymph node dissections of variable extent. The location of positive lymph nodes is rarely described, and reports of stage III renal cell carcinoma include patients with positive lymph nodes as well as those with renal vein and inferior vena cava involvement (1–3).

It is therefore necessary to review: (*a*) the lymphatic drainage of the kidney in normal and in pathologic situations; (*b*) the occurrence of lymph node metastases; (*c*) the cure rates of patients with histologically documented lymph node involvement, in order to evaluate the usefulness of lymphadenectomy in renal cell carcinoma and to determine the optimal extent of dissection.

NORMAL LYMPHATIC DRAINAGE OF THE KIDNEYS

The location of perinephric lymph nodes and the pathways involving lymphatic drainage of the kidneys were described as early as 1787 by Mascagni. Although there have been many studies on renal lymphatics, primary information on the extrarenal drainage of the renal lymphatics rests with the work of Poirier et al (4), Rouvière (5), and Parker (6). These studies were based on anatomic cadaveric dissections. In particular, Parker injected a modification of Gerota's Prussian blue medium in 50 kidneys and followed their extrarenal lymphatic drainage. Her work constitutes the primary basis for the present description of the extrarenal lymphatic drainage of the right and left kidneys.

Normal Lymphatic Drainage of the Right Kidney

The lymphatic drainage of the right kidney may be divided into posterior, anterior, and middle channels. The posterior channels leave the renal hilus, superior and posterior to the renal vessels, and end in the laterocaval, postcaval, and interaortocaval nodes from L1 to L3. There may be occasional lymphatics passing through the right diaphragmatic crus to the thoracic duct.

The anterior lymphatic channels leave the kidney anterior to the renal vessels and curve upward to join the posterior lymphatics, or they may course medially to end in the precaval nodes, or cross the inferior vena cava and end in the upper interaortocaval nodes.

The middle lymphatic vessels course between the artery and vein and join the posterior and anterior lymphatic channels. Therefore, the regional nodes of the right kidney are on the right side of the abdominal aorta. They are the laterocaval, precaval, postcaval, and interaortocaval nodes (Fig. 5.1). All of these nodes can be considered right para-aortic nodes.

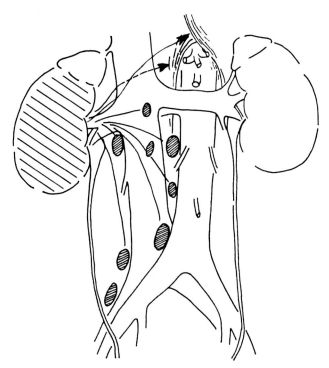

Figure 5.1. Regional anatomic lymphatic drainage of right kidney includes hilar, laterocaval, pre- and postcaval, interaortocaval nodes.

Once the regional lymph nodes are filled with dye, the interaortocaval nodes drain superiorly into the thoracic duct and inferiorly into the upper common iliac and sacral nodes. The laterocaval nodes tend to drain into the precaval, postcaval, interaortocaval, and, occasionally, common iliac nodes. Postcaval nodes can drain into the interaortocaval nodes, and then to channels extending up through the right crus of the diaphragm. From the precaval nodes, injected medium travels to interaortocaval and preaortic nodes. The lymphatic drainage from the regional lymph nodes of the right kidney is thus directed upward through the right diaphragmatic crus and downward to the right common iliac nodes. Contralateral drainage is uncommon.

Normal Lymphatic Drainage of the Left Kidney

The left renal lymphatics drain through anterior and posterior channels. The anterior group of lymphatics is anterior to the renal vein and divides into superior and inferior branches that drain along the abdominal aorta and may interconnect with the posterior group. The posterior group leaves the renal hilus posterior to the renal vessels. These lymphatics diverge at the left crus of the diaphragm into inferior and superior branches. Superiorly, they pass upward to the prediaphragmatic nodes, go through or around the left diaphragmatic crus, and end in the left retrocrural nodes from T11 to L1. Inferiorly, the lymphatics usually end in the left para-aortic nodes between the renal vessels and the lower pole of the kidney.

In other words, the lymphatic drainage of the left kidney includes all of the left para-aortic nodes from T11 to the level of the inferior mesenteric artery (Fig. 5.2). There are some nodes unique to the left kidney, including the left retrocrural nodes and several nodes in front of the left crus of the diaphragm posterior, medial, and proximal to the left adrenal vein. Once these nodes are injected, the medium travels into the thoracic duct. Left para-aortic nodes may drain inferiorly to the lower lymph nodes or superiorly to the diaphragmatic nodes and then to the thoracic duct. Preaortic and postaortic lymphatics also may be filled and, occasionally, the interaortocaval nodes may be involved.

In conclusion, the regional lymphatic drainage from the kidneys is mainly directed toward the ipsilateral para-aortic nodes. Beyond the regional nodes the lymphatic drainage becomes varied and potentially systemic.

According to the TNM (tumor-nodes-metastasis) classification, the regional lymph nodes are the para-aortic and paracaval nodes. The juxtaregional lymph nodes are the intrapelvic and the mediastinal nodes.

DISTRIBUTION OF LYMPH NODE METASTASES FROM RENAL CELL CARCINOMA IN SURGICAL SERIES

The location of metastatic lymph nodes from renal cell carcinoma was very carefully described by Hulten et al (7) in a small surgical series. The material comprised 22 consecutive patients operated upon for renal

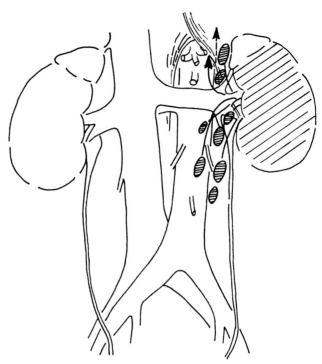

Figure 5.2. Regional anatomic lymphatic drainage of left kidney includes hilar, upper lateroaortic, pre- and postaortic nodes. There are additional nodes on the left crus of the diaphragm.

carcinoma. The tumor was right-sided in 9 cases, left-sided in 12, and bilateral in 1. Bilateral retroperitoneal lymphadenectomy from the diaphragmatic hiatus down to the bifurcation of the ipsilateral iliac artery, including lymph nodes and tissue around the aorta and the inferior vena cava, was carried out. This extensive lymph node dissection was omitted in 9 patients: in 6 the lymph node dissection was restricted to the ipsilateral side, and in 3 only local extirpation of lymph nodes was performed. In 15 cases mediastinoscopy with paratracheal lymph node biopsy was performed in addition to extirpation of supraclavicular lymph nodes.

A total of 1038 nodes was examined histologically, and in 7 of the 22 cases (32%), 24 metastases were found in lymph nodes or in lymph vessels. Of 4 patients with distant metastases, 3 (75%) also had lymph node involvement, which was homolateral in 2 cases and diffuse (bilateral retroperitoneal, mediastinal, and supraclavicular) in the third. Four of the 18 patients (22%) without any evidence of distant metastases had histologically proven lymphogenous spread: 1 had homolateral para-aortic lymph node metastases, and 3 had solitary metastases which were located near the homolateral iliac artery in 2 and in a supraclavicular lymph node in 1.

Giuliani et al (8) described the distribution of lymph node metastases according to the pathologic staging categories. Of 2 patients with pathologic stage T2 (pT2) tumors, metastases were located in the laterocaval

Table 5.1
Distribution of Retroperitoneal Lymph Node Metastases in 10 Cases of Renal Cell Carcinoma[a]

Patient	Side	TNM Category	Location in Kidney	Homolateral Iliac Nodes	Hilar Nodes	Para-aortic Nodes		Retrocrural Nodes	Mediastinal and Supraclavicular Nodes
						Homolateral	Contralateral		
ML	Right	pT2N2V0M0	Lower pole	0	+	+	0	0	0
GN	Left	pT3N1V2M0	Whole kidney	0	+	−	0	0	0
DE	Left	pT4N2V0M0	Whole kidney	+	−	−	−	0	0
TL	Right	pT3N1V0M0	Upper + central	0	+	−	0	0	0
BV	Right	pT4N4V0M0	Lower + central	+	+	+	+	+	+
PS	Right	pT2N1V0M1	Upper + central	0	+	−	0	0	0
FS	Right	pT2N1V1M1	Central	0	−	+	0	0	0
BR	Left	pT3N0V0M1	Lower + central	−	+	−	0	0	0
CL	Right	pT2N1V0M1	Central	0	−	+	0	0	0
ME	Right	pT3N2V0M1	Lower + central	−	−	+	−	0	0

[a] −, Histologically negative; 0, clinically negative; +, metastatic.

and mesenteric lymph nodes in 1 and in the parahilar lymph nodes in the other. Of 12 patients with pathologic stage T3 (pT3) tumors (perirenal fat involvement) metastases were located in the retrocaval and laterocaval lymph nodes in 4, parahilar and lateroaortic lymph nodes in 2, interaortocaval lymph nodes in 4, retroaortic lymph nodes in 1, and parahilar lymph nodes in 1. The patient with pathologic stage T4 (pT4) tumor had metastases in the precaval and interaortocaval nodes.

The author's group found retroperitoneal lymph node metastases in 10 patients (Table 5.1). One patient (BV) had widespread lymph node metastases to iliac, bilateral para-aortic, retrocrural, mediastinal, and supraclavicular nodes without any evidence of hematogenous spread, a very uncommon finding in renal carcinoma. Eight had hilar or homolateral para-aortic node involvement with a single lymph node metastasis in 6 cases. One patient (DE) had only involvement of the homolateral common iliac nodes. There was no correlation between tumor location in the kidney and distribution of the lymph node metastases.

Available data on the distribution of lymph node metastases in surgical specimens suggest that they are usually restricted to hilar, homolateral para-aortic, and homolateral common iliac nodes. Each of these lymph node groups may be the site of primary nodal involvement.

OCCURRENCE OF LYMPH NODE METASTASES IN RENAL CELL CARCINOMA

The occurrence of lymph node metastases in renal cell carcinoma may be studied in autopsy findings or in surgical specimens. Recently, Saitoh (9) analyzed the autopsy records of 1828 cases of renal adenocarcinoma. The lymph nodes were involved in 1001 of 1548 cases with metastases (65%), and lymph node involvement was second only to lung metastases. However, regional lymph nodes (hilar, para-aortic, and paracaval nodes) were involved in only 338 cases—34% of those with lymph node metastases and 18.5% of the whole series. It is outstanding that while lymph nodes were widely and frequently involved in the

Table 5.2
Occurrence of Lymph Node Metastases following Extensive Retroperitoneal Lymphadenectomy

Authors		Total No. of Cases	Retroperitoneal Metastases (%)	pT1-T2, M0		pT3-T4, M0		M1	
				No.	(%)	No.	(%)	No.	(%)
Robson et al	(1)	88	20 (21.7)	Not stated		Not stated		Not stated	
Hulten et al	(7)	22	6 (27.3)	Not stated		Not stated		3/4	(75.0)
Giuliani et al	(8)	104	Not stated	2/38	(5.3)	13/36	(36.1)	Not stated	
Carl et al	(10)	270	40 (23.5)	7/75	(9.3)	14/58	(24.2)	19/37	(51.3)

Table 5.3
Long Term Survival of Patients with Retroperitoneal Lymph Node Metastases

Authors	Total No. of N+ M0 Cases	5-Year Survival (%)	10-Year Survival (%)
Extensive lymphadenectomy			
Robson et al (1)	Not stated	(35)	(35)
Giuliani et al (8)	15	(35)	(23)
Regional lymphadenectomy			
Flocks and Kadesky (11)	21	3 (14)	2/12
Rapla (12)	14	3 (21)	1/12
Skinner et al (2)	19	3 (16)	1/12
Middleton and Presto (13)	7	2[a] (29)	0/2
Angervall and Wahlqvist (14)	3	2 (67)	
Waters and Richie (15)	8	1 (12)	
Siminovitch et al (16)	9	1 (11)	
Fuselier et al (17)	6	0 (0)	
Present series	4	1 (25)	

[a] One patient living with disease was excluded.

neck, the mediastinum, and the abdomen, regional lymph nodes were invaded in only approximately 20% of cases.

A review of the occurrence of lymph node metastases in surgical specimens is difficult, as findings depend on the extension of lymphadenectomy and on the stage of the disease.

Following extensive retroperitoneal lymph node dissection (1, 7, 8, 10), lymph node metastases were found in approximately 25% of cases (Table 5.2). Regional lymph node metastases were present in only 5 to 10% of intrarenal tumors (pT1-T2 categories), in approximately 30% of extrarenal tumors (pT3-T4 categories), and in over 50% of patients with distant metastases (M1 category).

Following regional lymphadenectomy, hilar and para-aortic lymph node metastases are reported to occur in approximately 15% of cases (2, 11–18).

SURVIVAL OF PATIENTS WITH LYMPH NODE METASTASES

The long term survival of patients with lymph node metastases from renal cell carcinoma is specifically reported only in a few series (1, 2, 8, 11–17). Results are depicted in Table 5.3, and the extent of lymphadenectomy is considered. The number of patients in every reported series is very small; however, it seems that following extensive retroperitoneal lymph node dissection, the projected 5-year survival in patients with positive nodes is 35% (1, 8) versus a cumulative 17% crude disease-free survival following regional lymphadenectomy (2, 11–17). The comparison may be faulty, because of the different methods of calculation. There is, however, a consistent disease-free survival rate in patients operated on for renal cell carcinoma metastatic to the retroperitoneal nodes. Only Petkovic (19) reported a large series of cases with lymph node involvement. Of 57 patients, only 5 (9%) survived 5 years, as compared to 20% of 88 cases of the same stage but without lymph node invasion. Furthermore, of 11 patients with only microscopic nodal metastases, 4 (37%) survived 5 years or longer, as compared to only 1 of 46 (2%) with gross nodal involvement or more than 5 metastases. The finding of microscopic disease at lymphadenectomy needs to be emphasized. In the series of Waters and Richie (15), 5 of 16 patients (30%) with lymph node metastases had microscopic disease, and in the series of Peters and Brown (3) 24 of 31 patients in stage III (77%) had microscopic nodal involvement only. These patients probably would have been assigned to stage II disease if node dissection had not been performed. Furthermore, in Peters and Brown's series (3), lymphadenectomy did not improve the 5-year survival in stage II (42% versus 40%), but did so in stage III (44% versus 26%).

In conclusion, lymph node invasion is a bad but not an absolutely adverse prognostic feature in patients undergoing curative nephrectomy for renal cell carcinoma. Microscopic metastases are removed only if lymphadenectomy is systematically performed, and approximately 35% of patients with microscopic disease can be cured. Lymph node metastases are usually found in 25% of cases following extensive lymphadenectomy and in 15% following a more limited regional dissection. As approximately 50% of metastases will be microscopic, lymphadenectomy will probably benefit 3% of patients who are operated on for category M0 renal cell carcinoma. The procedure is worthwhile if morbidity and mortality are not increased significantly.

MORBIDITY AND MORTALITY RELATED TO LYMPHADENECTOMY IN RENAL CANCER

Added morbidity and mortality of lymphadenectomy in addition to radical nephrectomy are difficult to evaluate. Robson et al (1) stated that morbidity was not a serious factor in his series of 88 patients who underwent radical thoracoabdominal nephrectomy with extensive lymphadenectomy, but hospital mortality consisted of 3 cases (3.4%). Giuliani et al (8), in their series of 104 patients undergoing a similar transperitoneal operation, reported 10 patients who died shortly postoperatively, without specifying whether they were surgical or cancer deaths. Skinner (2) compared the results of simple versus radical nephrectomy. Regional lymph node dissection was usually performed in the radical procedure. He reported only 1 operative mortality in 80 cases undergoing simple nephrectomy (1.25%) versus 6 of 149 (4%)

undergoing the radical operation for stage I to stage III disease. A similar operative mortality (4.9%) has been reported by Middleton and Presto (13) following thoracoabdominal radical nephrectomy with regional lymphadenectomy in 61 cases.

Even if most surgeons do not admit that lymphadenectomy adds significant morbidity and mortality to a curative nephrectomy for renal cell carcinoma, it likely did and does occur in several series, even in the most skilled hands. This author is unwilling to accept the increased morbidity and mortality in view of the limited gains of lymphadenectomy. Therefore, as suggested by deKernion (20), the author would limit the dissection to an extent which is both potentially useful and not dangerous to the patient. Using a regional lymphadenectomy, he had only 1 postoperative mortality due to myocardial infarction in a consecutive series of 70 patients operated on by transperitoneal radical nephrectomy for renal cell carcinoma.

REGIONAL LYMPH NODES FOR RENAL CELL CARCINOMA

Lymphadenectomy in renal cell carcinoma should remove possibly all of the regional microscopic lymph node metastases without increasing morbidity and mortality significantly.

When the tumor is confined to the renal parenchyma, the flow of lymphogenous metastases should correspond to the normal lymphatic drainage of the kidney (4–6). However, the little knowledge available on the distribution of lymph node metastases (7, 8) suggests that tumor cells might migrate through lymphatics in the renal capsule or perinephric fat, bypassing the theoretical first echelon of nodes near the hilum, even reaching the iliac nodes or the thoracic duct without any connection with the para-aortic nodes (7). On the other hand, contralateral para-aortic lymph node metastases have been only occasionally reported, usually in patients with widespread disease.

The surgeon cannot do anything to avoid the lymphogenous spread beyond the thoracic duct, but he can remove all of the regional nodes. For tumors of the right kidney, the regional nodes are all the right para-aortic nodes (laterocaval, pre- and retrocaval, interaortocaval nodes) from the right crus of the diaphragm down to the aortic bifurcation and the lateral border of the right iliac artery and vein.

The regional nodes for tumors of the left kidney are the left para-aortic nodes, from the precrural and retrocrural nodes, to the pre-, post-, and lateroaortic nodes, down to the lateral border of the left common iliac artery.

RECOMMENDED LYMPHADENECTOMY FOR RENAL CELL CARCINOMA

The transperitoneal approach with a subcostal xyphoumbilical flap (21) is the preferred routine procedure, because it is much less traumatic-

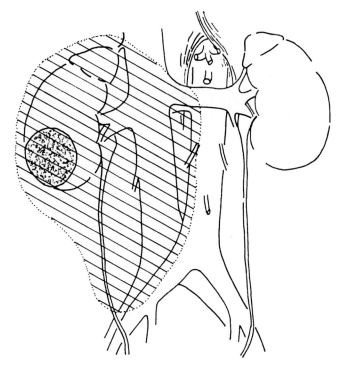

Figure 5.3. Extent of the dissection for right renal cell carcinoma. Interaorto-caval nodes are removed first; hilar and paracaval nodes are removed en bloc with the kidney; retrocaval and iliac nodes are removed at the end of the operation.

than the thoracoabdominal approach, which, in the author's view, should be restricted to large tumors of the upper poles.

Tumors of the Right Kidney (Fig. 5.3)

The right colon is reflected to the left, and the descending duodenum and the head of the pancreas are mobilized. The retroperitoneum is exposed from the superior mesenteric artery, along the aorta, down to the right iliac vessels. The left renal vein is identified, and intercavoaortic nodes are removed. The right renal artery is divided close to the aorta. Precaval and laterocaval nodes are detached from the inferior vena cava, and the right gonadic vein is divided. The inferior vena cava and the right renal vein come completely into view. This way, intravenous tumor thrombi can be safely removed. After dividing the right renal and suprarenal veins, extrafascial nephrectomy is completed en bloc with hilar, precaval, and laterocaval nodes. Retrocaval and lateral common iliac nodes are removed at the end of the operation, when the surgical field is completely free and wide open.

Tumors of the Left Kidney (Fig. 5.4)

The left colon is reflected to the right, and the body and the tail of the pancreas are elevated. The retroperitoneum is exposed from the diaphragm and superior mesenteric artery along the aorta down to the

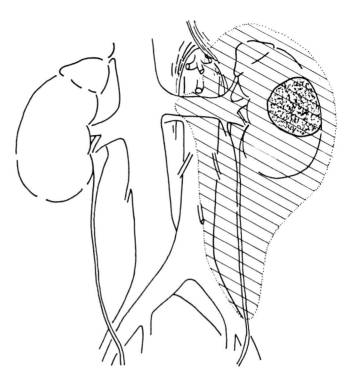

Figure 5.4. Extent of dissection for left renal cell carcinoma. Hilar and latero-aortic nodes are removed en bloc with the kidney. Prediaphragmatic, retrocrural, retroaortic, and iliac nodes are removed at the end of the operation.

inferior mesenteric artery and the left common iliac artery. If it seems that the tumor may be invading the colon or mesocolon, the renal vessels can be approached by dividing the peritoneal reflection over the lateral aspect of the duodenum. The inferior mesenteric vein will need to be retracted or divided between ligatures. Preaortic and left para-aortic nodes are detached from the aorta and the lumbar vessels. The left renal vein is elevated, and the left renal artery is divided close to the aorta. Then the renal vein is divided close to the vena cava. Extrafascial nephrectomy is completed en bloc with hilar and left para-aortic nodes. Precrural and retrocrural nodes, retroaortic nodes, and lateral iliac nodes are removed at the end of the operation, when the surgical field is clear.

Regional lymphadenectomy adds 1 hour or longer to extrafascial nephrectomy, but it is safely performed. A small aspirative drainage is left in the retroperitoneum and is removed after the patient starts to eat. Occasional chylous leak requires total parenteral alimentation for a few days and a delayed removal of the drainage. The posterior peritoneum is carefully closed along the paracolic gutter, in order to avoid postoperative adhesions and bowel obstructions.

SUMMARY

The lymphogenous spread of renal cell carcinoma seems to be relatively rare, unpredictable, and associated with a poor prognosis. However, it has been demonstrated that the ipsilateral retroperitoneal nodes, from the diaphragmatic crus down to the iliac artery, are primarily involved in approximately 20% of cases without distant dissemination. Nodal deposits are microscopic in 50% of these cases, and the long term survival of patients with microscopic lymph node metastases is approximately 35%. So far, a properly executed ipsilateral retroperitoneal lymph node dissection can theoretically improve the long term survival of category M0 renal cancer by approximately 3%. The procedure is worthwhile, if morbidity and mortality are not increased significantly.

Acknowledgment. This investigation was supported in part by grant 83.00915.96 from Progetto Finalizzato Controllo della Crescita Neoplastica, Consiglio Nazionale delle Ricerche (CNR), Rome, Italy.

REFERENCES

1. Robson CJ, Churchill BM, Anderson W: The results of radical nephrectomy for renal cell carcinoma. *J Urol* 101:297, 1969.
2. Skinner DG, Calvin RB, Vermillion CD, Pfeister RC, Leadbetter WF: Diagnosis and management of renal cell carcinoma. A clinical and pathologic study of 309 cases. *Cancer* 28:1165–1177, 1971.
3. Peters PC, Brown GL: The role of lymphadenectomy in the management of renal cell carcinoma. *Urol Clin North Am* 7:705–709, 1980.
4. Poirier P, Cunéo B, Delamère G: *The Lymphatics.* London, A Constable, 1903.
5. Rouvière H: *Anatomie des lymphatiques de l'homme.* Paris, Masson et Cie, 1932.
6. Parker AE: Studies on the main posterior lymph channels of the abdomen and their connections with the lymphatic of the genito-urinary system. *Am J Anat* 56:409, 1935.
7. Hulten L, Rosencrantz M, Seeman T, Wahlqvist L, Ahren C: Occurrence and localization of lymph node metastases in renal carcinoma. *Scand J Urol Nephrol* 3:129, 1969.
8. Giuliani L, Martorana G, Giberti C, Pescatore A, Magnani G: Results of radical nephrectomy with extensive lymphadenectomy for renal cell carcinoma. *J Urol* 130:664, 1983.
9. Saitoh H: Distant metastasis of renal adenocarcinoma in patients with a tumor thrombus in the renal vein and/or vena cava. *J Urol* 127:651–653, 1982.
10. Carl P, Klein U, Gebauer A, Schmiedt E: The value of lymphography for TNM classification of renal carcinoma. *Eur Urol* 3:286–288, 1977.
11. Flocks RH, Kadesky MG: Malignant neoplasms of the kidney: an analysis of 353 patients followed 5 years or more. *J Urol* 79:196–201, 1968.
12. Rapla S: Renal cell carcinoma. Natural history and results of treatment. *Cancer* 25:26–40, 1970.
13. Middleton RG, Presto AJ: Radical thoracoabdominal nephrectomy for renal cell carcinoma. *J Urol* 110:36–37, 1973.
14. Angervall L, and Wahlqvist L: Follow up and prognosis of renal carcinoma in a series operated by perifascial nephrectomy combined with adrenalectomy and retroperitoneal lymphadenectomy. *Eur Urol* 4:13–17, 1978.
15. Waters WB, Richie JP: Aggressive surgical approach to renal cell carcinoma: review of 130 cases. *J Urol* 122:306–309, 1979.
16. Siminovitch JP, Montie JE, Straffon RA: Lymphadenectomy in renal adenocarcinoma. *J Urol* 127:1090–1091, 1982.
17. Fuselier MA, Guice SL, Brannan W, Ochsner MG, Sangisetty KV, Beckman EN, Barnes CA: Renal cell carcinoma: the Ochsner Medical Institution experience. *J Urol* 130:445–448, 1983.
18. Pizzocaro G, Piva L, Salvioni R: Lymph node dissection in radical nephrectomy for renal cell carcinoma: is it necessary? *Eur Urol* 9:10–12, 1983.
19. Petkovic S: The value of tumor tissue penetration into the renal veins and lymph

nodes as anatomical classification and kidney tumor prognostic parameters. *Eur Urol* 6:289–293, 1980.

20. deKernion JB: Lymphadenectomy for renal cell carcinoma. Therapeutic implications. *Surg Clin North Am* 7:697–703, 1980.
21. Giuliani L, Carmignani G, Belgrano E: Subcostal xyphoumbilico flap: a new approach to the neoplastic kidney. *J Urol* (*Paris*) 87:441–443, 1981.

6

Lymphadenectomy for Renal Cell Carcinoma

Fray F. Marshall, M.D.

Should a regional lymphadenectomy be performed in conjunction with a radical nephrectomy for renal cell adenocarcinoma? If a lymphadenectomy is performed, what should be the extent of this dissection? These two questions have not been definitively answered, but there is an increasing body of knowledge that provides for reasonable recommendations at the present time (1). One recent review indicated that lymphadenectomy was not a necessary routine procedure with radical nephrectomy (2), but others have stated that lymphadenectomy should be an integral part of a radical nephrectomy (3–5). A limited regional lymphadenectomy has been recommended (6), but others have suggested a more extensive lymphadenectomy, including dissection of the iliac nodes (7).

Is there a way to reconcile these views, and can a reasonable consensus of opinion be achieved? Why should a lymphadenectomy be considered at all? First, a lymphadenectomy will more accurately stage the patient. If adjuvant therapy were present, patients could be selected for adjuvant treatment. Unfortunately, no effective adjuvant therapy exists. Radiation therapy, chemotherapy, and immunotherapy to date have proved largely disappointing, although there have been sporadic spectacular cases, but these cases may represent no more than the "freak rate" that is present with any tumor. This staging procedure, therefore, does not offer anything of significance at the present time.

On the other hand, if early spread of disease is confined to the lymph nodes, some patients may be cured of their tumor. Clearly, these patients are also at higher risk for the development of hematogenous metastases elsewhere, but some patients can be cured. This rationale is presently the primary reason for lymphadenectomy.

Most reports in the literature concerning positive lymph nodes and lymphadenectomy with renal cell carcinoma contain serious imperfections. The primary problem has been the inclusion of patients with both positive lymph nodes and renal vein involvement in stage III renal cell carcinoma (3, 4). The new TNM (tumor-node-metastases) classification does distinguish tumor in regional nodes and tumor in the renal vein

(8, 9). Nodal disease has been categorized from N1 to N4. N1 includes an ipsilateral node, and N2 includes multiple nodes that are easily resected. N3 represents fixed, enlarged nodes, and N4 represents disseminated nodal disease (9). Precise information on the incidence of positive nodes or their anatomic position is frequently unavailable in many reports. In the early reported series the surgical dissections varied tremendously. Rarely is the location of positive lymph nodes described. Only Hulten et al (7) described very accurately the precise anatomic location of positive lymph nodes, but no 5-year survival is reported.

Data concerning the lymphatic spread of renal cell adenocarcinoma and some of the clinical results of surgical management will be discussed in this chapter. In order to define the rational extent of a regional lymphadenectomy, the extrarenal lymphatic drainage of the kidney will be examined based on previous anatomic studies (1).

HISTORICAL PERSPECTIVE

Most early series of renal cell carcinoma describe patients undergoing simple nephrectomy rather than radical nephrectomy (10, 11). Although a more extensive operation was recommended as early as 1923 (12), it was not until much later that Chute et al (13) and Foley et al (14) described what is presently recognized as a radical nephrectomy which includes excision not only of the kidney but also the perinephric tissue, Gerota's fascia, and the ipsilateral adrenal gland. A few years later Flocks and Kadesky (15) recommended the grouping of patients with renal cell carcinoma into four stages. According to Flock's original recommendation, the stage III patient had only regional lymph node involvement without gross venous invasion. If this original stage III had been maintained by later surgeons, there would be more accurate information on the efficacy of regional lymphadenectomy for renal cell carcinoma.

Subsequently Petkovic also divided his patients with renal cell carcinoma into four groups or stages (16). His group C or stage III included patients with positive lymph nodes as well as renal venous involvement. Inclusion of both renal venous involvement and lymph node metastases in stage III patients has continued (3, 4). The TNM classification provides a more accurate description of patients that will provide for a better understanding of the management of this tumor.

CLINICAL DATA

The incidence of lymph node metastases and 5-year survival are summarized in Table 6.1. The incidence of positive lymph nodes varied from 6 to 32%; the highest incidence of 32% represented a study with probably the most careful pathologic investigation of all lymph node pathologic tissue (7). Sigel et al's study (22) emphasized the necessity for a formal lymph node dissection to determine the precise incidence of positive lymph nodes. In the 50 patients who underwent a lumbar nephrectomy, there was an incidence of positive lymph nodes of 4%. One hundred thirty patients underwent a nephrectomy without a sys-

Table 6.1
Summary—Lymph Node Metastases in Renal Cell Carcinoma

Reference	Incidence of Positive Lymph Nodes		5-Year Survival	
	Cases	%	Cases	%
Flocks and Kadesky (15)	137	25.0	3/21	14
Petkovic (16)	100	22.0	0–1/22	0.5
Robson et al (3)	88	22.7		42[a]
Hulten et al (7)	22	32.0		
Rafla (17)	190	8.0	3/14	21
Skinner et al (4)	309	6.0	3/19	16
Middleton and Presto (18)	62	11.0	3/7	43
Angervall and Wahlqvist (19)	41	22.0	2/3	67
Waters and Richie (20)	67	24.0		
Peters and Brown (5)	356	7.9		
Sigel et al (21)	50 lumbar	4.0		
	130 without formal node dissection	14.0		
	176 with node dissection	29.0		
Carl et al (22)	170	23.5		
Siminovitch et al (6)	102	9.0	1/9	11
Totals	2000	17.4%	15/95 (16%)	27% (Robson's series included)

[a] With positive nodes by correspondence.

tematic, formal node dissection, and the incidence of positive lymph nodes was 14%. A formal dissection was performed in 146 patients, and the incidence was 29% (21). The overall frequency of lymph node metastases varies according to the stage of the tumor. If the tumor was confined to the kidney within the renal capsule (T1 and T2) the incidence of positive lymph nodes was 9% in one series (22). In the T3 and T4 patients with extension beyond the renal capsule, the incidence of nodal metastases was 24% (22). In this series 12.4% of all tumors demonstrated positive lymph node metastases in the absence of other distant metastases. In all patients with lymph node metastases, the incidence of demonstrated distant metastatic disease was about 50% (22).

The 5-year survival rates were also quite variable. The number of patients is small with well defined regional lymph node metastases without obvious venous involvement or distant metastatic disease who underwent regional lymphadenectomy and have been followed 5 years. The series by Robson et al (3) represented excellent results with a 42% 5-year survival. The patients had a more extensive evaluation than many in the other series, and their evaluation also included mediastinoscopy. All of the patients in this series had a routine radical nephrectomy with a regional lymphadenectomy. Skinner et al. (23) had a 33% 5-year survival, but only a small number of patients were reported and these small numbers are typical of many series. In the larger series, many patients had only a simple nephrectomy (23). In order to underscore the importance of regional lymph node dissection, Waters and Richie's series (20) reveals that 5 of 16 patients (30%) had positive nodes with microscopic disease that might not have been appreciated unless the regional lymph node dissection was performed. These patients otherwise would have been assigned to stage II. Also, these patients would appear to be the most likely to benefit from regional lymphadenectomy rather than the patients with bulky disease. In Peters and Brown's series (5), the patients with stage III disease (positive lymph nodes and renal vein involvement) had a 44% 5-year survival when lymphadenectomy was performed and only a 26% 5-year survival if no lymphadenectomy was performed. The majority of patients with nodal disease had microscopic involvement of lymph nodes (77%), indicating again that many of these patients would have been understaged if a node dissection had not been performed.

The metastatic evaluation of a patient with renal cell carcinoma is improving dramatically with the advent of many new diagnostic techniques. These new techniques will clearly identify more patients with metastatic disease. With this careful selection process there is the likelihood for improvement in the survival rate because of more accurate preoperative staging.

For example, the bone scan is qualitatively more sensitive than the previously utilized radiographic bone survey. Pulmonary tomography identifies more patients with metastatic disease (10 to 37%) than a standard chest x-ray (24, 25). Computerized tomography (CT) has radically changed the evaluation of patients with renal cell carcinoma (26–28). CT can more accurately characterize the regional extent of tumor as well as involvement of the vena cava, regional lymph nodes, or extension to adjacent viscera. A CT scan will also evaluate the liver. The author is now utilizing CT in place of pulmonary tomography for evaluation of the chest because pulmonary lesions appear to be accurately characterized and mediastinal lymphadenopathy or tumor thrombus extension can often be appreciated. If there is any suspicion of neurologic findings, CT is also used to evaluate the brain. Relatively silent cerebral metastases have been demonstrated in several patients with initially very subtle neurologic findings. Large metastases can be accommodated in the parietal lobe with few neurologic findings. In the future, magnetic resonance imaging (29) or radioimmunoassays (30) may provide even greater identification of occult metastatic disease.

With this greatly increased technologic sophistication, the evaluation of patients with renal cell carcinoma will be enhanced. Subtle metastatic disease will be identified earlier, and management will be changed accordingly. Patients with distant metastatic disease will often be spared a radical nephrectomy or regional lymphadenectomy. On the other hand, patients with localized disease including regional lymphadenopathy may have an improved survival rate with radical nephrectomy and reginal lymphadenectomy because of improved patient selection. The patients with microscopic disease will probably derive the greatest benefit from regional lymphadenectomy.

REGIONAL LYMPHATIC DRAINAGE OF THE KIDNEY

The perinephric lymph nodes and regional lymphatics of the kidney were described as early as 1787 by Mascagni (31). Cadaveric studies were carried out by Poirier et al (32) at the turn of the century with careful anatomic dissections which demonstrated the lymphatics. Cadaveric dissections are often difficult especially with lymphatics, and many agents have been employed to study the lymphatics including mercury (injected through glass cannulas), Thorotrast, and neoprene (plastic) (31). In vivo techniques have been utilized with injection of thioflavine S into living animals, and the yellow dye was visualized as it passed through the walls of the vessels into lymphatics (33). Various colloidal solutions, including colloidal 198 gold and 99 m technetium antimony sulfide colloid, can be injected into the interstitial tissue of an organ under study (34–36). These colloidal solutions are preferentially taken up in the lymphatics, and the in vivo lymphatic spread can then be determined. At times there is a difference in the lymphatic uptake between separate organs in the same animal. The author's group made some preliminary studies in the utilization of antimony sulfide colloid in the canine kidney but there was very poor lymphatic uptake. The colloid appeared to enter the vascular system and a possible liver-spleen scan resulted. On the other hand, when the colloid was injected in the testis or other organs, there often did appear to be reasonable uptake within the lymphatics.

In the dog, the intrarenal and extrarenal lymphatics have been demonstrated with Evans blue dye (37) or India ink (38). Lymphatics were also demonstrated by ligation of the ureter which achieved pyelolymphatic backflow (40). Lymphatics were demonstrated by introducing radioactive Urokon with ureteral obstruction.

Most of the information on the extrarenal regional lymphatic drainage of the kidney is based on the work of Poirier and associates (32) and the excellent work of Alice Parker (40). In 1935 Parker studied the main lymphatic channels of the retroperitoneum and kidneys. She utilized Gerota's Prussian blue medium, which was injected through small glass needles. At times injections were made directly into lymphatics, but other injections were made directly into the parenchyma or into the lymph nodes. Sixty-five stillborn infants and 7 adult cadavers were utilized for her overall investigation of abdominal lymphatics. The work provides the most accurate description of the regional lymphatic drainage of the kidneys.

The regional lymphatic drainage of the right kidney is basically circumvena caval (Fig. 6.1). Lymphatic channels of the right kidney may be divided into posterior, anterior, and middle channels. Posterior channels leave the renal hilum superior and posterior to the renal vessels and drain into the postcaval and interaortocaval nodes from L1 to L3 and the upper lateral caval nodes. Occasionally, lymphatics can pass directly through the diaphragm to the thoracic duct. There are three to five anterior lymphatic vessels. They are anterior to the renal vessels and curve upward to join the posterior lymphatics, or they may curve immediately to end in the precaval nodes. They also may cross the vena cava and end in the upper interaortocaval nodes. The middle lymphatic vessels course between the artery and vein joining the anterior and posterior lymphatic chains. The regional lymph nodes of the right kidney

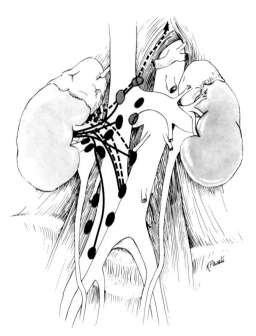

Figure 6.1. The regional lymph node drainage of the right kidney is demonstrated. A right radical nephrectomy and lymphadenectomy should include these nodes. (From Marshall FF: Anatomy of the retroperitoneum and adrenal. In Walsh PC, Gittes RF, Perlmutter AD, Stamey TA (eds): *Campbell's Urology*, ed 5. Philadelphia, WB Saunders, 1986, p 9.)

consist of the lateral caval nodes, the postcaval nodes, the precaval nodes, and the interaortocaval nodes.

The left renal lymphatics drain into a periaortic group of nodes, and there is no significant drainage to the interaortocaval area (Fig. 6.2). They drain into anterior and posterior groups of lymphatics. The anterior group is anterior to the renal vein. This group of lymphatics has superior and inferior branches that drain along the aorta and may also interconnect with the posterior group. The posterior group of lymphatics leaves the renal hilum posterior to the renal vessels. These lymphatics diverge at the left crus of the diaphragm into inferior and superior branches. Superiorly they pass to one or two diaphragmatic nodes through the diaphragm, and then postaortic nodes at T11, T12, and L1. Inferiorly the lymphatics usually end in the left lateral lumbar nodes between the lower pole of the kidney and the renal vein. The regional nodes of the left kidney include the left lateral lumbar, the preaortic, and the postaortic nodes. In addition, there are some nodes on the left crus of the diaphragm and several nodes at the left renal vein at the takeoff of the adrenal vein.

Once the regional lymph nodes are filled, the lymphatic drainage becomes diffuse. On the right side after the interaortocaval, lateral caval, postcaval, and precaval nodes are filled, the interaortocaval nodes drain superiorly into the thoracic duct and inferiorly to upper iliac and sacral nodes. The lateral caval nodes usually drain through pre- and postcaval nodes and occasionally down to iliac nodes as well as interaortocaval

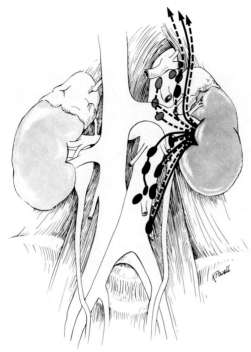

Figure 6.2. The regional lymph node drainage of the left kidney is demonstrated. A left radical nephrectomy should include these nodes. (From Marshall FF: Anatomy of the retroperitoneum and adrenal. In Walsh PC, Gittes RF, Perlmutter AD, Stamey TA (eds): *Campbell's Urology*, ed 5. Philadelphia, WB Saunders, 1986, p 9.)

nodes. Postcaval nodes can also have similar drainage and extend up through the right crus of the diaphragm as well. On the left side after the regional lymph nodes and diaphragmatic nodes are filled with injected medium, the lymphatics travel through around the left crus of the diaphragm into the thoracic duct. The lymphatics of the left lumbar nodes may drain inferiorly to the lateral lumber chain or superiorly to diaphragmatic nodes and then to the thoracic duct. Again, it should be emphasized that lymphatic drainage is fairly predictable to regional nodes, but beyond regional nodes the lymphatic drainage becomes highly variable and essentially systemic.

EXTENT OF REGIONAL LYMPHADENECTOMY

The rational limits of a regional lymph node dissection associated with a radical nephrectomy should include removal of the immediate primary lymphatic drainage of the kidney under normal conditions. A right radical nephrectomy should include a circumvena caval dissection with removal of the lateral caval, precaval, postcaval, and interaortocaval nodes (Fig. 6.3). This resection should start at the right crus of the diaphragm and extend inferiorly along the vena cava to the bifurcation of the vena cava and laterally on the psoas muscle because lymphatics often exist on the surface of this muscle.

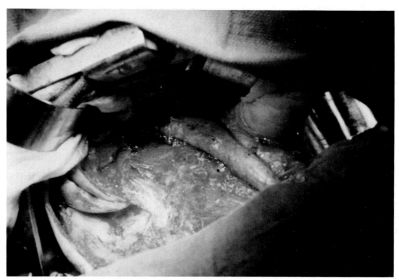

Figure 6.3. The vena cava and psoas muscle are visualized after right radical nephrectomy and regional lymphadenectomy.

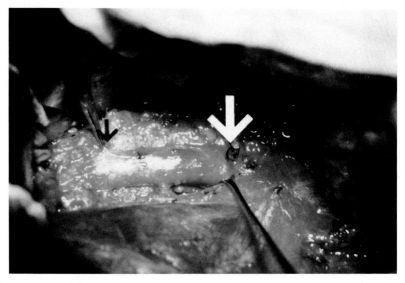

Figure 6.4. After a left radical nephrectomy and lymphadenectomy, the aorta is demonstrated; a vein retractor is under the left crus of the diaphragm, and a surgical clamp (*black arrow*) is at the level of the inferior mesenteric artery. A *white arrow* indicates the stump of the left renal artery.

A left radical nephrectomy and regional node dissection should include the left lateral lumbar nodes, the left diaphragmatic nodes, and the preaortic nodes (Fig. 6.4). In essence, the dissection is a periaortic node dissection, but there is no necessity for inclusion of the interaortocaval nodes. The upper postaortic nodes may be difficult to dissect because the left crus of the diaphragm prevents extensive dissection in this area (41). (Fig. 6.4). The dissection should start at the left crus of the diaphragm and extend inferiorly to the area of the bifurcation of the aorta, anterior and posterior to the aorta.

Important features to be emphasized include a retrocaval and inter-aortocaval dissection on the right which is much more important than an interaortocaval dissection with a left radical nephrectomy. If there is a tumor beyond the confines of the regional lymph nodes, the efficacy of a regional lymphadenectomy is doubtful. Large tumors may create abnormal lymphatic drainage with obstruction of the renal vein or ureteral obstruction with resultant change in the lymphatic spread. For example, Hulten et al. (7) described unusual apparent solitary metastases to the iliac region in one patient and a supraclavicular lymph node in another. Lymphatics follow blood vessels so that if there are multiple renal vessels a lymph node dissection should be altered accordingly. For example, if a lower pole accessory renal artery extends to the area of the aortic bifurcation, a proximal iliac node dissection should be performed.

RECOMMENDATIONS

Should a lymph node dissection be performed at all? The author thinks it should. In a collection of 2000 cases (see Table 6.1) 17% of the cases had positive lymph nodes, but the incidence was much higher when a systematic careful dissection was performed. It is therefore reasonable to assume that about 20 to 25% of patients will have positive lymph nodes. The collected 5-year survival was 27%, although the numbers are small. If those numbers are true, 5 to 10% of patients overall will benefit. Although this percentage is not huge, in the absence of adjuvant therapy, the author believes that regional lymphadenectomy is still justified.

Second, what is the rational extent of a regional lymphadenectomy? The limits of a regional lymph node dissection have been defined by the limits of normal extrarenal lymphatic drainage. A circumvena caval dissection is recommended on the right, and a periaortic dissection is performed on the left without an interaortocaval dissection.

REFERENCES

1. Marshall FF, Powell KC: Lymphadenectomy for renal cell carcinoma: anatomical and therapeutic considerations. *J Urol* 128:677, 1982.
2. McDonald MW: Current therapy for renal cell carcinoma. *J Urol* 127:211, 1982.
3. Robson CJ, Churchill BM, Anderson W: The results of radical nephrectomy for renal cell carcinoma. *J Urol* 101:297, 1969.
4. Skinner DG, Vermillion CD, Colvin RB: The surgical management of renal cell carcinoma. *J Urol* 107:705, 1972.
5. Peters PC, Brown GL: The role of lymphadenectomy in the management of renal cell carcinoma. *Urol Clin North Am* 7:705, 1980.
6. Siminovitch JP, Montie JE, Straffon RA: Lymphadenectomy in renal adenocarcinoma. *J Urol* 127:1090, 1982.
7. Hulten L, Rosencrantz M, Seeman T, Wahlqvist L, Ahren C: Occurrence and localization of lymph node metastases in renal carcinoma. A lymphographic and histopathological investigation in connection with nephrectomy. *Scand J Urol Nephrol* 3:129, 1969.
8. Javadpour N: *Principles and Management of Urologic Cancer.* Baltimore, Williams & Wilkins, 1979, pp 392–393.

9. Auvert J: Second Congress of the European Association of Urology. Lymphadenectomy in urological cancer. *Eur Urol* 4:149, 1978.
10. Foot NC, Humphreys GA, Whitmore WF: Renal tumors: pathology and prognosis in 295 cases. *J Urol* 66:190, 1951
11. Mintz ER, Gaul EA: Kidney tumors; some causes of poor end results. *NY State J med* 39:1405, 1939.
12. Stevens WE: Diagnosis and surgical treatment of malignant tumors of the kidney. *J Urol* 10:121, 1923.
13. Chute R, Soutter L, Kerr WS Jr: The value of the thoracoabdominal incision in the removal of kidney tumors. *N Engl J Med* 241:951, 1949.
14. Foley FEB, Mulvaney WP, Richardson EJ, Victor L: Radical nephrectomy for neoplasm. *J Urol* 68:39, 1952.
15. Flocks RH, Kadesky MC: Malignant neoplasms of the kidney: an analysis of 353 patients followed five years or more. *J Urol* 79:196, 1958.
16. Petkovic SD: An anatomical classification of renal tumors in the adult as a basis for prognosis. *J Urol* 81:618, 1959.
17. Rafla S: Renal cell carcinoma. Natural history and results of treatment. *Cancer* 25:26, 1970.
18. Middleton RG, Presto AJ III: Radical thoracoabdominal nephrectomy for renal cell carcinoma. *J Urol* 110:36, 1973.
19. Angervall L, Wahlqvist L: Follow-up and prognosis of renal carcinoma in a series operated by perifascial nephrectomy combined with adrenalectomy and retroperitoneal lymphadenectomy. *Eur Urol* 4:13, 1978.
20. Waters WB, Richie JP: Aggressive surgical approach to renal cell carcinoma: review of 130 cases. *J Urol* 122:306, 1979.
21. Sigel A, Chlepas S, Schrott KM, Hermanek P: Die operation des nierentumors. *Chirurg* 52:545, 1981.
22. Carl P, Klein U, Gebauer A, Schmidt E: The value of lymphography for TNM classification of renal carcinoma. *Eur Urol* 3:286, 1977.
23. Skinner DG, Colvin RB, Vermillion CD, Pfister RC, Leadbetter WF: Diagnosis and management of renal cell carcinoma. A clinical and pathologic study of 309 cases. *Cancer* 28:1165, 1971.
24. Bergman SM, Lippert M, Javadpour N: The value of whole lung tomography in the early detection of metastatic disease in patients with renal cell carcinoma and testicular tumors. *J Urol* 124:860, 1980.
25. Surya V, Clayman RV, Lange PH: Preoperative staging of renal cell carcinoma. Presented at annual meeting of the American Urological Association, Kansas City, MO, 1982, abstract 339.
26. Weyman PJ, McClennan BL, Stanley RJ, Levitt RG, Sagel SS: Comparison of computed tomography and angiography in the elevation of renal cell carcinoma. *Radiology* 137:417, 1980.
27. Pillari G, Lee WJ, Kumari S, Chen M, Abrams HJ, Buchbinder M, Sutton AP: CT and angiographic correlates: surgical image of renal mass lesions. *Urology* 17:296, 1981.
28. Levine E, Maklad NF, Rosenthal SJ, Lee KR, Weigel J: Comparison of computed tomography and ultrasound in abdominal staging of renal cancer. *Urology* 16:317, 1980.
29. Williams RD, London DA, Dombrovskis S, Davis PL, Crooks LE: Nuclear magnetic resonance (NMR) imaging: preclinical study in obstructed kidneys. Presented at annual meeting of the American Urological Association, Kansas City, MO, 1982, abstract 337.
30. Belitsky P, Ghose T, Path FR, Aquino J, Tai J, MacDonald AS: Radionuclide imaging of metastases from renal cell carcinoma by ^{131}I-labeled antitumor antibody. *Radiology* 126:515, 1978.
31. Haagensen CD, Feind CR, Grinnel RS, Herter FP, Hudson PB, Plentl AA, Weinberg JA: *The Lymphatics in Cancer.* Philadelphia, WB Saunders, 1972.
32. Poirier P, Cuneo B, Delamere G: *The Lymphatics.* London, Archibald Constable, 1903.
33. Schlegel JU: Demonstration of blood vessels and lymphatics with a fluorescent dye in ultraviolet light. *Anat Rec* 105:433, 1949.

34. Menon M, Menon S, Strauss HW, Catalona WJ: Demonstration of the existence of canine prostatic lymphatics by radioisotope techniques. *J Urol* 118:274, 1977.
35. Ege GN: Internal mammary lymphoscintigraphy. The rationale, technique interpretation and clinical application: a review based on 848 cases. *Radiology* 118:101, 1976.
36. Whitmore WF III, Blute RD Jr, Kaplan WD, Gittes RF: Radiocolloid scintigraphic mapping of the lymphatic drainage of the prostate. *J Urol* 124:62, 1980.
37. Sugarman J, Friedman M, Barrett E, Addis T: The distribution, flow, protein and urea content of renal lymph. *Am J Physiol* 138:108, 1942.
38. Peirce EC II: Renal lymphatics. *Anat Rec* 90:315, 1944.
39. Goodwin WE, Kaufman JJ: Renal lymphatics and hydronephrosis. *Surg Forum* 6:632, 1956.
40. Parker AE: Studies on the main posterior lymph channels of the abdomen and their connections with the lymphatics of the genitourinary system. *Am J Anat* 56:409, 1935.
41. Schmeller NT, Siegelman SS, Walsh PC: Anatomical considerations in suprahilar lymph node dissection for testicular tumors. *Urol Int* 36:341, 1981.

7

Treatment of Renal Cell Carcinoma Involving the Vena Cava and the Right Atrium

Christian Chatelain
Alain Jardin
M. O. Bitker
Y. Hammoudi

Venous dissemination is a characteristic feature of renal cell carcinoma. Neoplastic extension beyond the branches of the renal veins, involving the vena cava or even the right atrium, poses a number of specific therapeutic problems. At the present time, surgical resection is the only real therapeutic approach, and no complementary treatments have been found to be effective. The surgical procedure must therefore be designed and modified in terms of the involvement of the principal venous axis, as the prognosis, which has traditionally been considered to be very poor, is determined by the effectiveness of this resection.

MATERIALS AND METHODS

Between 1973 and 1984, 37 patients with renal cell carcinoma and involvement of the vena cava or the right atrium were admitted to the urologic department of Hôpital de la Pitié. Patients with tumor extending only as far as the junction of the renal vein with the vena cava were not included.

This series consisted of 27 men and 10 women with a mean age of 63 years (range: 26 to 79 years).

THE LESIONS

In 32 cases, the cancer involved the right kidney and in 5 cases, the left kidney. It involved the superior pole in 134 cases, the inferior pole in 10 cases, and was mediorenal or massive in 14 cases.

The tumor involved veins only (class IIIa, according to Robson's classification (1)) in 20 patients; veins and lymph nodes (IIIc) in 9 patients; adjacent organs (IVa) in 1 patient; and local invasion and metastases (IVb) in 7 patients (3 with lung metastases and 4 with hepatic metastases).

The upper limit of the cancer thrombus in the vena cava was located below the junction of the suprahepatic veins in 26 cases, retrohepatic and subdiaphragmatic in 7 cases, and in the right atrium in 4 cases. The subrenal vena cava was also involved in 4 cases, and bilateral iliac thrombosis was detected in 3 cases. One patient also had an associated thrombosis of the superior vena cava. All of these cases of "thrombosis" consisted of intracaval nodules of neoplastic cells, although in 2 cases, there was major fibrinothrombotic involvement.

TREATMENT

Six patients were not operated because the local, lymph node, and metastatic extension made any attempt at curative surgery unrealistic or because the cerebral or cardiovascular condition of the patient contraindicated any form of surgery.

Thirty-one patients were operated. Four patients were treated by simple exploratory laparotomy because the degree of local extension made resection impossible (these were among the earlier cases, for whom computerized tomography (CT) was not routinely available). Six patients underwent nephrectomy because of pain and hemorrhage, but the very extensive lesions were not completely excised. Twenty-one patients underwent complete resection of the lesions—extended nephrectomy and excision of the vena cava with or without lymphadenectomy.

The following surgical approaches were used: lumboabdominal approach (4 cases); anterior abdominal approach (median or Barraya) (12 cases); subcutaneous transverse abdominal approach (3 cases); thoracophrenolaparotomy (9 cases); large median abdominal median sternotomy (3 cases).

The surgical procedure on the inferior vena cava (24 cases) consisted of simple cavotomy with excision of the neoplastic tissue (6 cases); excision of the neoplastic tissue with partial cavectomy (16 cases); total cavectomy (2 cases) (associated with nephrectomy of a single kidney in 1 case). A selective thoracic approach to the right atrium was required in three cases.

ADJUVANT TREATMENTS

Fourteen patients underwent preoperative arterial embolization of the tumor. One inoperable tumor was also treated by means of embolization. Adjuvant chemotherapy or radiotherapy was used in 4 of the earliest cases, and hormonal treatment (progesterone) was administered in 15 patients (including 4 nonoperated patients).

RESULTS

Mortality

There was one intraoperative death as a result of massive embolism and cardiac arrest. Two patients died during the immediate postoperative period: one patient with chronic renal failure prior to the operation died after 48 hours due to a hemodialysis accident; the other patient died in acute renal failure on the fourth day after an extensive laparotomy; hemodialysis was not attempted.

The mortality in this series was therefore 10%.

Morbidity

Surprisingly, in view of the extent of the operation, the postoperative course was uncomplicated in 25 of the 31 operated patients (80%). The complications consisted of a wound abscess, a pulmonary embolism, and a transient confusional state with hemolysis.

Survival

Among the 6 nonoperated patients, 4 died within 1 year; 1 died after 27 months; and 1 is still alive after 23 months.

Among the 28 operated patients surviving the operation, 3 patients underwent only an exploratory laparotomy and died within 1 year. Four patients underwent "obligatory" nephrectomy with incomplete resection of the tumor, and all 4 patients died within 18 months.

In the remaining 21 patients, the operation was considered satisfactory. The 1-year survival was 47.62%; the 2-year survival was 28.62%; the 3-year survival was 29%; and the 5- to 7-year survival was 9.52%.

DISCUSSION

Frequency

Fortunately, renal cell carcinoma involving the vena cava is relatively uncommon. The incidence has been estimated to represent 4 to 6% (2), 7% (3), and 4 to 10% (4) of all renal cancers. In an earlier study, invasion of the intrarenal branches of the renal veins was found to be relatively common (16%), while invasion of the trunk of the renal vein was found to be less common (8%), and invasion of the vena cava was about 7% (5). This relative rarity makes statistical studies difficult and leads to the grouping of various series (4).

Symptoms and Preoperative Evaluation of the Invasion of the Vena Cava

Apart from a few exceptional cases, which presented with edema of the limbs, collateral circulation, a varicocele, repeated emboli, or impaired liver function, the patients did not present any symptoms suggestive of extension of the renal cancer into the vena cava. Thorough preoperative investigation is therefore very important. The present authors consider two examinations to be essential for adequate preoperative evaluation: the CT scan (Fig. 7.1), which is able to demonstrate any extension associated with the primary tumor, especially involving the lymph nodes; and cavography, which is essential to define the site of the cancer thrombus in the vena cava, particularly its upper limit. Computerized digital subtraction angiography may provide valuable additional information in this situation. Magnetic resonance imaging

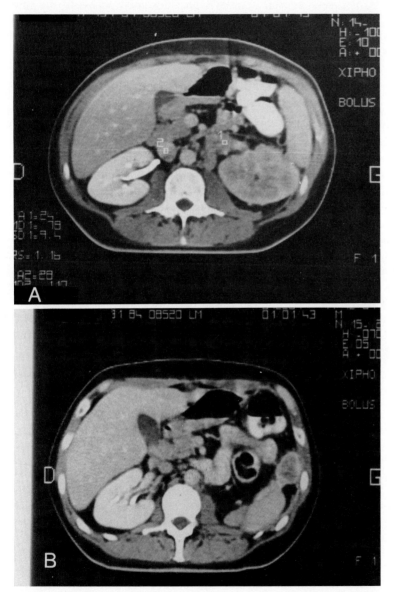

Figure 7.1. Male, 42 years old. Carcinoma of the left kidney with venous extension to the vena cava. *A*, Preoperative CT scan. *B*, Postoperative CT scan.

demonstrates the blood vessels without the need for contrast injection and may play an increasing role in vena caval assessment in the future.

An exact knowledge of the location of the thrombus is essential for the correct choice of the appropriate surgical approach.

Surgical Approach

The surgical approach to neoplastic involvement of the inferior vena cava should provide wide exposure. Thoracophrenolaparotomy provides good access to the sub- and retrohepatic vena cava, but poorer access to the diaphragmatic and supradiaphragmatic portion of the vena cava. The transverse subcostal approach provides good access to the retro- and suprahepatic vena cava. A median incision may be extended to include a median sternotomy, and the authors consider this approach to be the most effective in patients with extensive cancer thrombus.

Preoperative Arterial Embolization

Since the first application of selective arterial embolization to renal lesions by Almgard et al in 1973 (6) and its extension to the entire urogenital tract as a result of the work of Kuss et al (7), the techniques have been improved by the use of more effective embolizing agents (lipid synthetic polymers, releasable balloons) and by the control of the ischemic pain by means of continuous epidural anesthesia (8, 9).

This technique seems to be especially indicated in renal cell carcinomas with vena caval extension in order to collapse the dense collateral circulation which is always present in these cases, to retract the tumor, and to enable an easier surgical approach to the renal arterial axis. The authors believe that this technique is useful but not essential. They used this technique in 14 cases in this series, i.e., in about 50% of cases. However, it has been demonstrated that the only role of embolization is to facilitate the surgery (10). It causes pain and fever as a result of the partial devascularization of the tumor and may make the tumor more fragile (2).

Control of the Inferior Vena Cava

Whichever approach is used, it is generally accepted that it is essential to control the vena cava above and below the thrombus (11, 12). In cases with extensive retrohepatic thrombus, the authors control the vena cava in the hepatodiaphragmatic space after section of the triangular ligament.

The vena cava may be controlled superiorly by temporarily placing a plastic clip above the thrombus (3). However, this method of caval surgery carries a number of risks: the clamping of the vena cava involves a (low) risk of draining the cardiac pump, although temporary clamping of the aorta may correct this problem. Cavotomy requires the control of the major venous branches (left renal vein, right hemiazygous). Because of the shortness of the suprahepatic veins and the fragility of Spiegel's lobe, the retrohepatic approach to the vena cava is associated with certain difficulties.

The left renal vein can be ligated without any particular problems because of the great potential for collateral venous circulation. However, this is not the case for the right renal vein. Fortunately, the majority of cancers involving the inferior vena cava arise in the right kidney (a proportion of 6:1 in the authors' series).

For cancers of the left kidney, there are a number of possible techniques: renoportal anastomosis (2), venous patch graft from the superior mesenteric vein (2), use of prosthetic material (13), or use of a patch graft take from the pericardium (Faure).

Control of the Right Atrium

The authors use the following technique: median sternotomy, opening of the pericardium, access to the atrium, construction of a hemostatic pouch, auriculostomy, introduction of a finger which enables control of the inferior vena cava and allows the thrombus to be pushed inferiorly, where it is removed via a large inferior cavotomy. The authors have used this technique successfully in three cases without any complications (14–17). However, other authors prefer to clamp the atrium (18), while others prefer to use extracorporal circulation (19, 20) with (21, 22) or without hypothermia or circulatory arrest (23, 24) (Fig. 7.2).

Mortality-Morbidity

Surgery for neoplastic extension of renal cancer into the inferior vena cava carries a potential risk of mortality because of the possibility of migration of tumor fragments released during surgical manipulation. This is a real risk and can result in intraoperative pulmonary embolism (20, 25). The importance of correct control of the venous system above the thrombus prior to any manipulation is therefore obvious. The authors consider the techniques involving the use of Foley's or Fogarty's catheters to be dangerous.

The mortality has varied greatly over the years with the use of different techniques, ranging for 4 to 50% (20). On the other hand, the morbidity has generally been considered to be extremely low in most series, although some authors have been less optimistic (26).

Spontaneous Course of the Disease

Cases of spontaneous long term survival have been reported in patients with untreated renal cancer with vena caval extension, e.g., the patient reported by Schorn and Marberger (27), who survived 5½ years after the diagnosis of bilateral cancer with caval extension. Cases of acceptable survival have also been reported, such as the present authors' two cases with a 2-year survival. However, the great majority of patients die within 12 months.

Long Term Results

Extension of renal cell carcinoma to the inferior vena cava has been considered for a long time to be a sign of very poor prognosis. Attempts at surgical excision were thought to be dangerous and probably useless.

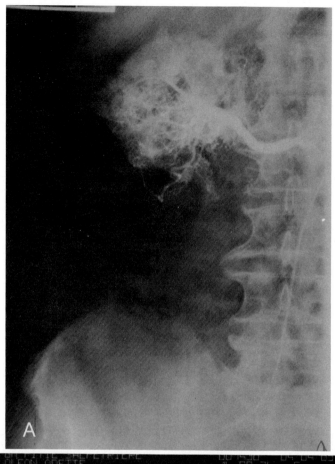

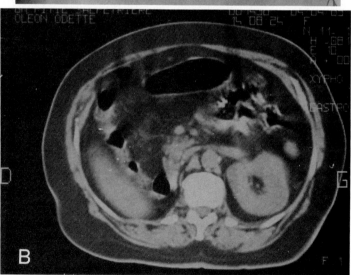

Figure 7.2. Female, 53 years old. Carcinoma of the right kidney. Radical nephrectomy and partial cavectomy (*A*). CT scan 7½ years later (*B*); patient still alive.

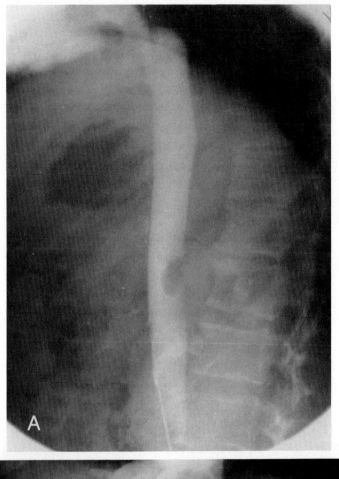

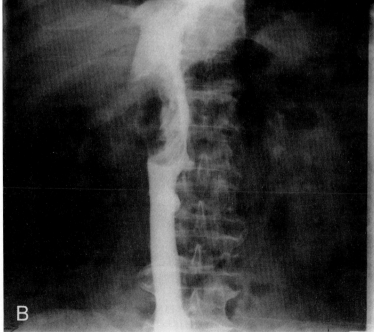

Figure 7.3. Male, 75 years old. *A*, Carcinoma of the right kidney invading the vena cava. *B*, Two years after radical nephrectomy and partial cavectomy, the patient is alive.

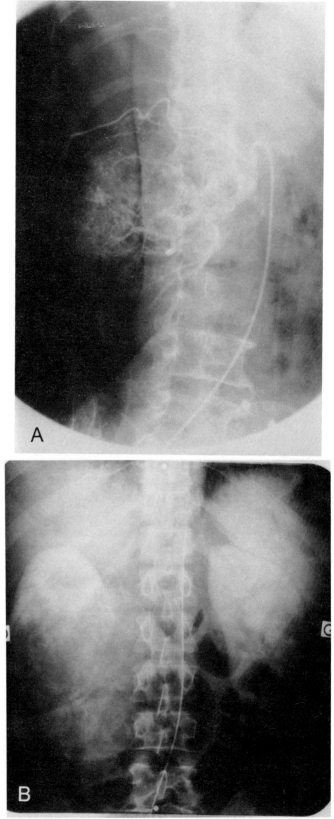

Figure 7.4. Male, 43 years old. Large right renal mass (*A* and *B*) with large vena caval neoplasic thrombosis (*C* and *D*). Removal under control of the right atrium. The patient had a normal life for 1 year, then died within 2 months with multiple metastases.

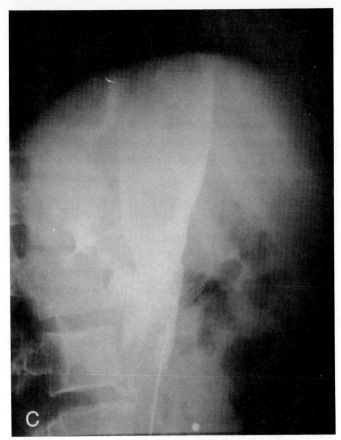

Figure 7.4. *C*

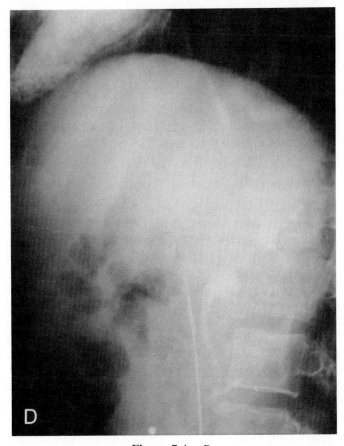

Figure 7.4. *D*

Only about 15 years ago, in a series of 11 operated patients, Marshall et al (28) reported 8 deaths within less than a year. In contrast, in 1972, in a series of 11 patients, Skinner et al (18) reported a 5-year survival in 6 patients and a 10-year survival in 5 patients, and they were therefore strongly in favor of an attempt at surgery. In 1982 Cherrie et al (4) studied a series of 27 patients and reviewed 46 cases in the literature. They concluded that extension into the inferior vena cava alone had only a limited impact on the prognosis, with a 2-year survival rate of 81%, a 5-year survival of 53%, and a mean survival of 81 months (4). To a lesser extent, extension into the perirenal fascia was also associated with a poor prognosis (2-year survival of 66%) (4).

However, a number of factors need to be taken into consideration in the analysis of these results.

Prognostic Factors

The presence or absence of distinct metastases is certainly the most important factor. In a series of eight patients with known metastases, Sogani et al (29) observed seven deaths within 12 months, while 50% of the eight patients without metastases obtained a mean disease-free survival of 93 months. In the series reported by Schefft et al (3), Clayman et al (30), and Kearney et al (26), there were no survivors out of eight patients with metastases after 24 months, with a mean survival of less than 1 year. In Cherrie et al's series (4), only 5% of the patients with metastases were alive after 2 years, and none of them survived for 5 years (mean survival: 8.5 months).

The present authors' series is no exception to the rule. However, they reported an unusual case of a patient with obvious bilateral pulmonary metastases at the time of operation which disappeared after excision of the renal cancer and the caval extension; the patient is presently alive with no signs of recurrence after 3½ years.

The site of the cancer thrombus in the vena cava also needs to be taken into consideration. Sosa et al (31) found a marked difference in the prognosis in a series of 24 patients, according to whether the thrombus remained below the suprahepatic veins (10 patients: 2-year survival rate of 80%, mean survival: 61.4 months) or whether it extended beyond this level (14 patients: 2-year survival rate of 21%, mean survival: 22.9 months).

The presence or absence of invasion of the wall of the vena cava is of great importance in the choice of surgical technique. However, the authors do not believe that it has a great impact on the prognosis, provided all of the invaded venous wall has been completely excised (Fig. 7.3).

The nature of the caval thrombus is a factor which has not been extensively studied. The authors found that even in patients with renal neoplastic extension, part of the mass present in the inferior vena cava may be fibrinothrombotic in various stages of organization (Fig. 7.4). This was the case in one particular patient, who presented thrombus extending as far as the right atrium; the base of this thrombus was composed of malignant cells, but the extremity adherent to the right atrium was found to contain only fibrous tissue. This male patient is alive 7½ years later with no signs of recurrence.

In the authors' series, all of the patients surviving for more than 2 years had "pure" venous invasion without associated lymph node involvement. However, the relatively good prognosis in these patients is dependent on complete excision of the neoplastic lesions.

Criticism of the Classification

In view of the above findings, it is obvious that Robson's classification, which is generally accepted, is inadequate for the staging of renal cell carcinoma, as it places lesions with entirely different prognoses in the same group III (venous extension, lymph node extension, or both types of extension). For this reason, Gouygou and Jardin (32), during the Congress of the International Society of Urology held in Johannesburg in 1976, proposed the use of a modified TNM (tumor-nodes-metastasis) classification, which becomes TVNM (tumor-veins-nodes-metastasis) in the case of renal cell carcinoma.

CONCLUSION

The extension of renal cell carcinoma into the inferior vena cava does not, in itself, indicate a poor prognosis nor does it constitute a therapeutic impossibility.

In the absence of any other effective treatment, only surgical excision is capable of providing a chance of prolonged survival. Extensive surgical procedures with en bloc resection of the tumor and the caval extension together with resection of part of the venous wall when required (sometimes involving intracardiac control of the vena cava) are therefore justified, despite their difficulty and their risks, in view of the good long term prognosis in patients with isolated venous invasion. The association of lymph node involvement and local extension results in a much poorer prognosis. When metastases are present, surgery does not appear to alter the short term fatal prognosis significantly and therefore is of doubtful value.

REFERENCES

1. Robson CJ, Churchill BM, Anderson W: The results of nephrectomy for renal cell carcinoma. *J Urol* 101:297, 1969.
2. Gittes RF: Locally extensive renal cell carcinoma. Current surgical management of invasion of vena cava, liver or bowel. In *Renal Tumors—Proceedings of the First International Symposium on Kidney Tumors.* New York, Alan R Liss, 1982, no. 497.
3. Schefft P, Novick AC, Straffon RA, Stewart BH: Surgery for renal cell carcinoma extending into the inferior vena cava. *J Urol* 120:28–31, 1978.
4. Cherrie RJ, Goldman DG, Lindner A, deKernion JB: Prognostic implications of vena caval extension of renal cell carcinoma. *J Urol* 128:910, 1982.
5. Chatelain C, Richard F: Pronostic des adenocarcinomes renaux etendus a la veine cave inferieure. *Actual Chirurg* 4:54–59, 1982.
6. Almgard LE, Fernstrom I, Haverlin GM, Ljungqvist A: Treatment of renal adenocarcinoma by embolic occlusion of the renal circulation. *Br J Urol* 45:474–479, 1973.
7. Küss R, Le Guillou M, Merland JJ, Lepage T, Bories J: L'embolisation en pathologie uro-genitale. *Ann Urol* 9:1–10, 1975.

8. Adrien G, Harari A, Viars P, Curet P, Richard F: Analgesie morphinique peridurale apres embolisation arterielle viscerale. *Nuv Presse Med* 10:431, 1981.
9. Grinnell VS, Hieshima GB, Mehringer CM, Fong T, Shaw S: Therapeutic renal artery occlusion with a detachable balloon. *J Urol* 126:233–237, 1981.
10. Kaisary AV, Williams G, Riddle PR: The role of preoperative embolization in renal cell carcinoma. *J Urol* 131:641, 1984.
11. Valvo JR, Cos LR, Altebarmakian VK, Khuri FJ, Cockett ATK: Surgery and immunotherapy in renal cell carcinoma involving inferior vena cava. *Urology* 20:359, 1982.
12. Beck AD: Renal cell carcinoma involving the inferior vena cava. Radiologic evaluation and surgical management. *J Urol* 118:533, 1977.
13. Katz NM: Reconstruction of the inferior vena cava with a polytetrafluoroethylene tube graft after resection for hypernephroma of the right kidney. *J Thorac Cardiovasc Surg* 87:791, 1984.
14. Camey M, Leduc A, Gandjback F, Chiche B: Chirurgie de l'envahissement cave. *J Urol Nephrol* 80:150, 1974.
15. Chatelain C: Results of radical nephrectomy without lymphadenectomy in renal cell carcinoma. In *Renal Tumors—Proceedings of the First International Symposium on Kidney Tumors.* New York, Alan R Liss, 1982, no. 475.
16. Cinqualbre J, Py JM, Bollack C: Renal cell carcinoma extending into the inferior vena cava. Technical problems. In *Renal Tumors—Proceedings of the First International Symposium on Kidney Tumors.* New York, Alan R Liss, 1982, no. 529.
17. Gandjbakhch I, Guiraudon G, Cabrol C, Leduc A, Jardin A, Chatelain C, Küss R: Traitement chirurgical du cancer du rein etendu a la veine cave inferieure. Aspects techniques. *Actual Chirurg* 4:52–54, 1982.
18. Skinner DG, Pfister RF, Colvin R: Extension of renal cell carcinoma into the vena cava: the rationale for aggressive surgical management. *J Urol* 107:711, 1972.
19. Klein FA, Vernon Smith MJ, Greenfield LJ: Extracorporeal circulation for renal cell carcinoma with supradiaphragmatic vena caval thrombi. *J Urol* 131:880, 1984.
20. Richaud C, Breton F, Jouven JC, Casanova P, Kohler JL: L'extension cave des cancers du rein. Problemes Chirurgicaux. *J Urol (F)* 88:505, 1982.
21. Paul JG, Rhodes DR, Skow JR: Renal cell carcinoma presenting as right atrial tumor with successful removal using cardio-pulmonary bypass. *Ann Surg* 181:471, 1975.
22. Marschall FF, Reitz BA, Diamond DA: A new technique for management of renal cell carcinoma involving the right atrium: hypothermia and cardiac arrest. *J Urol* 131:103, 1984.
23. Abdelsayed MA, Bissada NK, Finkbeiner AE, Redman JF: Renal tumors involving the inferior vena cava: plan for management. *J Urol* 120:153, 1978.
24. Prager RL, Dean R, Turner B: Surgical approach to intracardiac renal cell carcinoma. *Ann Thorac Surg* 33:74, 1982.
25. Cukier J, Berrada F, Dibo S: Le pronostic des envahissements veineux et lymphatique dans les cancers du parenchyme renal traites par nephrectomie elargé. *J Urol (F)* 89:643, 1983.
26. Kearney GP, Waters WB, Klein LA, Richie JP, Gittes RF: Results of inferior vena cava resection for renal cell carcinoma. *J Urol* 125:769, 1981.
27. Schorn A, Marberger M: Long term survival of untreated bilateral renal cell carcinoma with supradiaphragmatic vena caval thrombus. *J Urol* 131:108, 1984.
28. Marshall VF, Middleton RG, Holswade GR, Goldmith ET: Surgery for renal cell carcinoma in the vena cava. *J Urol* 103:414, 1970.
29. Sogani PC, Herr HW, Bains MS, Whitmore WF: Renal cell carcinoma extending into inferior vena cava. *J Urol* 130:660, 1983.
30. Clayman RV, Gonzalez R, Fraley EE: Renal cell cancer invading the inferior vena cava. Clinical review and anatomical approach. *J Urol* 123:157, 1980.
31. Sosa RE, Muecke EC, Vaughan ED, McCarron JP: Renal cell carcinoma extending into the inferior vena cava: the prognostic significance of the level of vena caval involvement. *J Urol* 132:1097, 1984.
32. Gouygou C, Mazeman F, Jardin A: Bases Actuelles d'Approche d'unf Classification des Tumeurs Renales. Presented at the International Society of Urology meeting, Johannesburg, 1976, T1, pp 15–32.

8

Renal Cell Cancer with Extension into the Vena Cava

Richard Bihrle, M.D.
John A. Libertino, M.D.

The management of renal cell cancer with extension into the vena cava is both controversial and challenging. Variable results, which have been reported by different investigators, have added to the confusion (Table 8.1). Proper patient selection and meticulous attention to surgical technique will improve clinical results and make this difficult problem less controversial in the future.

The reported incidence of renal cell adenocarcinoma in the United States is 3.5/100,000 population/year (4). Although renal cell carcinoma has been reported in patients at all ages from infancy to old age, the median age at the time of diagnosis has variously been reported as between 55 and 57 years. Despite numerous trials with single and multidrug chemotherapeutic regimens, radiation therapy, and hormonal manipulation, surgical extirpation remains the mainstay for curative treatment of renal cell cancer.

In a review of 309 patients treated by radical nephrectomy between 1935 and 1965, Skinner et al (1) reported an operative mortality rate of 5%, with an overall survival rate of 45% at 5 years and 33% at 10 years. Excluding patients who had metastasis when first evaluated, the 5- and 10-year survival rates were 57% and 44%, respectively.

STAGING

In an effort to evaluate results of treatment and the prognosis of individual patients better, Flocks and Kadesky (6) proposed a pathologic staging system that was subsequently modified by Robson and associates (7, 8).

The staging system for renal cell carcinoma that is currently in use is as follows:

Stage I: Tumor is confined to the kidney without involvement of the perinephric fat.

Table 8.1
Results

Year	Author	No. of Patients	Survival (%)	Mean Follow-up (months)	Operative Mortality (%)
1972	Skinner et al (1)	11	45.0	60	Not available
1978	Schefft et al (2)	21	28.5	21	14.3
1981	Kearney et al (3)	24	16.6	21	4.0
1983	Lahey Clinic	24	62.5	36	4.0

Stage II: Tumor involves the perinephric fat (confined to Gerota's fascia).

Stage III: Tumor involves the renal vein or the regional nodes or both with or without involvement of the vena cava or perinephric fat.

Stage IV: Distant metastasis or histologic involvement of contiguous visceral structures.

When survival rates were assessed according to this staging system, Skinner and associates (5) reported that of 102 patients with stage I cancer, 65% survived 5 years and 56% survived 10 years; of 22 patients with stage II cancer, 47% survived 5 years and 20% survived 10 years; of 108 patients with stage III cancer, 51% survived 5 years and 37% survived 10 years; and of 77 patients with stage IV cancer, 8% survived 5 years and 7% survived 10 years.

A shortcoming of this staging system is apparent when critical analysis of stage III disease is made. Patients with renal vein or caval involvement, but without nodal or perinephric involvement, have had survival rates that are similar to patients with stage I disease (1, 7, 9, 10). In a recent review of the present authors' experience with 25 patients with vena caval extension from renal cell cancer treated by thoracoabdominal radical nephrectomy and partial vena caval resection, survival rates were excellent when involvement of nodes or perinephric fat was absent.

Intracaval tumor thrombus is usually a manifestation of advanced renal cell carcinoma but occasionally may be associated with Wilms' tumor and adrenal carcinoma. Approximately 5% of patients undergoing radical nephrectomy for renal cell carcinoma have extension of tumor thrombus into the inferior vena cava. The level of extension varies from a small tongue of thrombus at the level of the renal vein to an extensive thrombus into the right atrium. A recent classification of extension of the tumor into the vena cava is depicted in Figure 8.1.

In the authors' 25 patients, the tumor extended into the vena cava at the level of the renal vein in 16.7% of patients, above the renal veins but infradiaphragmatic in 62.5%, supradiaphragmatic but not into the atrium in 12.5%, and into the right atrium in 8.3%. Extended survival was achieved in all patients, regardless of whether the tumor was supradiaphragmatic or infradiaphragmatic.

SYMPTOMS AND SIGNS

Most patients present with symptoms and signs typical of renal carcinoma with hematuria, flank or abdominal pain, and a flank or

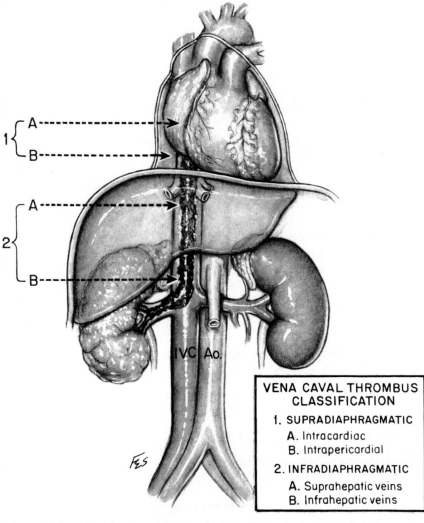

Figure 8.1. Classification of vena caval thrombus extension. *IVC*, inferior vena cava; *Ao*, aorta. (From Libertino JA: Renal cell cancer with extension into vena cava. In McDougal WS (ed): *Rob and Smith Operative Surgery: Urology*, ed 4. London, Butterworths, 1984.)

abdominal mass predominating. However, one-third to one-half of patients demonstrate signs or symptoms directly referable to vena caval involvement. The diagnosis of vena caval extension should be suspected when bilateral lower extremity edema, right varicocele or left varicocele of recent onset, dilated superficial abdominal wall veins, caput medusae, pulmonary embolus, or proteinuria is noted in association with a renal tumor.

PREOPERATIVE TESTS

Since renal cell carcinoma is primarily a radiologic diagnosis and since the presence or absence of metastases is paramount in treatment decisions, all patients should be evaluated with intravenous pyelography, computed tomography (CT), lung tomography, bone scan, liver function tests, and selective renal arteriography. Vena caval extension must be considered (and consequently inferior venacavography is indicated) when a perihilar mass associated with a nonfunctioning kidney is seen on intravenous pyelography, filling defects are noted on the venous phase of the arteriogram, and renal vein or caval involvement is suspected on the CT scan.

Superior venacavography is indicated in the presence of total occlusion of the vena cava or when the uppermost limit of caval extension cannot clearly be determined by inferior venacavography. In addition to superior venacavography, a right heart study may be warranted in patients demonstrating complete occlusion of the inferior vena cava. Preoperative studies must delineate the proximal and distal limits of the tumor thrombus so that the appropriate surgical approach is employed.

The preoperative evaluation of a patient with vena caval tumor thrombus cannot be overemphasized. The presence of perihilar nodal involvement as well as distant visceral and bony metastasis must be excluded for any hope of cure. The level of caval involvement must also be known so that the surgeon can plan a safe operative approach and anticipate any special maneuvers that may be required during resection.

SURGICAL TECHNIQUE

In performance of vena caval surgery for renal cell tumor thrombus, certain principles apply regardless of where the tumor thrombus extends. First, this is primarily a vena caval operation, and therefore the operative approach should be from the right side even if the tumor thrombus extends from a left renal tumor. Second, as in all cancer surgery, manipulation of the renal vein and vena cava should be kept to a minimum until a DeWeese clip is temporarily placed on the vena cava above the tumor thrombus to avoid dislodgment and dissemination of tumor emboli. Third, if a venacavotomy is required, the surgeon must gain control of the vena cava above and below the tumor thrombus. Finally, knowledge of the venous drainage of the kidneys is essential in planning this operative procedure.

While the right kidney has very little collateral venous drainage, the left kidney is endowed with abundant collateral drainage through the gonadal, adrenal, and lumbar veins (Fig. 8.2). This assumes surgical significance when radical nephrectomy with partial or total vena caval resection is contemplated. No problems are encountered when a right radical nephrectomy is performed in association with complete caval resection. The left renal vein can usually be divided with relative impunity, relying on the left kidney's extensive venous collateral network for drainage. However, the authors always ascertain the integrity of the venous collateral system by cross-clamping the left renal vein and occluding the right ureter. Failure to observe bluish discoloration of the urine 10 to 12 minutes after the intravenous injection of 1 ampule of methylene blue precludes ligation of the left renal vein. Cross-clamping the left renal vein rarely proves to be problematic when this phenomenon is observed.

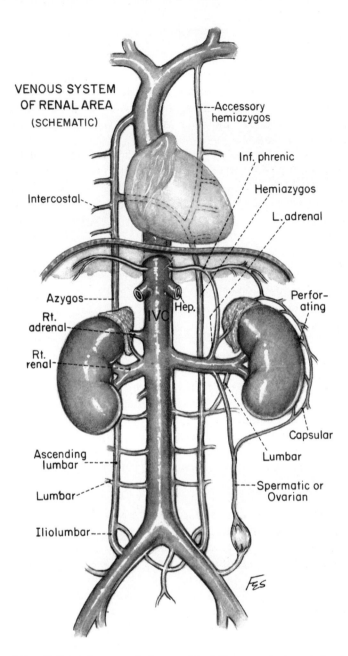

Figure 8.2. Collateral venous drainage of the kidneys and adrenal glands. *IVC*, inferior vena cava. (From Libertino JA: Renal cell cancer with extension into vena cava. In McDougal WS (ed): *Rob and Smith Operative Surgery: Urology*, ed 4. London, Butterworths, 1984.)

Complete vena caval resection in conjunction with left radical nephrectomy poses a more difficult problem that requires more elaborate surgical maneuvers. In this instance, the surgeon must create venous outflow for the right kidney by interposing a segment of saphenous vein either from the right renal vein to the vena cava above the point of resection or to the portal vein.

RENAL CANCER WITH EXTENSION INTO VENA CAVA   115

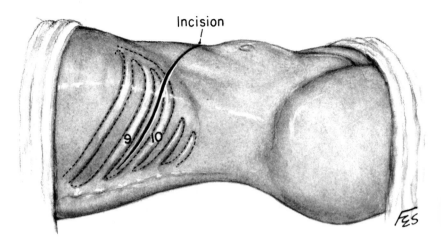

Figure 8.3. Thoracoabdominal incision. (From Libertino JA: Renal cell cancer with extension into vena cava. In McDougal WS (ed): *Rob and Smith Operative Surgery: Urology*, ed 4. London, Butterworths, 1984.)

A right eighth or ninth intercostal thoracoabdominal incision is employed because this primarily vena caval operation is best approached and controlled through the right chest. For a left-sided tumor, the abdominal portion of the incision is extended across the midline beyond the lateral border of the left rectus muscle (Fig. 8.3). The abdominal portion is opened initially to assess operability and to rule out the presence of liver metastasis, invasion of the mesocolon, the presence of involved perihilar nodes, or extension of the tumor into the posterior musculature. The presence of any of these conditions precludes an extensive vena caval operation because the patient has a poor prognosis. If the abdominal exploration proves negative, the thoracic extension of the incision is completed.

Two-thirds of renal tumors involving the vena cava arose from the right kidney in the authors' series. For right-sided tumors, the right colon is mobilized from the hepatic flexure to the cecum, as is the small bowel mesentery to the ligament of Treitz. A Kocher maneuver is used to mobilize the second portion of the duodenum and head of the pancreas. The colon and small bowel are elevated out of the abdomen, inserted into a moistened Lahey bag, and placed on the chest wall. In the performance of this maneuver, the superior mesenteric artery is elevated; this affords excellent visualization and access to the left renal vein as it crosses over the aorta just inferior to the superior mesenteric artery. Undue tension placed on the superior mesenteric artery may have a disastrous effect on the blood supply to the small bowel.

Before dissection, a DeWeese clip is placed on the vena cava, and the right renal artery is ligated and divided. The origin of the right renal artery from the aorta is located directly behind the left renal vein (Fig. 8.4). The vein is gently elevated, and the artery is ligated at its origin from the aorta. Preoperative embolization may be employed for a large tumor to reduce the kidney's size and to allow easier access to the vena caval portion of the procedure. The right renal vein is isolated but, of course, is not divided at this time.

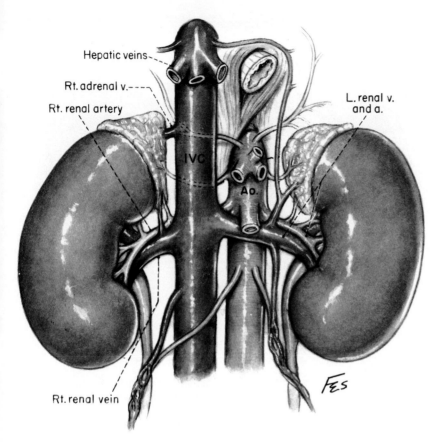

Figure 8.4. Vascular supply of the kidneys and adrenal glands. *IVC*, inferior vena cava; *Ao*, aorta. (From Libertino JA: Renal cell cancer with extension into vena cava. In McDougal WS (ed): *Rob and Smith Operative Surgery: Urology,* ed 4. London, Butterworths, 1984.)

If the tumor involves only the renal vein or is a small protruding tongue into the vena cava, the tumor may be milked proximally into the renal vein far enough to allow placement of a C-shaped Satinsky clamp incorporating the renal vein and a portion of vena cava. This allows removal of the kidney with a cuff of vena cava while obviating the need to clamp the left renal vein, vena cava, or lumbar veins.

If the tumor thrombus extends into the vena cava to a level where it cannot be resected in this manner, the entire vena cava must be mobilized to a level above the tumor thrombus. In this event, access to the vena cava is best achieved by performing a Langenbeck maneuver by dividing the right triangular ligament and coronary ligament and rotating the right lobe of the liver medially (Figs. 8.5–8.7). With careful dissection, the minor and major hepatic veins are isolated. The minor veins, usually two in number, are divided to avoid disrupting them inadvertently during the procedure and causing unnecessary and troublesome bleeding.

Again, before the vena cava is mobilized, a DeWeese clip is placed above the tumor thrombus to prevent the possibility of a tumor pulmonary embolus. This clip is left in place until the operation is com-

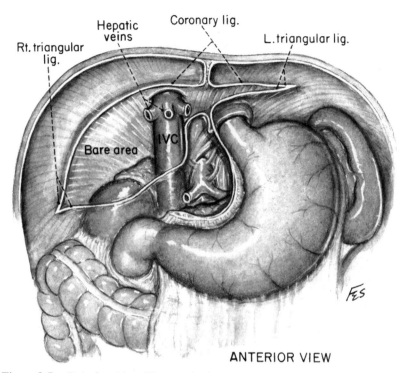

Rt. triangular lig.

Hepatic veins

Coronary lig.

L. triangular lig.

Bare area

IVC

ANTERIOR VIEW

Figure 8.5. Relationship of liver and triangular and coronary ligaments to the vena cava. *IVC*, inferior vena cava. (From Libertino JA: Renal cell cancer with extension into vena cava. In McDougal WS (ed): *Rob and Smith Operative Surgery: Urology*, ed 4. London, Butterworths, 1984.)

pleted, and then it is either removed or placed below the left renal vein depending on whether the patient has the propensity for the development of a pulmonary embolus.

Once the DeWeese clip is secured, umbilical tapes are passed around the vena cava above and below the tumor thrombus and around the left renal vein (Fig. 8.8*A*). The lumbar veins are ligated and divided whenever possible. Depending on the collateral venous outflow, the left renal artery may need to be occluded temporarily with a microvascular bulldog clamp before occluding the left renal vein and vena cava. The Rummel tourniquets are then cinched down, and the inferior vena cava is opened longitudinally (Fig. 8.8*B*). The tumor thrombus is extracted by blunt dissection with an elevator or Penfield dissector. Often the most distal portion of the tumor thrombus is actually blood clot, which is easily dissected from the caval wall. When tumor invades the vena cava, it usually is limited to the ostium of the renal vein. To ensure complete removal of tumor, a cuff of vena cava is excised in continuity with the right kidney (Fig. 8.9*A*). The venacavotomy is closed with a continuous 5-0 suture (Fig. 8.9*B*). Just before the closure is completed, the distal caval clamp is released to fill the vena cava and to lessen the chance of an air embolus. The tourniquets are then removed in the following order: the distal caval tape, the proximal caval tape, the left renal vein tourniquet, and finally the left renal artery tourniquet.

When the tumor extends above the level of the hepatic veins or is in

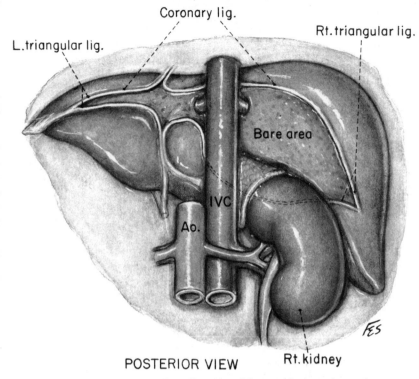

Coronary lig.

Rt. triangular lig.

L.triangular lig.

Bare area

IVC

Ao.

FES

POSTERIOR VIEW   Rt. kidney

Figure 8.6. Posterior view of relationship of liver and triangular and coronary ligaments to the vena cava. *IVC*, inferior vena cava; *Ao*, aorta. (From Libertino JA: Renal cell cancer with extension into vena cava. In McDougal WS (ed): *Rob and Smith Operative Surgery: Urology*, ed 4. London, Butterworths, 1984.)

the intrapericardial portion of the vena cava, the DeWeese clip must be placed at this level. In addition, it may be necessary to place a Fogarty vascular clamp on the porta hepatis (Pringle maneuver) to control the arterial and venous inflow into the liver and also across the major hepatic veins to prevent back bleeding when the venacavotomy is created.

When the tumor thrombus extends into the supradiaphragmatic vena cava, the operative approach is determined by the presence or absence of intra-atrial tumor. In the absence of intra-atrial tumor, a DeWeese clip is placed about the intrapericardial inferior vena cava, and the tumor thrombus is extracted from below the diaphragm using the method previously described. Cardiopulmonary bypass is not needed in this situation.

CARDIOPULMONARY BYPASS

The presence of tumor within the right atrium requires the use of atriotomy and cardiopulmonary bypass. In this select group of patients, a chevron incision combined with median sternotomy provides the best exposure. Cardiopulmonary bypass is not performed until the entire kidney has been mobilized, being attached only by the renal vein. This

RENAL CANCER WITH EXTENSION INTO VENA CAVA   119

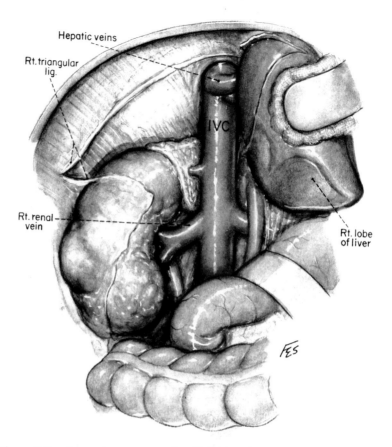

Figure 8.7. Access to vena cava by the Langenbeck maneuver. *IVC,* inferior vena cava. (From Libertino JA: Renal cell cancer with extension into vena cava. In McDougal WS (ed): *Rob and Smith Operative Surgery: Urology,* ed 4. London, Butterworths, 1984.)

portion of the procedure must be carried out before systemic heparinization, required for cardiopulmonary bypass, is instituted to avoid excessive bleeding.

For cardiopulmonary bypass, the heart is cannulated with the arterial return by means of the ascending aorta and the venous drainage by means of the superior vena cava and the right common femoral vein. Bypass is then instituted, the right atrium is opened, and the intra-atrial portion of the tumor is removed. Attention is next directed to the infradiaphragmatic portion of the procedure using the technique described earlier. After complete removal of the tumor thrombus, the atriotomy and vena cava are sequentially closed, and the patient is removed from cardiopulmonary bypass.

SURVIVAL

Using these methods, the authors have attained results that are comparable or superior to previous reports (2, 3). In the overall group of patients who have undergone thoracoabdominal radical nephrectomy with excision of caval thrombus, the authors have achieved an unad-

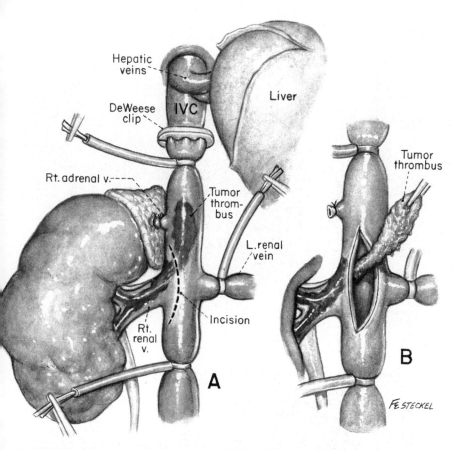

Labels in figure:
Hepatic veins
Liver
DeWeese clip
IVC
Rt. adrenal v.
Tumor throm-bus
L. renal vein
Incision
Rt. renal v.
A
Tumor thrombus
B
FE STECKEL

Figure 8.8. *A* and *B*, Vascular control of vena cava, cavotomy, and tumor thrombectomy. *IVC*, inferior vena cava. (From Libertino JA: Renal cell cancer with extension into vena cava. In McDougal WS (ed): *Rob and Smith Operative Surgery: Urology*, ed 4. London, Butterworths, 1984.)

justed 5-year survival rate of 45.7% ± SE 13.3% with a median survival time of 53.2 months. They found a statistically significant correlation between pathologic staging and survival. Of the patients with unfavorable disease, that is, patients with metastatic disease discovered at the time of operation or with positive nodes or both, only one of six patients (17%) has survived, with a group median survival time of 14.0 months. Of patients free of nodal or metastatic disease, 14 of 18 (78%) have thus far survived, with a group median survival time of 146+ months. Ten of 11 patients (91%) who were free of metastatic, nodal, or perinephric fat involvement are currently alive and free of evident disease for an unadjusted 5-year disease-free rate of 85.7% ± SE 13.2% and a median disease-free time of 146+ months. Six of these 11 patients have survived beyond 5 years.

Chronic renal failure requiring chronic dialysis did not develop in any patient in the authors' series. This is in contradistinction to several other reported series (2, 3) and may be attributed to meticulous technique, which includes every effort to avoid occlusion of the venous outflow of the contralateral kidney and favors partial rather than complete caval resection.

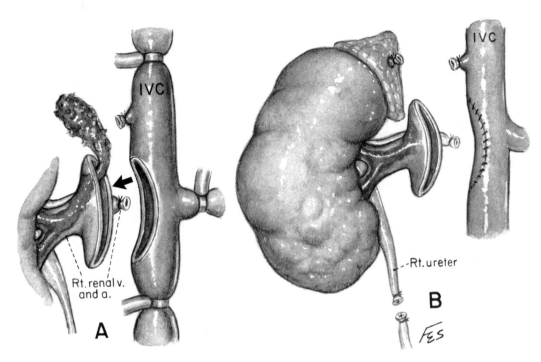

Figure 8.9. *A* and *B*, Partial vena caval resection and vena caval closure. *IVC,* inferior vena cava. (From Libertino JA: Renal cell cancer with extension into vena cava. In McDougal WS (ed): *Rob and Smith Operative Surgery: Urology,* ed 4. London, Butterworths, 1984.)

COMMENT

Based on the authors' experience with 25 patients, they believe that extended surgery for renal cell cancer with vena caval involvement is warranted and provides reasonable long term survival in carefully selected patients. It is imperative to make every effort to exclude the presence of metastatic disease or regional node involvement before proceeding with such radical extirpative surgery. The presence of metastatic disease or nodal involvement, on the basis of the authors' experience, precludes consideration of vena caval surgery.

REFERENCES

1. Skinner, DG, Pfister RF, Colvin R: Extension of renal cell carcinoma into the vena cava: the rationale for aggressive surgical management. *J Urol* 107:711–716, 1972.
2. Schefft P, Novick AC, Straffon RA, Stewart BH: Surgery for renal cell carcinoma extending into the inferior vena cava. *J Urol* 120:28–31, 1978.
3. Kearney GP, Waters WB, Klein LA, Richie JP, Gittes RF: Results of inferior vena cava resection for renal cell carcinoma. *J Urol* 125:769–773, 1981.
4. MacDonald EJ: Present incidence and survival picture in cancer and promise of improved prognosis. *Bull Am Coll Surgeons* 33:75–93, 1948.
5. Skinner DG, Colvin RB, Vermillion CD, Pfister RF, Leadbetter WF: Diagnosis and management of renal cell carcinoma: a clinical and pathologic study of 309 cases. *Cancer* 28:1165–1177, 1971.
6. Flocks RH, Kadesky MC: Malignant neoplasms of the kidney: an analysis of 353 patients followed five years or more. *J Urol* 79:196–201, 1958.

7. Robson CJ: Radical nephrectomy for renal cell carcinoma. *J Urol* 89:37–42, 1963.
8. Robson CJ, Churchill BM, Anderson W: The results of radical nephrectomy for renal cell carcinoma. *Trans Am Assoc Genitourin Surg* 60:122–129, 1968.
9. Middleton RG, Presto AJ III: Radical thoracoabdominal nephrectomy for renal cell carcinoma. *J Urol* 110:36–37, 1973.
10. Ochsner MG, Brannan W, Pond HS III, Goodier EH: Renal cell carcinoma: review of 26 years of experience at the Ochsner Clinic. *J Urol* 110:643–646, 1973.

9

The Treatment of Bilateral Renal Cell Carcinoma or Renal Cell Carcinoma in the Solitary Kidney

Robert B. Smith, M.D.

Bilateral renal cell carcinoma or renal cell carcinoma in the solitary kidney represents a challenge to the clinician. Surgery remains the only currently available treatment alternative with a realistic chance to cure patients with renal adenocarcinoma. Renal adenocarcinoma is chemotherapy resistant and is not radiosensitive. Other systemic forms of therapy, including immunotherapy, are experimental and are not effective when utilized for cure. Complete surgical removal of this neoplasm represents the only hope for patients with renal cell carcinoma.

An increasingly aggressive approach to the problem of bilateral renal cell carcinoma or renal cell carcinoma in a solitary kidney is evident when one reviews the literature (1–8). In the past, bilateral renal cell carcinoma, especially with synchronous presentation, was believed to indicate an ominous prognosis. Recent experience seems to contraindicate these previously held concepts. Bilateral renal cell carcinoma occurs with a frequency as high as 3%. Other patients will present with renal cell carcinoma in a solitary kidney because of a prior contralateral nephrectomy for benign disease or contralateral renal agenesis. The therapeutic options include: (*a*) no treatment, (*b*) medical or radiation treatment, (*c*) local excision of the tumor, or (*d*) conventional radical nephrectomy. All have potential disadvantages. Wickham (9), in his review, found that patients without definitive surgical therapy did poorly. His review also showed clearly, that patients who received no treatment had short survival times, with 75% of these patients succumbing to their disease with a mean follow-up period of 24 months. Sixteen patients in his review, who had bilateral synchronous tumor and who had no surgical treatment, died within 5 months of diagnosis.

He also reported that renal cell carcinoma in a solitary kidney carried a 2-fold better prognosis when the contralateral kidney had been removed for benign disease than when the contralateral kidney had been removed for renal cell carcinoma. Synchronous lesions in his review carried an even more ominous prognosis. However, only seven patients in his "malignant group" were treated with potentially curative resection, whereas 23 of 25 patients in his "benign group" were treated with potentially curative resections. In those cases in each group where curative surgical resection could be accomplished, the survival was similar. Thus it appeared that an aggressive approach was justified whether the disease was solitary or bilateral.

Patients with solitary kidneys treated by radical nephrectomy suffer potentially grave consequences as the result of this therapy, despite the fact that this operative procedure offers the opportunity of eradicating local disease. The patient is subjected to the numerous complications of chronic renal failure, including dialysis, in addition to the possibility of primary tumor recurrence. Also, the possibility that immunosuppression for subsequent renal transplant might interfere with the host's defense mechanisms against tumor is an important consideration. Penn (10) reported on 26 patients with adenocarcinoma treated by radical nephrectomy (making the patient anephric) followed by subsequent renal transplantation. Nine of 26 survived in the study, whereas 10 of these 26 patients developed either metastatic disease or a new primary tumor. Fifteen of these patients received transplants within 1 year of being placed on chronic hemodialysis, and 11 were on dialysis 1 year or longer prior to transplantation. The survival rates of these two groups are 14% (mean follow-up 24 months) and 64% (mean follow-up 31.6 months), respectively. Thus, it is obvious that no patient should be transplanted prior to 1 year following radical nephrectomy. The complications of dialysis in patients in the sixth decade of life are well known, including cardiovascular and infectious complications. Since most patients are in this age group, the chance of them doing well on dialysis is poor. Also, there is ample evidence that the uremic state is immunosuppressive and compromises the patient's immune system, enhancing the possibility of tumor recurrence. Thus in this select group of patients, consideration must be given not only to tumor eradication, but also to renal preservation. Since approximately 80% of renal adenocarcinoma originate from the apical or basilar pole of the kidney, partial nephrectomy with nephron salvage is almost always feasible. Even centrally located tumors can be approached satisfactorily, even when they penetrate deeply into the renal hilum. The availability of current techniques of renal preservation, including in situ cooling and ex vivo surgical techniques, has dramatically broadened surgical horizons and has allowed for the current aggressive approach to patients with these problems.

Partial nephrectomy for the removal of renal tumor, whether it is done in situ or ex vivo, usually requires interruption of the renal circulation for a variable period of time. At normal body temperature, the kidney will begin to undergo permanent functional impairment after 30 minutes of ischemia. Most cases of resection of renal tumor with subsequent renal reconstruction require longer than 30 minutes. Some form of short term renal preservation is necessary to avoid permanent renal damage. For the rare case where ex vivo partial nephrectomy is needed, an intracellular perfusate (Collins solution) is utilized instead of ex vivo perfusion with a Belzer or Water's machine. The use of pulsatile perfusion is expensive, cumbersome, and requires the availability of a technician and machine. Clearly, the ischemia times necessary for ex vivo tumor resection are well covered by Collins solution. Surface cooling with renal artery occlusion and packing the kidney in ice offer excellent renal preservation for shorter periods of time. This technique is satisfactory for all cases of in situ resection. As the tumor resection progresses, ice should be packed within the cut surfaces of the kidney to decrease the core temperature. Only rare instances of acute tubular necrosis have been seen in in situ resection with kidneys preserved in such a manner.

SURGICAL TECHNIQUE

Ex Vivo Partial Nephrectomy

The incision utilized for ex vivo partial nephrectomy varies with the choice of the surgeon. It is the author's preference to have the patient placed in the supine position to use a midline transabdominal incision or a large flank incision, utilizing the torque-flank position. Other surgeons favor two separate incisions, using an upper transverse abdominal incision to perform the radical nephrectomy and a standard Gibson incision for renal implantation. This "two hole" technique mandates the transection of the ureter, which is unnecessary with a single incision.

A standard radical nephrectomy with regional lymphadenectomy is performed, paying particular attention to detail in dissection of the renal pedicle in order to secure a renal artery and vein that will be suitable for implantation. Excessive hilar dissection should be avoided if possible for fear of compromise of ureteral vascularity. This is much more important if the ureter is transected and reimplanted than if the ureter is left intact. After radical nephrectomy has been performed, the kidney is perfused with an intracellular perfusate (Collins solution), and tumor excision and reconstruction are performed on a workbench. With the use of intracellular perfusate, the tumor excision and subsequent reconstruction can be performed in a meticulous manner without undue concern about ischemic damage. In the author's view, the ureters should be left intact if possible, to lessen the likelihood of urologic complications. Large central tumors often mandate hilar dissection, which may compromise ureteral vascularity in those cases where the ureter has been transected. If the ureter has been left intact, the ureter should be occluded with a noncrushing clamp, as ureteral blood flow may cause some renal warming, increasing the possibility of ischemic renal damage. If the contralateral kidney and adrenal gland have been removed previously for malignant disease, the ipsilateral adrenal gland should be retained or the patient will develop adrenal insufficiency. The adrenal gland is removed only if it is involved grossly with tumor. Prior to occluding the artery, the patient should be given mannitol (25 g) or furosemide (Lasix, 40 mg) intravenously to ensure good renal function prior to vascular interruption. Optical magnification and the use of microsurgical instruments aid in the ex vivo resection of tumor. Since all tumors removed in an ex vivo fashion should be central, dissection should begin by mobilization of the renal artery with all of its branches. The renal vein with its branches is dissected next. Arteries and veins that are seen to enter directly into the area of tumor are individually ligated and divided. It is precisely this dissection which can compromise ureteral vascularity. Careful study of the preoperative angiogram helps greatly in this portion of the procedure. After the hilar structures have been controlled, the tumor should then be excised, taking care not to enucleate the tumor. A rim of normal parenchyma is essential to ensure total removal. The only cases of local recurrence in the University of California at Los Angeles (UCLA) series involved cases that were enucleated. Microinvasion of the tumor capsule with tumor cells is not uncommon. Questionable areas should be examined by frozen section to ensure that they are free of tumor.

Topley et al (11) recently presented a combined series from the Mayo Clinic and Cleveland Clinic in which 33 patients were treated by enucleation with only 2 cases of local recurrence. It may be possible to distinguish such cases that are amenable to enucleation by angiogram and CT scan, but it is still safer to obtain a margin of parenchyma when possible. The "capsule" around the renal cell carcinoma is a pseudocapsule composed of compressed renal parenchyma which may contain tumor. Certainly, in the majority of lesions which are polar (80%), enucleation should not be performed. In cases of complex central lesions, enucleation can simplify the procedure and lessen the chance of operative complications. It may also be of use in cases of multiple lesions with a solitary kidney. Despite this recent favorable report of Topley et al (11), enucleation should rarely be used in this author's opinion.

Following removal of the tumor, the kidney should be flushed and moved to a clean operative environment to minimize the possibility of tumor seeding during reconstruction. A new set of instruments should be used, and the surgical team should change gowns and gloves. The collecting system defects can be visualized by injecting normal saline into the renal pelvis. Defects in the collecting system should be closed with fine chromic catgut suture (5-0 or 6-0). Defects in the arterial or venous system can similarly be demonstrated by infusion of the artery and vein with Collins solution. Arterial bleeders are controlled generally with figure-of-eight sutures of 5-0 or 6-0 chromic material. Any holes in the veins which seem major can be closed with a running 6-0 or 7-0 cardiovascular silk. The large defect in the midportion of the kidney should be filled with a pedicle of omentum, and the poles should then be folded back on themselves, taking care not to cause a kink in the collecting system or in the artery. The approximated poles should then be secured with horizontal mattress sutures and tied carefully over bolsters of fat or Surgicel. The use of Avitene is of considerable benefit in securing hemostasis. It is the author's preference not to implant the omentum or approximate the poles of the kidney until the kidney has been autotransplanted to ensure that the major vessels indeed have been controlled. The kidney is autotransplanted into the ipsilateral iliac fossa, using standard transplantation techniques. The renal vein is sewn end-to-side to the common iliac artery. If multiple vessels exist, either a pantaloon type of repair is used (if double renal arteries are of similar size), or if a polar vessel is present, this is anastomosed end-to-side to the main renal artery when the kidney is cooled and on the workbench. Final hemostasis is then achieved with the use of additional sutures, if necessary, and Avitene. A pedicle of omentum is then placed over the raw surface of the kidney, and the poles are approximated. The following case illustrates these principles.

CASE REPORT

This patient is a 59-year-old male with a solitary left kidney. His right kidney had been removed 13 years previously, because of a renal artery aneurysm. A routine periodic physical examination revealed a creatinine of 1.8 compared to a value of 1.2 mg/100 ml a year previously. An intravenous pyelogram was obtained, which showed a large central mass lesion of the left kidney (Fig. 9.1A and B). Ultrasound demonstrated a large central solid mass. Renal angiogram revealed a relatively avascular mass with a double renal artery (Fig. 9.1C and D). Metastatic evaluation was negative. On November 7, 1977, a radical nephrectomy was performed with the kidney being perfused with Collins solution. Ex vivo resection of the tumor was performed (Fig. 9.1E) with reconstruction of the collecting system with 5-0 and 6-0 chromic catgut and 5-0 chromic catgut figure-of-eight sutures for exposed artery and veins. The upper pole artery was anastomosed end-to-side to the main renal artery, while the kidney was ex vivo, utilizing interrupted 7-0 material (Fig. 9.1E and F). The kidney was autotransplanted to the left iliac fossa using standard transplantation techniques (Fig. 9.1G). A running 5-0 Tycron suture was used for the end-to-side anastomosis of the renal vein to the external iliac vein, and interrupted 5-0 Tycron was used for the end-to-side anastomosis of the renal artery to the internal iliac artery. The ureter was left intact. The total ischemia time was 2 hours and 45 minutes. Prompt urine output was noted. The serum creatinine peaked on the third postoperative day (3.2 mg/100 ml) and was at the preoperative level by the seventh postoperative day, when an intravenous pyelogram was performed (Fig. 9.1H). His follow-up intravenous pyelogram 5 years later revealed a satisfactory result (Fig. 9.1I). At the present time, the patient is disease free 7 years later with a serum creatinine of 1.7 mg/100 ml.

Advantages of ex vivo surgery include better visualization and access to the tumor, reduced possibility of tumor spill, more complete excision of regional lymph nodes and lymphatics, and less intraoperative blood loss. Disadvantages include the complexity of the technique and the need for arterial and venous anastomoses with attending complications and increased operating time. Also, there is an increased possibility of ischemic renal damage. While the combined frequency of vascular complications in renal transplantation should be less than 3%, vascular complications, especially thrombosis of the renal vein, seem to be more prevalent in patients who have undergone ex vivo resection of renal tumors followed by autotransplantation. In a report by Gellin (12), 20% (3 of 15) of his patients experienced renal vein thrombosis. *Most lesions are best managed by in situ partial nephrectomy.*

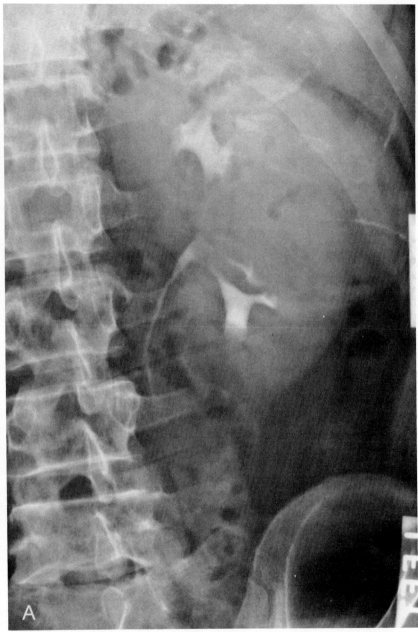

Figure 9.1. *A*, Intravenous pyelogram. Solitary left kidney; right kidney had been removed 14 years earlier for renal artery aneurysm. The intravenous pyelogram was obtained because of an increase in serum creatinine from 1.2 mg/100 ml in 1976 to 1.8 mg/100 ml in 1977.

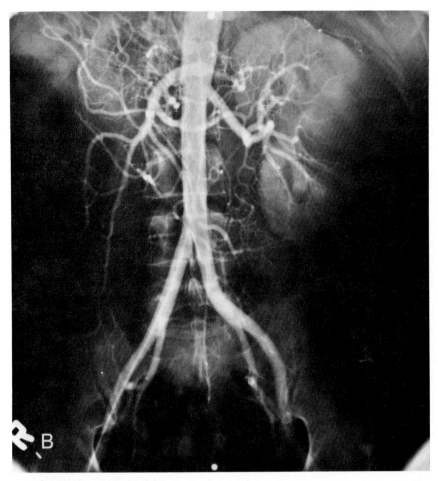

Figure 9.1. *B*, Flush angiogram. Note upper pole accessory renal artery. The lesion is distending the hilar vessels.

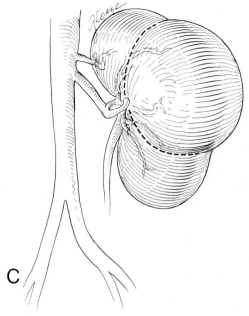

Figure 9.1. *C*, Artist's depiction of the size of the lesion. (From Smith RB, deKernion JB, Ehrlich RM, Skinner DG, Kaufman JJ: Bilateral renal cell carcinoma and renal cell carcinoma in solitary kidney. *J Urol* 132:450–454, 1984.)

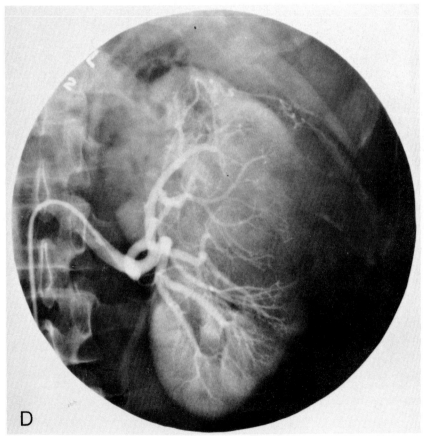

Figure 9.1. *D*, Selective angiogram.

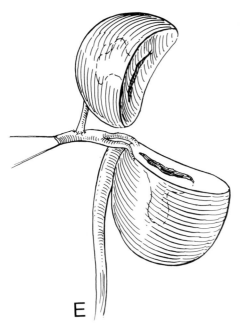

Figure 9.1. *E*, Diagram of surgical procedure. Ex vivo central resection was performed. The upper polar artery was sewn end-to-side to the main renal artery. The upper pole infundibulum was sewn to the renal pelvis. Total ischemia time was 2 hours and 45 minues.

E

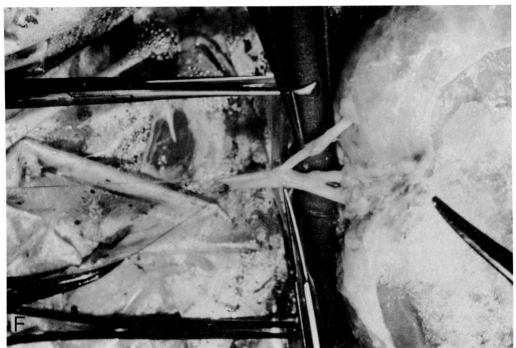

Figure 9.1. *F*, Photograph of reconstructed kidney.

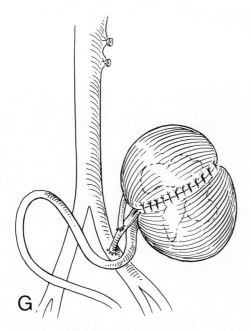

Figure 9.1. *G,* Diagram of autotransplanted kidney. (From Smith RB, de-Kernion JB, Ehrlich RM, Skinner DG, Kaufman JJ: Bilateral renal cell carcinoma and renal cell carcinoma in solitary kidney. *J Urol* 132:450–454, 1984.)

In Situ Partial Nephrectomy

Excellent surgical exposure is essential in performing in situ partial nephrectomy for cases of renal cell carcinoma in the solitary kidney. Generally, a tenth or eleventh interspace extrapleural incision is utilized for these procedures. For large upper pole lesions, a thoracoabdominal incision should be utilized. Some surgeons favor an anterior transperitoneal incision, but in the author's view, this affords a less than optimal exposure, especially for upper pole lesions. Surgical principles involved in in situ partial nephrectomy include separation of the kidney from Gerota's fascia, except for the area directly overlying the tumor. The adjacent perinephric fat with Gerota's fascia should be removed with the tumor. Resection of regional lymphatics and lymph nodes is performed if feasible, and the wound is excluded with a barrier to lessen the likelihood of tumor spill and also facilitate renal cooling. The renal pedicle is occluded only when necessary. Mannitol infusion (25 g) or furosemide (Lasix, 40 mg) is administered prior to the occlusion of the pedicle. Some surgeons do not favor the use of mannitol because of the theoretic undesirable swelling of the renal parenchyma. This has rarely been a problem in this author's experience. Renal cooling is used if the ischemia time is expected to exceed 30 minutes. Protection of renal function is important during the dissection, taking care not to put excessive traction on the renal hilum, which may cause significant renal vasospasm prior to the initiation of vascular occlusion, which in effect lengthens the ischemic interval. Prior to the occlusion of the pedicle, the patient should have hypovolemia corrected and a brisk ongoing diuresis. A sterile sheet of plastic filled with ice-saline slush is packed

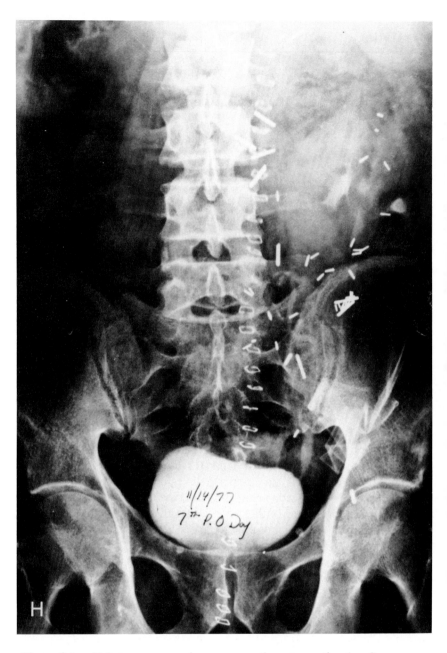

Figure 9.1. *H*, Intravenous pyelogram, seventh postoperative day. Serum creatinine peaked at 3.2 mg/100 ml on the third postoperative day. Creatinine was 1.8 mg/100 ml on postoperative day 7. (From Smith RB, deKernion JB, Ehrlich RM, Skinner DG, Kaufman JJ: Bilateral renal cell carcinoma and renal cell carcinoma in solitary kidney. *J Urol* 132:450–454, 1984.)

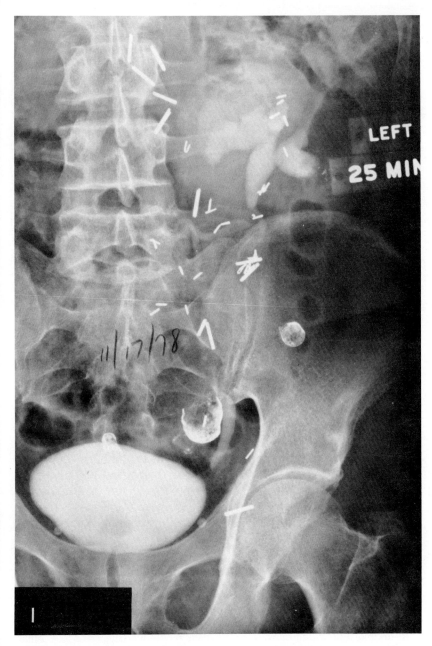

Figure 9.1. *I*, Intravenous pyelogram, 1 year postoperatively. The patient remains disease free 8 years following surgery.

around the kidney prior to the renal artery occlusion. The line of resection should be chosen to ensure that a margin of kidney is taken around the tumor. Most renal cell carcinomas amenable to partial nephrectomy are encapsulated. While it is tempting to perform enucleation on these lesions, this should not be done, especially in polar lesions. Segmental renal arteries entering the tumor directly are ligated. Arteries not adjacent to the collecting system can be managed with the use of small Ligaclips, which decreases operative time.

The collecting system can then be distended after gentle noncrushing ligation of the ureter. Defects in the collecting system are closed with 5-0 chromic catgut sutures. The renal artery and vein are then released, and bleeding sites are controlled directly with suture ligatures of 5-0 and 6-0 chromic catgut. Large venous holes can be closed with either 6-0 absorbable suture or 6-0 silk. If nonabsorbable silk is used, care must be taken to ensure that this is not close to the collecting system so that a stitch is placed in the collecting system. This may form a nidus for subsequent stone formation. As in ex vivo resection, Avitene is of great aid with hemostasis. Generally, in cases such as this, enough capsule is not remaining to cover the raw parenchyma surface. A flap of retained retroperitoneal perinephric fat can be used to cover this defect, or if none is present, a pedicle flap of omentum can be brought through a defect in the peritoneum to serve the same purpose. Large mattress sutures are not used because they may cause further damage to surrounding parenchyma. After resection and reconstruction are complete, intravenous Lasix is given if the kidney does not promptly resume function. Progressive doses of Lasix can be given up to 600 mg, but rarely is this necessary. The retroperitoneum should be drained adequately because temporary urine leaks are not uncommon. It is the author's belief that suction drains (Jackson-Pratt or Hemovac drains) are not necessary and, in fact, may prolong the healing process of the fistula. Simple Penrose drains to the site of resection have been quite satisfactory in the author's experience. The following case illustrates these principles.

CASE REPORT

A 62-year-old man presented with a large right renal cell carcinoma (Fig. 9.2A and B). The contralateral kidney had recently been removed for nonmalignant disease. The retrograde pyelogram revealed a dilated collecting system occluded with clots. The patient was on dialysis at the time of presentation. Only the superior infundibulum and caliceal system originating from this infundibulum were uninvolved by tumor (Fig. 9.2E). A renal angiogram revealed the typical neovascularity of a renal cell carcinoma. Only a single branch of the renal artery was uninvolved by tumor (Fig. 9.2D and E). A renal venogram was performed, which demonstrated a superior branch of the renal vein to be salvageable (Fig. 9.2F). Metastatic evaluation was negative.

The patient was taken to surgery, where an in situ resection was accomplished. The renal pelvis and lower caliceal structures were amputated from the upper infundibulum, and the collecting system was closed with a longitudinal suture line (Fig. 9.2G). The solitary arterial branch going to the upper pole and the venous tributary to the upper pole were salvaged. The remainder of the kidney was resected. Arterial occlusion was necessary for only 15 minutes. The patient had immediate urine output, with the creatinine falling to a low of 2.6 mg/100 ml postoperatively. At the present time, the patient is

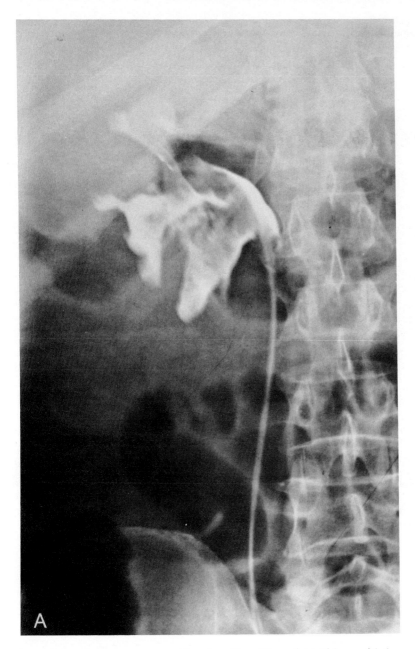

Figure 9.2. *A*, Sixty-two-year-old male with solitary right kidney with large tumor involving lower 75%. His left kidney had been removed for a benign condition. The patient was on dialysis with collecting system obstructed with clots.

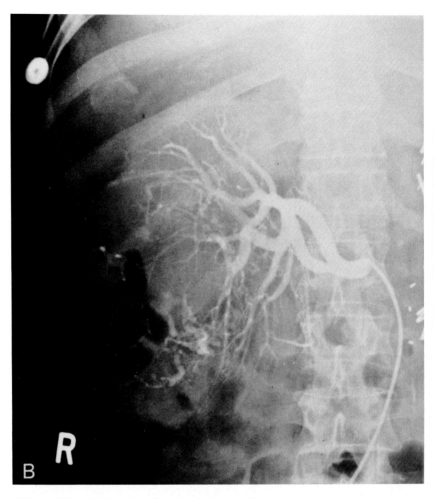

Figure 9.2. *B*, Renal angiogram demonstrating extent of lesion. A superior branch of the renal artery supplies the salvageable upper pole.

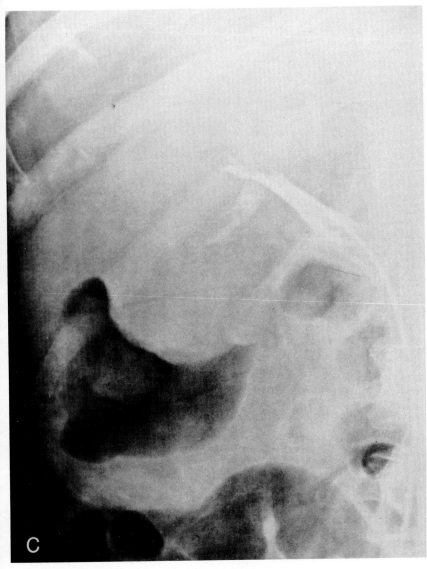

Figure 9.2. *C*, Renal venogram. The superior branch of the renal vein is not involved with tumor.

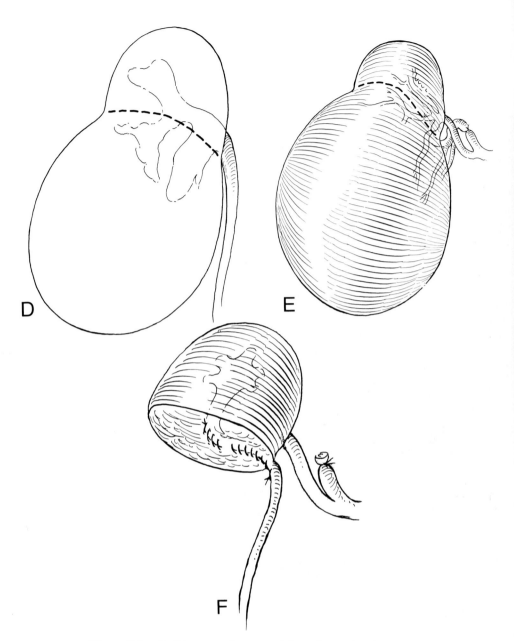

Figure 9.2. *D*, Diagram of proposed line of resection in relation to collecting system. *E*, Diagram of proposed line of resection in relation to arterial supply. *F*, Diagram of resected specimen. Only the superior infundibulum was retained. The renal pelvis was resected and the medial portion of this was closed to form an upper "ureter" connecting to the upper infundibulum. This was done in situ. Ischemia time was 15 minutes. The patient did not require postoperative dialysis. (*D–F* from Smith RB, deKernion JB, Ehrlich RM, Skinner DG, Kaufman JJ: Bilateral renal cell carcinoma and renal cell carcinoma in solitary kidney. *J Urol* 132:450–454, 1984.)

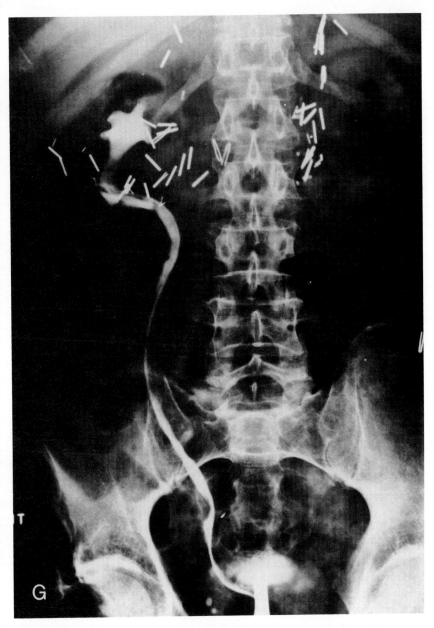

Figure 9.2. *G*, Postoperative retrograde pyelogram. The patient is now over 2 years free of disease. Creatinine leveled at 2.5 mg/100 ml postoperatively, but is now 4.2 mg/100 ml because of interstitial nephritis, secondary to a course of postoperative antibiotics. (From Smith RB, deKernion JB, Ehrlich RM, Skinner DG, Kaufman JJ: Bilateral renal cell carcinoma and renal cell carcinoma in solitary kidney. *J Urol* 132:450–454, 1984.)

2 years postoperative without evidence of metastatic or recurrent local disease. (Figure 9.2*H* is a retrograde pyelogram demonstrating the reconstructed collecting system.)

This case illustrates that even an extensive lesion can be managed with in situ resection. The overutilization of workbench ex vivo surgery is not warranted. The need to perform ex vivo workbench surgery in the author's experience is rare.

UCLA EXPERIENCE

Forty-five cases of bilateral renal cell carcinoma or renal cell carcinoma in a solitary kidney have been seen at UCLA. Forty-one of the 45 patients underwent a potentially curative resection, 38 of 41 having a nephron-salvaging procedure. Four cases early in this series underwent exploration only.

There were 17 cases where the contralateral kidney had been removed for benign disease (solitary lesion) and 26 cases of bilateral renal cell carcinoma, 13 of which were synchronous in presentation. Two cases were included in the solitary group where the contralateral kidney was present but could not support life without dialysis. As in most cases, a higher incidence of nephron-salvaging procedures was possible with solitary lesions than with bilateral lesions. Partial nephrectomy was possible in 16 of 17 solitary lesions, whereas 6 of 26 patients with bilateral lesions were not amenable to partial nephrectomy. Four patients had exploration only (early in the surgeons' experience), and 2 patients had radical nephrectomy with subsequent dialysis in the bilateral group. Of the 4 patients with exploration only, 3 had renal artery ligation and infarction, and 1 patient had radiation therapy. Survival times of these 4 patients were 6, 12, 18, and 26 months. These patients were not included in subsequent survival data presented; only patients with *potentially curable resections* are included. Patients that presented with solitary or bilateral lesions with distant metastatic disease are not included in this series.

Thirty-eight patients had partial nephrectomy, 34 of which were performed in situ. Only 4 cases required ex vivo partial nephrectomy, and in retrospect, 2 of these probably could have been done in situ. There were 3 radical nephrectomies in this series (Fig. 9.3). There were 2 operative deaths; 1 death secondary to myocardial infarction on the first postoperative day, and the second to pneumonia on the fifth postoperative day. Follow-up in this series ranges from 15 to 132 months. The overall crude survival in this series is 64%. Only patients who were followed longer than 12 months were considered in these survival figures. Only 8 patients in this series, however, died of disease (20%; 2 patients did survive with disease). If patients dying of other causes are excluded, the disease-free survival is 68% (26 of 38). Figure 9.4 depicts a Kaplan-Meyer curve for the entire series. There are no statistical differences in survival between solitary and bilateral lesions through 65 months ($p = 0.267$). After this period in the author's series,

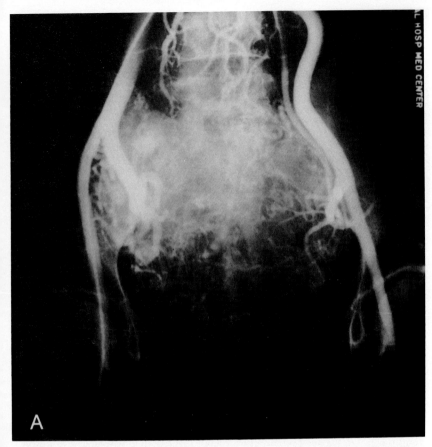

Figure 9.3. Patient presented with frequency of urination and a large pelvic mass. *A*, Angiogram of solitary pelvic kidney with obvious neovascularity suggestive of renal cell carcinoma.

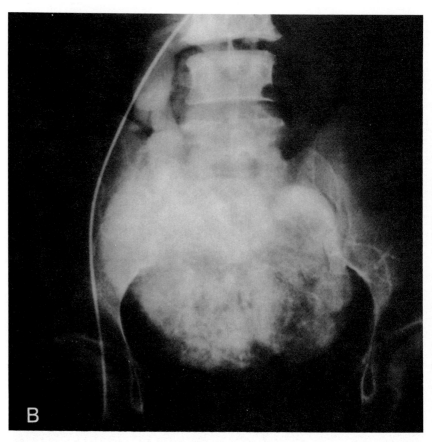

Figure 9.3. *B*, Delayed nephrogram phase. Entire pelvic kidney was involved with renal cell carcinoma. Serum creatinine was 3.0 mg/100 ml. Note filling of large renal vein.

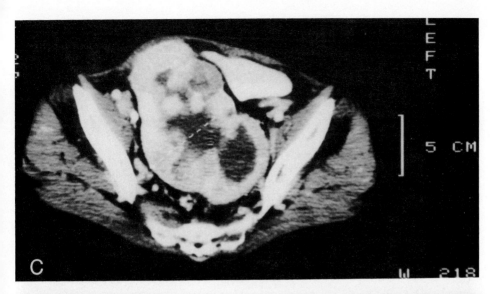

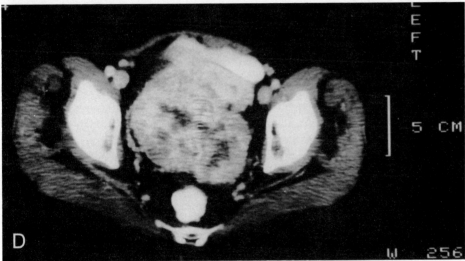

Figure 9.3. *C* and *D*, Pelvic CT scan. Note displacement of rectum and bladder. Radical nephrectomy was performed. The patient is now disease free 2½ years after surgery and is being considered as a possible renal transplant candidate.

the number of cases is so small that statistical evaluation is meaningless. Even though the natural history of renal cell carcinoma is variable, the author believes that these statistics through 65 months are meaningful. In a previously reported series, of the patients who developed metastatic disease after "curative radical nephrectomy," 71% did so within 1 year (13).

The similarity of survival between solitary and bilateral lesions is even more remarkable when one notes the disparity in incidence of stage I lesions in the bilateral group compared to the solitary group. Only 5 of 22 patients (22%) with resectable bilateral renal carcinoma had stage I lesions, whereas 12 of 17 (71%) of the solitary lesions were stage I. Only

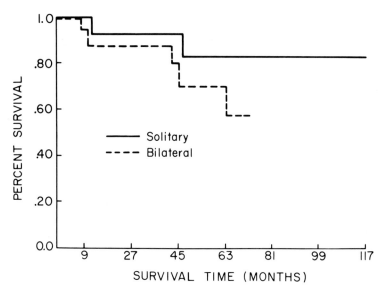

Figure 9.4. Survival in months of patients with solitary and bilateral renal cell carcinoma by Kaplan-Meyer method. The difference in survival is more apparent than real, since only 22.7% of bilateral lesions were stage I, compared to 70.6% of solitary lesions. (From Smith RB, deKernion JB, Ehrlich RM, Skinner DG, Kaufman JJ: Bilateral renal cell carcinoma and renal cell carcinoma in solitary kidney. *J Urol* 132:450–454, 1984.)

1 patient with a stage I lesion has died of disease. Lower survival rates are seen with higher stages, as expected (Fig. 9.5). Although it is difficult to compare the solitary and bilateral groups with regard to survival related to stage, because of the difference in numbers in each stage, there appears to be no difference in survival, stage for stage, between the two groups. Where histologic grade can be determined in this series, the majority of the author's cases were relatively well differentiated, clear cell lesions. The rare instances of poorly differentiated or spindle cell variety fared poorly.

Simultaneous renal cell carcinoma has occurred 13 times in this series. The approach to such simultaneous lesions varies in the literature. Possible treatment options include primary partial nephrectomy, operating on the least involved kidney first, allowing for the worst side to remain in place to lessen the need for postoperative dialysis. Some surgeons feel that the most involved side should be attacked first, making certain that it is resectable, later followed by partial nephrectomy of the contralateral kidney. This approach also allows for some functional compensatory hypertrophy of the contralateral kidney, thus perhaps increasing the likelihood of being able to perform a nephron salvage procedure. There is some evidence that a solitary kidney tolerates periods of ischemia better than if a contralateral kidney is present. A simultaneous approach is possible with either bilateral partial nephrectomy, combination radical and partial nephrectomy, or bilateral nephrectomy. All approaches are acceptable and have been used in this series. Of the 13 cases, there have been 2 primary partial nephrectomies, 7 primary radical nephrectomies, 3 simultaneous partial and radical

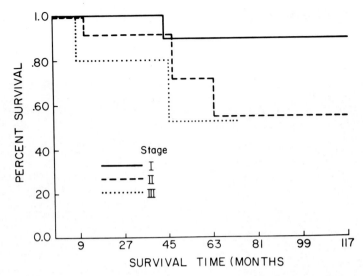

Figure 9.5. Survival in months related to stage of lesion at presentation. Stage for stage, there was no difference in survival between patients with solitary and bilateral lesions.

nephrectomies, and 1 staged bilateral nephrectomy. In Jacobs et al's review (2) of synchronous bilateral renal cell carcinoma, 12 patients had primary partial nephrectomy, 10 patients had primary radical nephrectomy, and 23 patients had a simultaneous approach. Survival did not seem to depend on which surgical approach was used. Also in Jacob et al's review of 51 nephron salvage procedures, 34 were done in situ and 17 were done ex vivo. The survival rate is similar in those patients having ex vivo resections (82%) and those having in vivo procedures (76%). This emphasizes the fact that ex vivo partial nephrectomies should be reserved for large central complex lesions.

It is the author's belief that if the patient is a satisfactory operative risk, this simultaneous approach to both kidneys is the best option (Fig. 9.6). If the lesions are complex, then a staged approach is best, doing the radical nephrectomy first on the most involved side to make sure that it is resectable (Fig. 9.7).

Only 2 of 13 patients with synchronous bilateral renal cell carcinoma in the author's series have died of disease. An additional patient is alive with evidence of disease. Two additional patients have died disease free. The survival rates of patients with bilateral renal cell carcinoma did not seem to vary in regard to the tumor-free interval between the time when the renal cell carcinoma in the first kidney was removed and the second appeared. Survival of patients with synchronous lesions compared favorably to that of those with metachronous bilateral lesions.

Of the eight cancer deaths in this series, five were failures secondary to distant metastatic disease. There were three incidences of local recurrence; enucleation procedures were performed on all three patients.

Schiff and associates (1), in a literature review, found 62 patients undergoing curative resection for both bilateral and solitary lesions. Seventy-five percent were alive with an average follow-up of 45.7

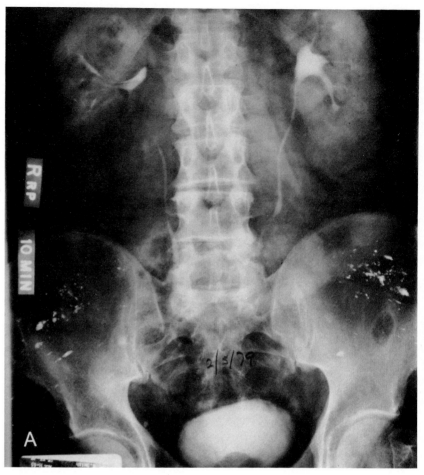

Figure 9.6. *A*, Forty-four-year old male with bilateral synchronous renal cell carcinoma. The intravenous pyelogram showed a central lesion on the right and a lower polar lesion on the left.

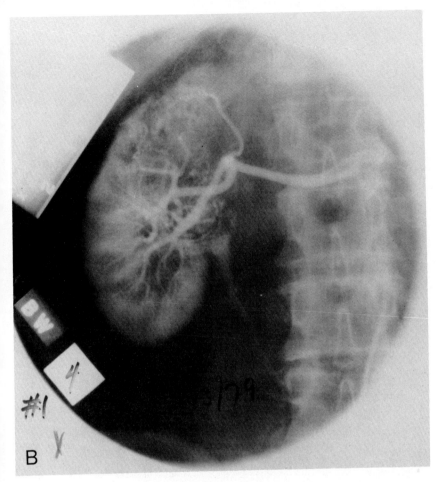

Figure 9.6. *B*, Right selective angiogram.

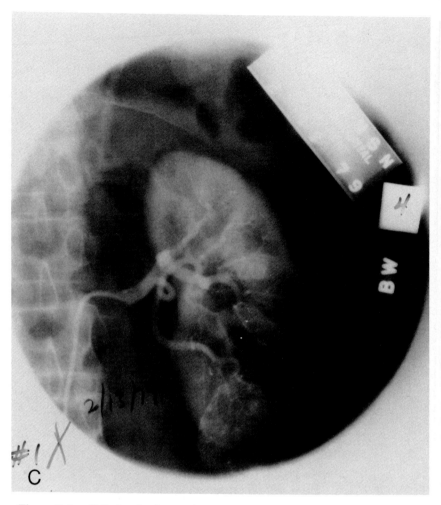

Figure 9.6. *C*, Left selective angiogram. The patient was treated with simultaneous right radical nephrectomy and left partial nephrectomy. The patient is now disease free 6 years after surgery.

months. There were no survival differences between those with bilateral disease and the solitary kidney group. Jacobs et al (2) reviewed 61 cases of synchronous bilateral renal cell carcinoma in the literature and found a 60% survival at 5 years. Only a 10% local recurrence rate was noted. The author's current series concurs with the review of Jacobs et al (2) and Schiff et al (1) in that patient survival seems dependent on adequacy of tumor resection and not on the fate of the contralateral kidney. Survival, however, is dependent on the stage of the lesion at presentation.

SUMMARY

Survival rates of bilateral renal cell carcinoma and renal cell carcinoma in the solitary kidney justify an aggressive surgical approach. Survival rates stage for stage approximate that for radical nephrectomy for unilateral disease when the contralateral kidney is present. If results

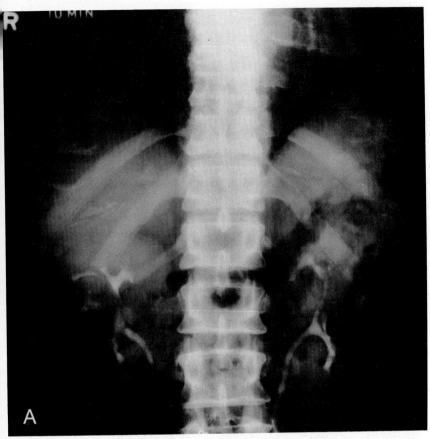

Figure 9.7. Forty-two-year-old male with bilateral synchronous renal cell carcinoma. *A*, Intravenous pyelogram. The right kidney was treated with radical nephrectomy as first stage due to hilar involvement.

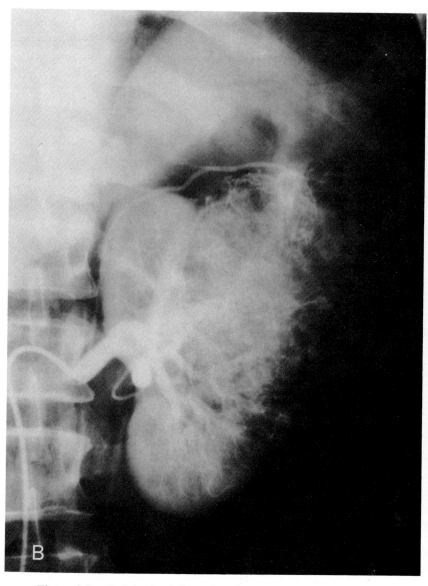

Figure 9.7. *B*, Selective left renal angiogram. Note hilar invasion.

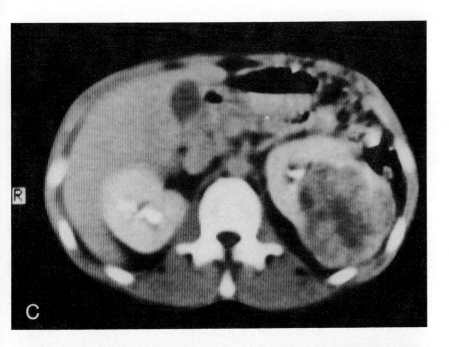

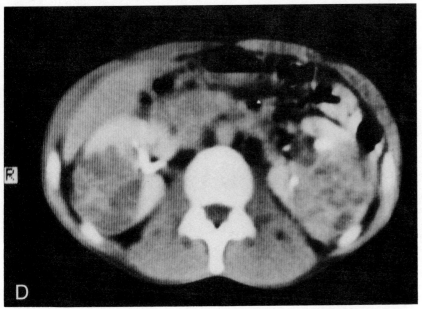

Figure 9.7. *C* and *D*, CT scan. Note extreme hilar invasion.

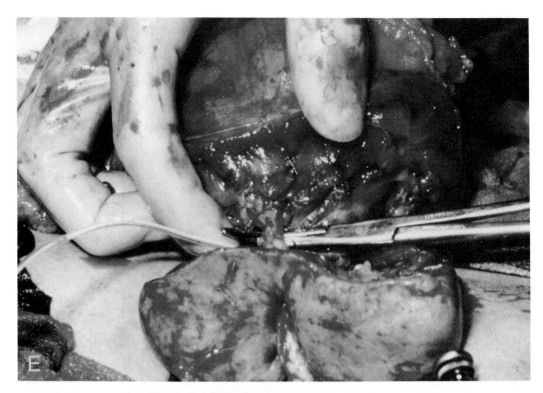

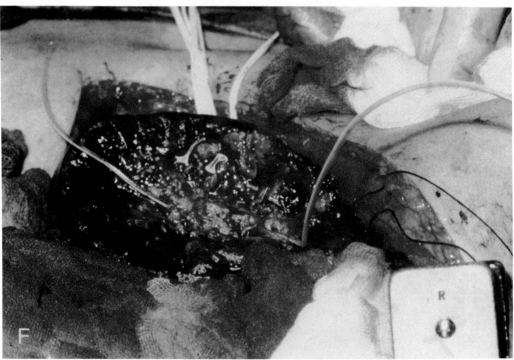

Figure 9.7. *E* to *G*, In vivo resection (*E*). Individual ligation of major central feeding vessels (*F*). Remaining kidney with the "rim of parenchyma" surrounding hilar fat. Stents are in open upper and lower infundibula (*G*). The resected specimen. The patient is now disease free 32 months after surgery. Serum creatinine is 2.4 mg/100 ml.

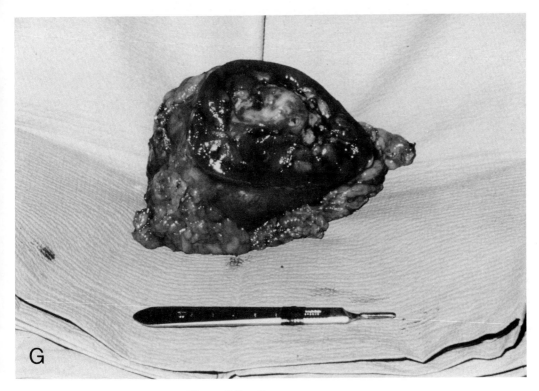

Figure 9.7. *G*

with stage I lesions treated with partial nephrectomy are similar after a 10-year follow-up, an argument could be made for utilization of techniques of partial nephrectomy for stage I renal cell carcinoma even when a normal contralateral kidney is present, especially if the lesion is polar.

Most lesions are amenable to partial nephrectomy by established in vitro techniques. Ex vivo surgery should be reserved for complex central lesions. The author cautions against enucleation of these lesions, even though a definite capsule may be present, as microinvasion of the tumor into the capsule is common. Certainly, enucleation should never be done for simple polar lesions, but it may be necessary in cases of multiple lesions or in large central lesions impinging upon the hilum. This current report, along with results of two reviews (1, 2), challenges the prior concept that patient prognosis depends on the fate of the contralateral kidney (i.e., worst prognosis if it had been removed for carcinoma). This prognosis depends more on the adequacy of tumor resection and tumor stage than on the fate of the contralateral kidney.

REFERENCES

1. Schiff M Jr, Bagley DH, Lytton B: Treatment of solitary and bilateral renal carcinomas. *J Urol* 121:581, 1979.
2. Jacobs SC, Berg SI, Lawson RK: Synchronous bilateral renal cell carcinoma: total surgical excision. *Cancer* 46:2341, 1980.
3. Novick AC, Stewart BH, Straffon RA, Banowsky LH: Partial nephrectomy in the treatment of renal adenocarcinoma. *J Urol* 118:932, 1977.

4. Palmer JM, Swanson BA: Conservative surgery in solitary and bilateral renal cell carcinoma: indications and technical considerations. *J Urol* 120:113, 1978.
5. Viets DH, Vaughn ED Jr, Howards SS: Experience gained from the management of 9 cases of bilateral renal cell carcinoma. *J Urol* 118:937, 1977.
6. Beraha D, Block NL, Politano VA: Simultaneous surgical management of bilateral hypernephroma: an alternative therapy. *J Urol* 115:648, 1976.
7. Finkbeiner A, Moyad R, Herwig K: Bilateral simultaneously occurring adenocarcinoma of the kidneys. *J Urol* 116:26, 1976.
8. Zincke H, Swanson SK: Bilateral renal cell carcinoma: influence of synchronous and asynchronous occurrence on patient survival. *J Urol* 128:913, 1982.
9. Wickham JEA: Conservative renal surgery for adenocarcinoma: the place of bench surgery. *Br J Urol* 47:25, 1975.
10. Penn I: Transplantation in patients with primary renal malignancies. *Transplantation* 24:424, 1977.
11. Topley M, Novick A, Montie JE: Long-term results following partial nephrectomy for localized renal adenocarcinoma. *J Urol* 131:1050, 1984.
12. Gellin I: Extracorporeal surgery for renal problems. *Surg Ann* 9:351, 1977.
13. deKernion JB, Ramming KP, Smith RB: The natural history of metastatic renal cell carcinoma: a computer analysis. *J Urol* 120:148, 1978.

10

Conservative Surgery for Renal Adenocarcinoma

Michael Marberger, M.D.

Radical, perifascial nephrectomy with primary control of the renal vessels and regional lymphadenectomy is today considered the standard treatment of renal adenocarcinoma (RC) without nonresectable metastases. With RC in solitary kidneys or bilateral RC this results in the need for chronic hemodialysis and renal allotransplantation with excessive morbidity and poor results (1–6). Therapeutic attempts in this situation have therefore focused on parenchyma-sparing surgical excision of the lesions.

Improved in situ and workbench techniques, regional hypothermia, and optical magnification yield surprisingly favorable results. In 1981 the author reported on a joint retrospective study of the European Intrarenal Surgical Society (EIRSS) on this topic (3).* Seventy-two patients, of whom 23 were submitted by the author, were treated by surgical excision of the tumor only. Five-year survival rates of 78% were achieved for RC in solitary kidneys, if the contralateral kidney was congenitally absent or lost because of benign disease (= unilateral RC), of 48% for bilateral synchronous RC, and of 38% for bilateral asynchronous RC (i.e., the contralateral kidney was removed for RC previously) (Fig. 10.1). As expected, prognosis correlated clearly with the extent of the disease. In the most favorable group with unilateral RC, excisional surgery provided survival rates for pT1 and pT2 RC that appear similar to the results of radical nephrectomy for RC in the presence of a normal contralateral kidney (2, 6–8) (Fig. 10.2). Although a bias in patient selection cannot be excluded in studies of this type, other authors have presented comparable data (9–12). A local tumor

---

* Participating urologists: J Auvert, Hôpital Henri Mondor, Créteil, France; H Bertermann, Universitätskliniken Kiel, Federal Republic of Germany; A Constantini, Università degli Studi, Florence, Italy; PA Gammelgaard, Kobenhavens Amtssygehus i Herlev, Denmark; M Marberger, Universitätskliniken Mainz, Federal Republic of Germany, and Rudolfstiftung, Vienna, Austria; S Pettersson, Sahlgrenska Sjukhuset, Gothenburg, Sweden; JEA Wickham, St Peter's Hospitals, London, England; Reference pathologist: RCB Pugh, St Peter's Hospitals, London, England.

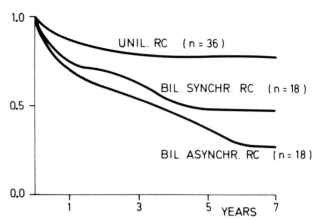

Figure 10.1. Survival of patients with RC treated by conservative surgery (smoothed Kaplan-Meier curves). (From Marberger M, Pugh RBC, Auvert J, Bertermann H, Constantini A, Gammelgaard PA, Pettersson S, Wickham JEA: Conservative surgery of renal carcinoma: the EIRSS experience. *Br J Urol* 53:528, 1981.)

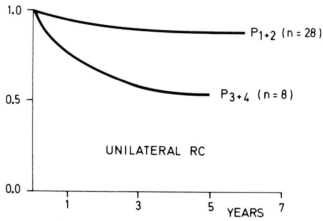

Figure 10.2. Survival of patients with unilateral renal carcinoma correlated with pT category (UICC, 1974). (From Marberger M, Pugh RCB, Auvert J, Bertermann H, Constantini A, Gammelgaard PA, Pettersson S, Wickham JEA: Conservative surgery of renal carcinoma: the EIRSS experience. *Br J Urol* 53:528, 1981.)

recurrence of 9% was observed in the EIRSS series, but this occurred only in large <PT3 or multilocular lesions, many of which required bench surgery. Other authors give a similar experience with recurrence rates varying from 6 to 13% (1, 11).

The excellent results of excisional surgery of small, peripheral RC question the need for radical nephrectomy when tumors of this type are diagnosed in the presence of a normal contralateral kidney. Because of today's wide availability of sonography and computerized tomography, they are found far more frequently and usually in asymptomatic patients. Autopsy studies have shown up to 21% of the kidneys to have solid peripheral nodules, mainly adenomas and benign mesenchymal tumors (13, 14). With the refinement of imaging techniques an increasing number of harmless benign lesions are now also detected in vivo, but they usually cannot be distinguished from small RC. Fine needle aspiration biopsy may be helpful in defining the dignity of the tumor, but in the author's experience the nodules are easily missed and negative cytology does not rule out malignancy (Fig. 10.3). Even frozen section examination of small cortical tumors is frequently difficult (Fig. 10.4), and it may be impossible to distinguish between renal adenoma and low grade adenocarcinoma.

Should every solid parenchymal mass, regardless of tumor size and position, be subjected to radical nephrectomy, with primary division of the renal vessels and without opening Gerota's fascia (8)? The author firmly believes that this principle developed in the era of intravenous

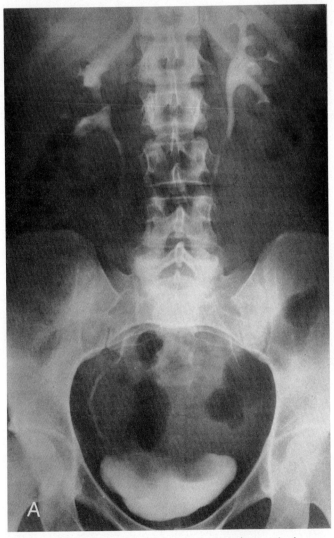

Figure 10.3. Twenty-three-year-old female undergoing urologic examination after hemorrhagic cystitis. A perihilar mass was suspected on the intravenous pyelogram (*A*), but sonography (*B*) and computerized tomography (*C*) only showed a solid nodule 2 cm in diameter at the upper pole. A fine needle biopsy suggested an adenoma, and this was confirmed by conservative surgery.

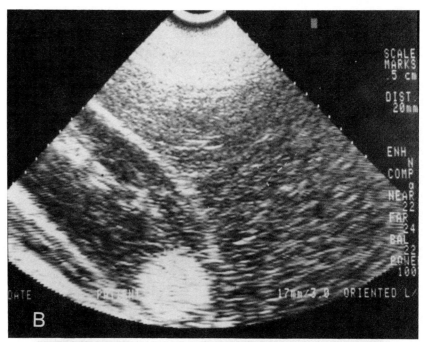

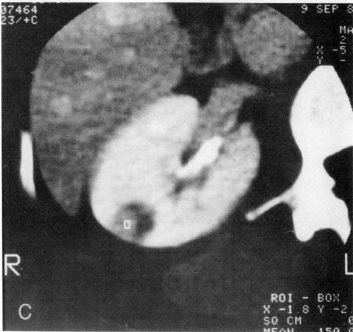

Figure 10.3. *B* and *C*

pyelography and renal angiography has lost some of its validity with the progress in renal imaging techniques. In selected cases a cautious, conservative approach with excisional surgery is justified. This is substantiated by the facts that at serial autopsies up to 14% of the peripheral solid nodules are found bilaterally (13), tumors with a hereditary background occur always in both kidneys (5), and up to 3% of all patients

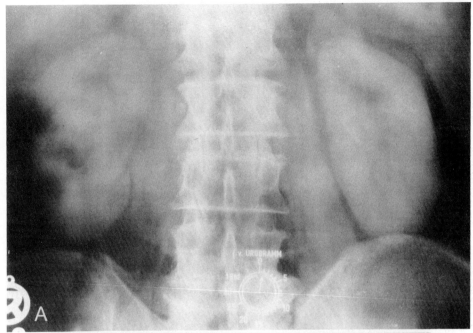

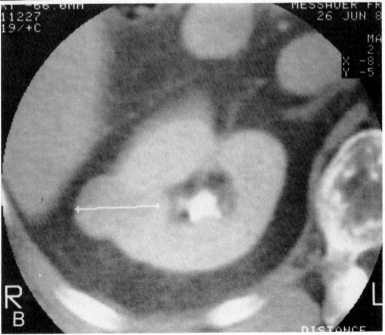

Figure 10.4. Seventy-four-year-old male undergoing urologic examination because of benign prostatic hyperplasia. The routine intravenous pyelogram (A) suggested a peripheral nodule in the right kidney, which was confirmed to be a solid tumor 2 cm in diameter at sonography, computerized tomography (B) and surgery (C). It was removed by wedge resection and on frozen sections classified as heterotopic adrenal tissue (D). At definite histologic examination the diagnosis was changed to a low grade RC. (Microscopic sections courtesy of Dr D Kosak, Department of Pathology, Rudolfstiftung. 100×, hematoxylin and eosin.)

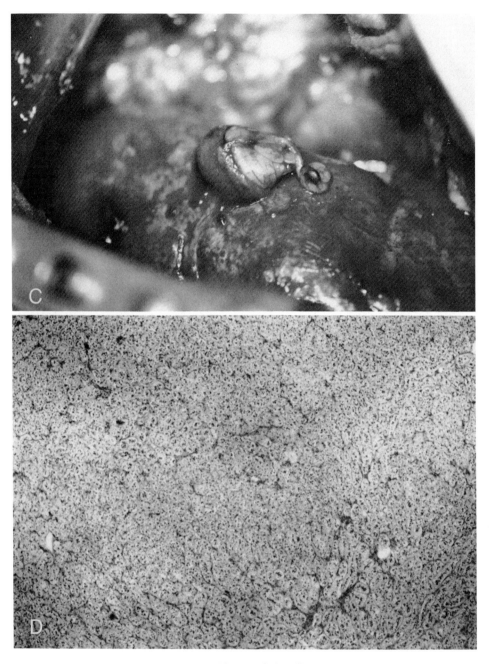

Figure 10.4. *C* and *D*

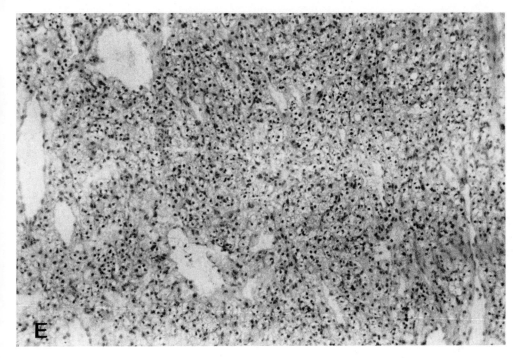

Figure 10.4. *E*

Table 10.1
Tumor Extension of Unilateral RC in Solitary Kidneys at Surgery (EIRSS Study)

	Tumor Diameter (No. of Patients)			
	< 4 cm (n = 6)	4–6 cm (n = 12)	6–8 cm (n = 9)	> 8 cm (n = 9)
Invasion of renal vein				1
Invasion of renal capsule			2	5
Multifocal tumor				1
Lymph node metastasis			1	

with RC eventually develop a tumor in the contralateral kidney (1, 2, 4, 15).

The size, i.e., the diameter, of the tumor can easily be determined preoperatively and therefore represents the most valuable parameter for selecting a patient for conservative surgery. Naturally, excisional surgery is safer the smaller and more localized the tumor is. In an attempt to define the limitations of conservative surgery, the data of the EIRSS study were re-evaluated in this respect. With bilateral synchronous or asynchronous RC the possibility of a contralateral metastasis and therefore metastatic spread cannot be ruled out. The study was therefore limited to unilateral RC in solitary kidneys.

The survival data of 36 patients were available. Table 10.1 correlates the tumor stage to the diameter. Only one tumor just over 6 cm in diameter had hilar lymph node metastases; although they were excised and clear margins were obtained around the tumor, the patient died

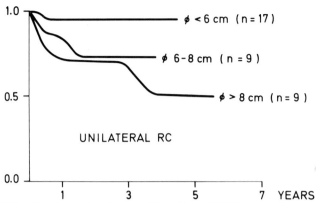

Figure 10.5. Survival of patients with unilateral RC treated by conservative surgery, correlated to diameter of tumors (EIRSS study).

after 14 months of diffuse tumor spread. Invasion of the renal vein and multifocal tumors were also ominous findings, as both of these patients died from the tumor within 1 year. The position of the tumor within the kidney had no significant influence on survival, but this may result from a bias in patient selection. In 26 patients the tumor was located in polar regions of the kidney. Lymph node and vascular involvement was only observed among the 10 tumors in the central/hilar region, which usually were larger than 6 cm in diameter. Figure 10.5 correlates the tumor diameter to the survival data. The only patient who died in the group who had tumors < 6 cm succumbed to a complication of chronic hemodialysis subsequent to renal artery thrombosis after bench surgery and renal autotransplantation for a central tumor; he was found tumor free at autopsy. A local recurrent tumor or metastases were never observed in this group.

The specimens of 27 patients were still available for pathologic re-evaluation by Dr. RCB Pugh of St Peter's Hospital, London. In the EIRSS study he had shown a significant correlation between survival and tumor grade, vascular invasion, and the appearance of spindle cells. Although oncocytic elements or the predominance of clear cells did not have a significant impact on survival, some authors attribute a lower grade of malignancy to tumors of these types than to tumors with predominantly granular cells (16). Regardless of the classification used, however, all unilateral RCs that were < 6 cm were uniformly of low grade malignancy (Table 10.2).

Due to compression of the surrounding renal parenchyma RC tends to form a pseudocapsule of lamellar collagen fiber bundles, which macroscopically separates the tumor from the remaining parenchyma (Fig. 10.6) and forms a good plane of cleavage. Even very large tumors may be "shelled out" by blunt dissection along it (Fig. 10.7), and this type of enucleative surgery has been recommended as standard technique (17–20). With this approach the integrity of the pseudocapsule as the outermost limit of tumor growth is, of course, essential.

Rocca Rossetti and Muto (21) noted a continuous pseudocapsule in 80% of all RCs > 7 cm in diameter; only 23.5% of larger tumors had an unperforated capsule. In a most detailed study, however, Rosenthal

Table 10.2
Histology of Unilateral RC in Solitary Kidneys (EIRSS Study)

	Tumor Diameter (No. of Patients)			
	< 4 cm (n = 6)	4–6 cm (n = 9)	6–8 cm (n = 7)	> 8 cm (n = 7)
Predominantly clear cells	3	6	2	1
Predominantly granular cells			3	4
Oncocytic elements	1		2	
Spindle cell elements				2

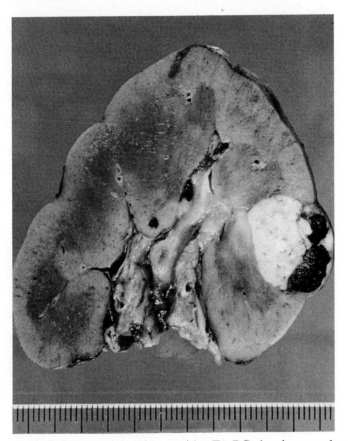

Figure 10.6. Section through kidney with pT1 RC showing pseudocapsule and sharp demarcation of tumor against the adjacent parenchyma.

et al (22) demonstrated the pseudocapsule of virtually all tumors to be microscopically invaded by neoplastic cells which frequently reach the pericapsular parenchyma, even around very small tumors (Fig. 10.8). With enucleation the pseudocapsule is separated bluntly between the tumor-attached and tumor bed-associated layers. Regardless of tumor size the neoplasma may reach the surface of the enucleate at one or several sites, so that tumor cells are left behind in the tumor bed. Using microangiography techniques they also demonstrated that tumors > 6 cm usually lose their radial vascular pattern, develop large areas of central necrosis, and have multiple arteries and veins perforating the

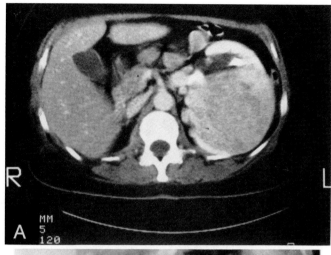

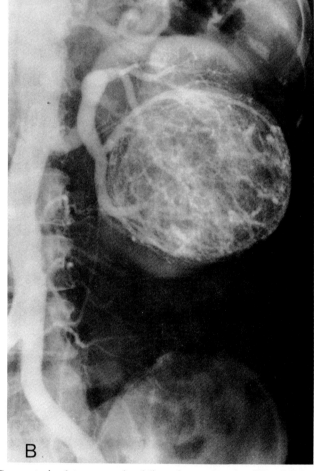

Figure 10.7. Computerized tomography (*A*) and aortography (*B*) of RC 12 cm in diameter in solitary kidney of a 62-year-old female. The tumor was removed completely along the pseudocapsule in ischemia and regional hypothermia; a major part of the collecting system was infiltrated and also had to be removed (*C*). As demonstrated by intravenous pyelography 7 days later (*D*) renal function remained virtually unchanged; the patient is still tumor free 3 years later.

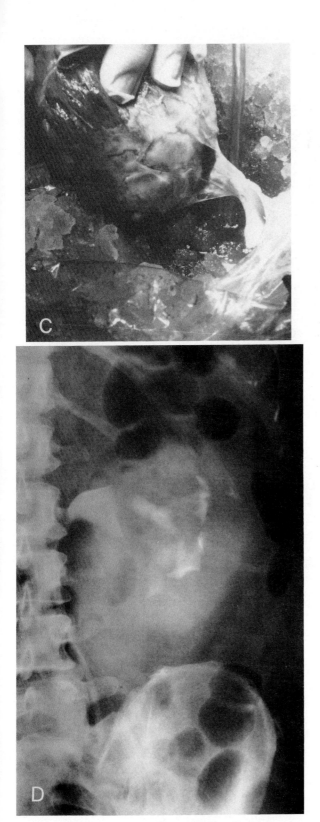

Figure 10.7. *C* and *D*

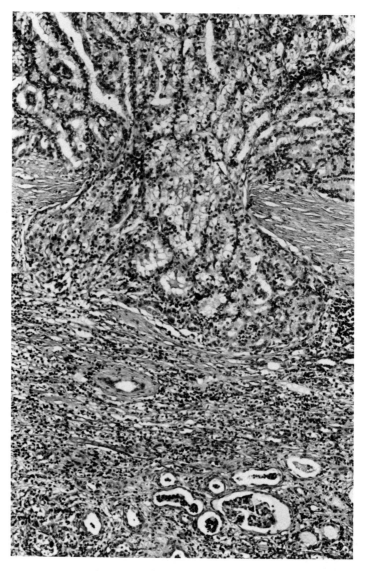

Figure 10.8. Pseudocapsule of RC 1.8 cm in diameter, showing perforation and tumor infiltration of adjacent renal parenchyma (125×, hematoxylin and eosin.) (From Rosenthal CL, Kraft R, Zingg EJ: Organ-preserving surgery in renal cell carcinoma: tumor enucleation versus partial kidney resection. *Eur Urol* 10:222, 1984.)

pseudocapsule (Fig. 10.9). The study revalidates the absolute need for removing a margin of at least 1 cm of renal parenchyma with the tumor, as Vermooten had already postulated in 1950 (23). According to the results of Rosenthal et al (22), only RC < 6 cm in diameter appears amenable to conservative surgery, a figure which corresponds to the author's data derived from the EIRSS study.

When selecting a patient with RC for conservative surgery it must be kept in mind that surgical removal is the only effective therapy presently available for this neoplasm. Whereas with RC in solitary kidneys or bilateral RC the need to preserve renal function facilitates the decision,

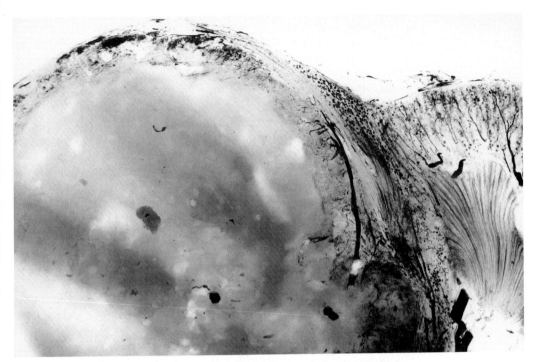

Figure 10.9. Microangiography of RC > 6 cm in diameter showing perforation of the pseudocapsule by large vessels and extensive areas of necrosis within the tumor. (From Rosenthal CL, Kraft R, Zingg EJ: Organ-preserving surgery in renal cell carcinoma: tumor enucleation versus partial kidney resection. *Eur Urol* 10:222, 1984.)

the surgeon carries a considerably higher responsibility in the presence of a normal contralateral kidney. Incomplete tumor excision is a fatal error for the patient. Based on the studies outlined above and given an empirical extra safety margin of 2 cm, the author today limits conservative surgery to solid peripheral tumors < 4 cm in diameter. These are almost always asymptomatic lesions diagnosed by chance or even found unexpectedly at open surgery for another reason (see Fig. 10.3). Frequently these solid masses are benign tumors that cannot be distinguished from RC at the time of surgery. If definite histology proves them to be RC, properly performed conservative excision eradicates them with high probability. The author is aware of anecdotal reports of RCs < 3 cm in diameter with metastases (24), but in these cases survival would in no way have been altered by a radical nephrectomy rather than excisional surgery.

The correct surgical technique is essential. After excluding visceral and lymph node metastases, the kidney is carefully mobilized, but the perirenal fat immediately adjacent to the tumor is not stripped off. The renal artery and vein are then clamped with soft bulldog clamps. A plastic intestinal bag, the sealed end of which has been opened, is placed around the kidney so that its tie string can be closed around the renal pedicle. Sterile soft ice is now positioned around the renal kidney for regional cooling, leaving the tumor area exposed. Renal ischemia and hypothermia may appear unnecessary for small tumors, but they certainly facilitate delineation of the tumor margins and precise frozen section studies without causing the surgeon to be hurried. The tumor is excised sharply with a margin of at least 1 cm of healthy renal tissue. Tumors in an apical or basilar position are best removed by a guillotine partial nephrectomy; peripheral tumors in the central portion of the kidney require a wedge resection. If a good margin of healthy tissue cannot be obtained without endangering hilar vessels, the case is unsuited for conservative surgery and a radical nephrectomy should be performed. In the presence of a normal contralateral kidney there is no place for bench surgery, problematic in situ kidney reconstruction, or compromises in the completeness of tumor removal. While collecting system and transected vessels on the nephrotomy plane are carefully sutured with the help of optical magnification, the tumor and multiple biopsies from the tumor bed are examined by frozen section. If the margins are not tumor free, the kidney is removed without another attempt to gain free margins. Otherwise the defect in the kidney is closed with a running suture of the capsule or, if the margins cannot be adapted, with a free graft of peritoneum patched onto the defect with fibrinogen tissue adhesive.

This concept of cautious, conservative surgery of solid peripheral tumors was utilized in 21 patients at the Rudolfstiftung (Vienna, Austria) in the last 5 years. During the same period another 141 patients underwent standard tumor nephrectomy for RC, so that 13% were selected for the conservative approach. In 4 patients a solid nodule was found unexpectedly at renal surgery for another reason. In the others diagnostic workup, including sonography and computerized tomography in all patients, fine needle aspiration biopsy in 11 patients, and angiography in 4 patients, had not reliably ruled out RC. Table 10.3 lists the final histologic diagnosis and treatment. Three kidneys were removed: one for a rather central RC with positive margins of resection, one poor kidney with multilocular, infected cysts, and one kidney with segmental arterial infarction. All other kidneys were preserved with good function, as documented by postoperative excretory urograms. None of the patients has any evidence of a local recurrent tumor or metastases. In an earlier study the author evaluated a similar group of patients (25). Although arteriography was used routinely in these patients rather than computerized tomography and the groups are therefore not strictly

Table 10.3
Final Histology of 21 Patients Subjected to Conservative Surgery for an Apparently Solid, Small, and Peripheral Renal Mass at the Rudolfstiftung, Vienna, 1981–1985[a]

Cystic (calcified/hemorrhagic) lesion	4 (1)
Angiomyolipoma	2
Adenoma	8
Genuine hypernephroma (7)	1
Renal adenocarcinoma	5 (1)
Segmental arterial infarction	1 (1)
	21 (3)

[a] Number of nephrectomies in parentheses.

Table 10.4
Final histology of 23 patients subjected to explorative surgery for a solid, small, and peripheral renal mass of doubtful dignity at the Department of Urology, University of Mainz Medical School, 1969–1977[a]

Cystic (calcified) lesions	3 (2)
Angiomyolipoma	3 (3)
Cavernous lymphangioma	1 (1)
Hemangiopericytoma	2 (2)
Adenoma	7 (5)
Mesoblastic nephroma	1
Renal adenocarcinoma	6 (6)
	23 (19)

[a] From Marberger M: Benign tumors of the kidney. Presented at the Third Annual Meeting of the European Intrarenal Surgical Society, Berne, 1978.
Number of nephrectomies in parentheses.

comparable, the histologic diagnoses appear almost identical (Table 10.4). These patients were still treated adhering to the principle that any solid tumor suspected to be RC requires radical nephrectomy without prior manipulation of the tumor. As shown in Table 10.4, this resulted in a nephrectomy rate of 19 of 23, although benign tumors again prevailed. In neither group has a metastasis of RC or a local recurrent tumor been observed during follow-up to date.

CONCLUSION

In solitary, peripheral renal tumors smaller than 4 cm in diameter excision of the entire tumor with a margin of at least 1 cm of healthy renal parenchyma provides adequate treatment. These lesions are today diagnosed far more often due to the liberal use of sonography and computerized tomography. They are frequently benign tumors and can only be distinguished from RC by histologic examination. RC of this size is usually circumscript and of low grade. Clinical evidence is presented that kidney-preserving excision as pointed out provides cure rates similar to those of radical nephrectomy.

REFERENCES

1. Jacobs SC, Berg SI, Lawson RK: Synchronous bilateral renal cell carcinoma: total surgical excision. *Cancer* 46:2341, 1980.
2. Marberger M, Hohenfellner R: Das Nierenkarzinom. *Nieren Hochdruckkr* 6:253, 1979.
3. Marberger M, Pugh RCB, Auvert J, Bertermann H, Constantini A, Gammelgaard PA, Pettersson S, Wickham JEA: Conservative surgery of renal carcinoma: the EIRSS experience. *Br J Urol* 53:528, 1981.
4. Palmer JM, Swanson DA: Conservative surgery in solitary and bilateral renal carcinoma: indications and technical considerations. *J Urol* 120:113, 1978.
5. Pearson JC, Weiss J, Tanagho EA: A plea for conservation of kidney in renal adenocarcinoma associated with von Hippel-Lindau disease. *J Urol* 124:910, 1980.
6. Penn I: Transplantation in patients with primary renal malignancies. *Transplantation* 24:424, 1977.
7. Herrlinger A, Schott KM, Sigel A, Giedl J: Results of 381 transabdominal radical nephrectomies for renal cell carcinoma with partial and complete en-bloc lymph-node dissection. *World J Urol* 2:114, 1984.

8. Skinner DG, Vermillion CD, Colvin RB: The surgical management of renal cell carcinoma. *J Urol* 107:705, 1972.
9. Marshall F, Walsh P: In situ management of renal tumors: renal cell carcinoma and transitional cell carcinoma. *J Urol* 131:1045, 1984.
10. Roehl L, Dreikorn K, Horsch R: Erfahrungen und Ergebnisse in der in situ- und extrakorporalen Exstirpation von Solitärnieren und bei Patienten mit bilateralen Nierentumoren. *Verh Dtsch Ges Urol* 32:187, 1980.
11. Topley M, Novick AC, Montie JE: Long-term results following partial nephrectomy for localized renal adenocarcinoma. *J Urol* 131:1050, 1984.
12. Zincke H, Swanson SK: Bilateral renal cell carcinoma: influence of synchronous and asynchronous occurrence on patient survival. *J Urol* 128:913, 1981.
13. Apitz K: Die Geschwülste und Gewebsmißbildungen der Nierenrinde. *Virchow's Arch (Pathol Anat)* 311:258, 1944.
14. Newcomb WD: The search for truth, with special reference to the frequency of gastric ulcer-cancer and the origin of Grawitz tumors of the kidney. *Proc R Soc Med* 30:113, 1936.
15. Schiff MD, Bagley DH, Lytton B: Treatment of solitary and bilateral renal carcinoma. *J Urol* 121:581, 1979.
16. Hermanek P, Sigel A, Chlepas S: Histological grading of renal cell carcinoma. *Eur Urol* 2:186, 1976.
17. Carini M, Selli C, Muraro GP, Tripitelli A, Masini G, Truini D: Conservative surgery for renal cell carcinoma. *Eur Urol* 7:19, 1981.
18. Graham SD, Glenn JF: Enucleative surgery for renal malignancy. *J Urol* 122:546, 1979.
19. Johansson S, Wahlqvist L: Conservative surgery in renal carcinoma: total surgical excision. *Scand J Urol Nephrol Suppl* 60:25, 1981.
20. Marberger M, Stackl W: Renal hypothermia in situ. In Resnick MI (ed): *Current Trends in Urology.* Baltimore, Williams & Wilkins, 1981, vol 1, p 70.
21. Rocca Rossetti S, Muto G: Possibilità e limiti della therapia conservativa del carcinoma renale. Atti dall' 3° Congresso dell' Società Italiana di Chirurgia Onchologica, 1980, p 461.
22. Rosenthal CL, Kraft R, Zingg EJ: Organ-preserving surgery in renal cell carcinoma: tumor enucleation versus partial kidney resection. *Eur Urol* 10:222, 1984.
23. Vermooten V: Indications for conservative surgery in certain renal tumors: a study based on a growth pattern of the clear cell carcinoma. *J Urol* 64:200, 1950.
24. Bell ET: *Renal Diseases*, ed 2. Philadelphia, Lea & Febiger, 1950, p 435.
25. Marberger M: Benign tumors of the kidney. Presented at the Third Annual Meeting of the European Intrarenal Surgical Society, Berne, 1978.

3
Section

Treatment of Metastatic Disease

11

Angioinfarction in Renal Adenocarcinoma

Grant Williams, M.S., F.R.C.S.

Since Almgard et al (1) described 19 patients with renal carcinoma treated by angioinfarction, there has been a steady flow of reports and developments on this technique. The high hopes generated by early reports must now be viewed skeptically (2). Unfortunately, there have been few randomized trials (3) to test and delineate the criteria for the use of this therapeutic modality, or to decide on which embolic material should be used.

Presumably the aims of angioinfarction and possible subsequent nephrectomy are as follows:

1. Improved access to the renal pedicle;
2. Palliative local control of pain or hemorrhage;
3. Prolonged survival;
4. Remission of metastases;
5. Production of some immunologic enhancement.

TECHNIQUES

Since the earlier communications of Almgard (1), using autologous muscle suspended in contrast material, it was known that these techniques were not without complication. Lalli et al (4) even reported complications from infarction with dextran—composed of cross-linked macromolecules of polysaccharides. It soon became known that embolization with autologous clot did not in fact completely infarct the kidney. Presumably the initial embolization produced some arteriolar spasm, which later opened up, or parasitic blood supply from perinephric fat, or even lumbar arteries had not been occluded.

Attempting to deal with these problems, a variety of techniques proliferated. Autologous clot and muscle were followed by Gelfoam (5) and a variety of particulate agents. These included lyophilized dura mater, Ivalon and microspheres—some of which later have even been conjugated with chemotherapeutic agents, such as mitomycin C (6) or radioactive agents (7), a technique which was suggested 15 years previously by Lang (8). However, there continues to be considerable evidence that these particulate angioinfarct agents do not produce complete infarction of the kidney. Animal studies have shown that revascularization occurs, sometimes within 3 weeks of the original procedure (9), and this observation of partial infarction and recanalization occurs with virtually all agents with the exception of barium sulfate paste.

This was not a particularly surprising observation, and attempts had already been made to produce internal obstruction of the renal artery and its main branches, leading to the development of metal springs (10) and cyanoacrylate adhesives, used originally by Dotter et al (11) and later by Kerber et al (12) for spinal vascular abnormalities. Carmignani et al (13) have later used this for other urologic abnormalities.

However, all of these techniques are not without complication and the postinfarction syndrome of pain, pyrexia, and paralytic ileus has now been reported in most published series, with distal emobilization, contralateral acute tubular necrosis, and spinal infarction adding an occasional morbidity to a possibly dying patient (14, 15).

Two variants of these occlusive techniques must be mentioned: First is balloon catheter occlusion in the immediate preoperative period. Mee and Heap (16) used a Swan-Ganz balloon-tipped catheter to produce immediate preoperative arterial occlusion. This allowed immediate vascular access to the renal vein, avoiding the occasional difficulties encountered when the usually posteriorly located renal artery was obscured by tumor or nodes. This is particularly a complication of transabdominal radical nephrectomy, seldom being a problem when the thoracoabdominal approach is used.

Obviously this balloon catheter technique avoids the postinfarction syndrome, may reduce the vascularity of the tumor, and allows immediate approach to the renal vein—a desirable aim if there is tumor in the renal vein or inferior vena cava. However it is not surprising that Mee (17) reported that the prognosis in metastatic disease treated with balloon infarction and nephrectomy was the same as that for patients who were treated with nephrectomy alone.

The second technique which must be mentioned as an occlusive agent is alcohol. This obviates some of the complications of particulate embolizations, in that unintentional distal embolization should not be deleterious as the bolus of alcohol would be diluted rapidly by blood. Absolute ethanol and propyl alcohol seem to have been mostly used and work by causing intimal damage to glomerular endothelial, epithelial and mesangial cells, with renal artery thrombosis occurring as a secondary phenomenon (18, 19). However this technique is also not without hazard because bowel infarction has now been reported as a complication (20), and this, like all reported techniques, usually produces patchy infarction. Possibly infarction in excess of 50% may be all that is necessary to produce the speculative antigenic release which is sought after, as long as the main renal artery remains occluded and allows early access to the renal vein.

It remains to mention that ferromagnetic infarction as described by Turner et al in 1975 (21) has been re-evaluated by Sako et al (22), but this work has not born much fruit. Neither have there been any developments on pharmacoangioinfarction with epinephrine, suggested from the observations of Abrams et al in 1962 (23), and developed by Turini and colleagues in 1976 (24).

There is therefore an *embarrasse de richesse* of techniques for angioinfarction of renal cell carcinoma, but the purpose and the effect of the procedure on the patient are not always immediately clear.

AIMS OF ANGIOINFARCTION

Access to the Renal Pedicle

It is unarguable that any nephrectomy, whether simple or radical, requires primary ligation of the renal artery. The blood supply to the kidney may be from a single renal artery; but multiple renal arteries are commonplace, and major vascular contribution from lumbar arteries may also occur. These considerations must be borne in mind when staging by computerized tomography or ultrasound is proposed as a valid alternative to angiography. Obviously, angioinfarction is ideally performed at the same time as the staging angiogram, although delaying angioinfarction for 24 hours after diagnostic angiography may prevent renal failure associated with high volume contrast material (25).

Renal cell carcinoma is notoriously highly vascular in many cases (26), and any approach to the renal artery is fraught with disaster. While immediate nephrectomy after embolization allows immediate access to the renal vein, delayed nephrectomy has technical advantages. In one series (27) the interval from embolization to nephrectomy varied from 4 to 8 days. This has usually led to a useful area of edema around Gerota's fascia with an impressive shutdown of troublesome vessels from the perinephric fat to lumbar vascular pedicles, which can be rapidly approached through this plane for ligation and division with ease. Of course, the familiar pulsating renal artery should not be palpable, and this can cause anxiety to the uninitiated because the embolized renal artery will frequently be encased in acute inflammatory tissue. In the author's experience this expected advantageous plane of edema was not present if the nephrectomy was performed too early, and certainly it had resolved if surgery was performed too late.

Even the acknowledged patchy infarction previously noted and confirmed by the author's group (15, 27) surprisingly does not cause any bleeding problems. The dissection can safely proceed to the vena cava where meticulous dissection of venous tributaries combined with en bloc lymphadenectomy can be performed. This leaves the final procedure as the division of the renal arteries. If Gianturco coils have been used in the infarction they can be removed with ease by the judicious relaxation of a Satinsky vascular clamp at the aortic level.

Some surgeons do claim that preoperative infarction makes the operation more difficult. A survey by Ritchie and Chisholm (28) reported that 81 of 134 British urologists responding to a questionnaire used preoperative arterial embolization, but that 16 of those 81 urologists had tried the technique but abandoned it. It is possible that as 34% delayed the nephrectomy for 24 or 48 hours only, that was their difficulty. In the author's experience, performing the nephrectomy very early or very late conferred no technical advantages at all.

Palliative Local Control

The technical advantage of reduced vascularity has already been alluded to, and most reported series include a number of patients who were considered inoperable but were embolized to control local symptoms. Of the 102 patients reported by Wallace et al (25), 25 patients were embolized without nephrectomy. Similarly, 8 of the 19 patients reported by Almgard (1) did not receive an adjuvant nephrectomy. There continued to be reports of patients who were treated by infarction only (29, 30), but follow-up information is not available. In fact, these inoperable patients with uncontrollable symptoms are few. Johnson and Swanson (31) make the point that nephrectomy alone seldom relieves local symptoms which cannot be achieved as easily with simpler procedures, such as angioinfarction. In the author's series (27), they did not proceed to nephrectomy in six patients but, apart from occasionally stopping hematuria, they noted a tendency to substitute one set of iatrogenic symptoms for the original symptoms, and palliative infarction is not always a therapeutic triumph.

Prolonged Survival

Whether preoperative infarction per se prolongs survival has not been tested in any prospective trial. The earlier communications on this subject are not specific on the histologic grade of their tumors or which patients also received adjuvant therapy, such as medroxyprogesterone. The well known actuarial survival figures between the sexes are missing from many retrospective studies because the sex of the patient is frequently omitted. For what it is worth, the author found that 5% of stage I, 33% of stage II, and 60% of stage III patients developed metastases, and six of the seven patients developing metastases did not develop them for a median period of 20 months. This compares with the observations of Lokich and Harrison (32) where metastases developed within 1 year in 19% of their patients treated by nephrectomy alone for localized disease. Possibly the author's rate of 6 of 32 patients (19%) with a median period of 20 months before developing metastases is a move in the right direction. However, there has been no study to test the role of angioinfarction in delaying the appearance of metastases or in altering the interval between emergence of metastases and demise.

Any discussion on prolongation of survival following angioinfarction must examine three factors: (*a*) interval to development of metastases; (*b*) interval from development of metastases to demise; and (*c*) prolongation of survival in de novo metastatic disease.

This situation is complicated by the well known phenomena of spontaneous remission and long surviving static disease. Fairlamb (33) could only find 67 documented cases of spontaneous remission, and most papers record this phenomenon in less than 1% of all patients with metastatic disease. While this has seldom been recorded when the primary tumor is still in situ, there are now multiple publications decrying the practice of adjuvant nephrectomy in the presence of metastatic disease.

Two recent publications indicate that angioinfarction and adjuvant nephrectomy can be followed by remission of metastases. Swanson et al (34) reported on 100 patients treated this way. Seven patients developed complete remission, although six of them developed new metastases from which they died. Patients in their series recorded with stable disease are surviving for similar lengths of time as patients treated without angioinfarction, and, in any case, 88 of their 100 patients also received progesterones. The earlier reports from the MD Anderson Hospital in Houston (25) discussed 36 of 102 patients who survived beyond 4.5 months, and they then reported that the median survival was 17 months against 6 months for a control group. In that series six patients gained complete remission of metastases for periods in excess of 6 months. Presumably the 49 patients with metastatic disease in the 1979 series from the MD Anderson Hospital are included in the 100 patients reported in 1983 from the same institution, and again the survival with metastatic disease shows prolongation of survival, a point confirmed by the author's group (27), where survival in stage IV disease was prolonged for periods beyond 18 months in 20% of patients. Two of the author's patients have had metastatic remission or static disease for over 2 years after angioinfarction.

If protagonists of angioinfarction in stage IV disease continue to report remission of metastases following this procedure, then this must be seen within the context of spontaneous remission. Fairlamb (33) could only find 67 cases of spontaneous remission and this paper is frequently quoted, but it is probably a much commoner phenomenon. Ritchie and Chisholm (28), surveying 134 British urologists, found 53 surgeons who had seen metastatic regression in 106 instances. When details of 60 of these 106 instances were examined, there were 11 treated on angioinfarction programs. Two of these 11 received angioinfarction only, while 9 had angioinfarction, delayed nephrectomy, and occasionally progesterones.

MODE OF ACTION

If angioinfarction increases patient survival, then it may be relevant in stages I to III by reducing tumor dissemination at the time of surgery, but if it leads to metastases regression or prolongation of life, it presumably can only do so by an immunologic phenomenon, the potentiation of progesterones used, or even the two together.

Early studies of immune competence before and after infarction using delayed hypersensitivity with a variety of recall antigens have not been very helpful (27). Other studies have included total peripheral T and B cell numbers and T cell transformation (35), but these types of studies tend to be nonspecific and could be a simple response to the inflammatory response of infarction. These T cell responses can even be dependent on the type of anesthesia used (36, 37). In other surgical procedures (36, 37) studies have shown that there is a difference in T cell behavior when inhalation anesthesia is used that is not present when spinal anesthesia is used. It is therefore possible that all of the immune competence studies on angioinfarction and delayed nephrectomy could easily have been the result of inhalation anesthesia. There has not yet been a prospective study of changes in immune competence, whether by delayed hypersensitivity, T cell responses, or monocyte maturation in renal carcinoma where there is a control group of nephrectomy alone for benign disease.

With these provisos concerning lack of controls it is interesting that monocyte to macrophage maturation studies (35, 38) have shown that declining levels of macrophage in renal carcinoma surgery have been associated with a poor prognosis, whereas increasing and maintained levels after angioinfarction have been associated with a good prognosis, but these studies do not indicate that the angioinfarction produced the good prognosis.

One study on total lymphocyte transformation (39) has shown that there is no significant difference between lymphocyte transformations before and after angioinfarction alone, but if the patients underwent a delayed nephrectomy within 5 weeks of the angioinfarction, then the levels of transformations were maintained at statistically significantly higher levels than the preinfarction levels. However, it must be remembered that Nakano et al's patients received chemotherapy, progesterones, and immunotherapy after the nephrectomy and also their studies were on total lymphocyte transformation. Therefore, the studies of Ritchie et al (40), examining lymphocyte subsets with monoclonal antibodies, are more than welcome. They have demonstrated that T cell deficiency in renal carcinoma is, in fact, due to a deficit of the helper-inducer phenotype Leu-3a+, but this deficiency is restored by nephrectomy alone. As one of the actions of Leu-3a+ is thought to be on B cell differentiation and specific antibody production, then restoration of the frequently noted leukocyte deficit should be advantageous. If the Leu-3a+ subset deficiency is, in fact, due to entrapment within the tumor, then angioinfarction should correct that deficit, but that does not occur. In fact, the T cell subset number continues to drop after angioinfarction. If, therefore, angioinfarction precipitates some as yet unknown antibody-mediated effect, then it is most unlikely to be caused by T cell-B cell interaction. Search along the monocyte-macrophage axis might be more productive, especially as macrophages are abundantly present in the postinfarction nephrectomy specimen.

POSTINFARCTION SYNDROME

Angioinfarction with a delayed nephrectomy usually produces unpleasant side effects. These symptoms begin almost immediately and last for 3 to 4 days. There may be fever up to 40°C, severe loin pain, and paralytic ileus. The pain will frequently require large narcotic sedation, and during these worrisome few days there are the occasional mishaps of unintentional distal embolization. Abscess formation with bacterial colonization is now well recorded, and this possibly should deter from too great a delay in the proposed nephrectomy. However, the possibility that angioinfarction is, in fact, a rather complicated and hazardous way of producing a nebulous effect must be considered. If fever is the desirable trigger mechanism, then fever can certainly be associated with changes in lymphocyte transformation. Pain is undoubtedly associated with increased cortisol excretion, and lymphopenia should follow.

CONCLUSIONS

The advent of angioinfarction has generated a steady flow of noncontrolled studies on the management of renal carcinoma. It is not yet clear whether reports of therapeutic efficacy with this modality, in fact, fall within spontaneous remission rates of this fascinating tumor and whether the desirable antibody-mediated response is really a manifestation of a simpler phenomenon.

Before angioinfarction can be accepted as a standard treatment, a detailed study is vital. This study must have controls which include radical nephrectomy without preoperative infarction for renal carcinoma and also nephrectomy for benign diseases; the ideal control would be donor nephrectomy in related living renal transplantation. Somehow the effect of anesthesia on immune competence must be excluded. This study must have clearly defined parameters which include the following: (*a*) in stages I, II, and III, the interval from nephrectomy to advent of metastases; (*b*) the interval between the advent of metastases and patient demise; and (*c*) in stage IV, prolongation of survival.

Such an initial study must exclude chemotherapy, progesterones, and immunotherapy, and immunologic studies must be specific and indicative of changes in immune competence. Monocyte to macrophage maturation or T cell subsets would appear helpful, while delayed hypersensitivity or crude lymphocyte proliferation would preferably be excluded. Finally, a strict standardization of the embolization technique and of the infarction to nephrectomy interval must be examined.

Until that study is performed the whole concept of angioinfarction of renal tumors must remain sub judice.

REFERENCES

1. Almgard LE, Fernstrom I, Haverling M, Ljungquist A: Treatment of renal carcinoma by embolic occlusion of the renal circulation. *Br J Urol* 45:474–479, 1973.
2. Teasdale C, Kirk D, Jeans WD, Penry JB, Tribe CT, Slade N: Arterial embolization in renal carcinoma. *Br J Urol* 54:616–619, 1982.
3. Kurth KH, Cinqualbre J, Oliver RTD, Schulman CC: Embolization and subsequent nephrectomy in metastatic renal cell carcinoma. In Kurth KH, Debruyn FMJ, Schroeder FH, Splinter TAW, Wagener TDJ (eds): *Progress and Controversies in Oncological Urology.* New York, Alan R Liss, 1984, pp 423–436.
4. Lalli AF, Petersen N, Beckstein JJ: Roentgen guided infarction of kidneys and lungs. *Radiology* 93:434–435, 1969.
5. Bree RL, Goldstein HM, Wallace S: Transcatheter embolization of the internal iliac artery. *Surg Gynecol Obstet* 143:597–601, 1976.
6. Kato T, Nemoto R, Mori H, Takahashi M, Tamakawa Y: Transcatheter arterial chemo-embolization of renal cell carcinoma with microencapsulated mitomycin C. *J Urol* 125:19, 1981.

7. Lang EK, Sullivan J, deKernion JB: Transcatheter embolization of renal cell carcinoma with radioactive infarct particles. *Radiology* 147:413–418, 1983.
8. Lang EK: Superselective arterial catheterization as a vehicle for delivering radioactive infarct particles. *Radiology* 98:391–399, 1971.
9. Cho KJ, Nishiyama RH, Shields JJ, McGormick JL, Forrest ME: Experimental renal infarcts. *AJR* 136:493–496, 1981.
10. Gianturco C, Anderson JH, Wallace S: Mechanical development for arterial occlusion. *AJR* 124:438, 1975.
11. Dotter CL, Goldman ML, Rosch J: Instant selective arterial occlusion with isobutyl 2 cyanoacrylate. *Radiology* 114:227–230, 1975.
12. Kerber CW, Cromwell LD, Sheptak PE: Intra-arterial cyanoacrylate. An adjunct in the treatment of spinal/paraspinal arteriovenous malformations. *AJR* 103:99–103, 1978.
13. Carmignani G, Belgrano E, Puppo P, Cichero A, Giuliani L: Transcatheter embolization of the hypogastric arteries in cases of bladder hemorrhage from advanced pelvic cancers. *J Urol* 124:196–200, 1980.
14. Kaisary AV, McIvor J, Williams G: Conservative management of unintentional distal embolization following intravascular occlusive therapy. *Br J Surg* 69:422, 1982.
15. McIvor J: Embolization of renal carcinoma. Correspondence. *Clin Radiol* 35:335–336, 1984.
16. Mee AD, Heap SW: Pre-operative balloon occlusion of the renal artery for radical nephrectomy. *Br J Urol* 50:153–156, 1978.
17. Mee AD: Prognosis after radical nephrectomy for carcinoma. The influence of pre-operative balloon occlusion. *Br J Urol* 54:201–203, 1982.
18. Ellman BA, Green CE, Eigenbrodte E, Garriot JB, Curry TS: Renal infarction with absolute ethanol. *Invest Radiol* 15:318–322, 1980.
19. Buchta K, Sands J, Rosenkrantz H, Roche WD: Early mechanism of action of arterially infused alcohol V.A.P. in renal devitalization. *Radiology* 145:45–48, 1982.
20. Mulligan BD, Espinosa GA: Bowel infarction: a complication of ethanol ablation of a renal tumour. *Cardiovasc Intervent Radiol* 6:55–57, 1983.
21. Turner RD, Rand RW, Bentson JR, Mosso JA: Ferromagnetic silicone necrosis of hypernephromas by selective vascular occlusion of the tumor—a new technique. *J Urol* 113:455, 1975.
22. Sako M, Yokogawa S, Sakamoto K, Adach S, Hirota S, Okada S, Murad S: Transcatheter microembolization with ferropolysaccharides. *Invest Radiol* 17:573–582, 1982.
23. Abrams HL, Boijsen E, Borgstrom KE: Effect of epinephrine on the renal circulation: angiographic observations. *Radiology* 79:911, 1962.
24. Turini D, Nicita G, Fiorelli C, Selli C, Villari N: Selective transcatheter arterial embolization of renal carcinoma. *J Urol* 116:419–421, 1976.
25. Wallace G, Chuang V, Green B, Swanson DA, Bracken RB, Johnson DE: Diagnostic radiology in renal carcinoma. In Johnson DE, Samuels ML (eds): *Cancer of the Genito-urinary Tract.* New York, Raven Press, 1979, p 33.
26. Folin J: Angiography in renal tumors. *Acta Radiol (suppl)* 267:7–91, 1967.
27. Kaisary AV, Williams G, Riddle PR: The role of pre-operative embolization in renal cell carcinoma. *J Urol* 131:641–646, 1984.
28. Ritchie AWS, Chisholm GD: Management of renal carcinoma. *Br J Urol* 55:591–594, 1983.
29. Ekelund L, Mannson W, Olsson AM, Stigsson L: Palliative embolization of arterial renal tumor supply. Results in 10 cases. *Acta Radiol Diagn* 20:323–336, 1979.
30. Macerlean DP, Owens A, Bryan PJ: Hypernephroma embolization—is it worthwhile? *Clin Radiol* 31:297–300, 1980.
31. Johnson DE, Swanson DA: The role of nephrectomy in metastatic renal carcinoma. In Johnson DE, Samuels ML (eds): *Cancer of the Genito-urinary Tract.* New York, Raven Press, 1979, pp 27–31.
32. Lokich JJ, Harrison JH: Renal cell carcinoma. Natural history and chemotherapeutic experience. *J Urol* 114:371–374, 1975.
33. Fairlamb DJ: Spontaneous regression of metastasis of renal cancer. *Cancer* 47:2102, 1982.

34. Swanson DA, Johnson DE, von Essenbach AC, Chuang VP, Wallace S: Angioinfarction plus nephrectomy for metastatic renal cell carcinoma. *J Urol* 130:449–452, 1983.
35. Mebust WK, Weigel JW, Lee KR, Cox GG, Jewell WR, Krishnan EC: Renal cell carcinoma—angioinfarction. *J Urol* 131:231–235, 1984.
36. Ryhanen P: Effects of anesthesia and operative surgery on the immune-response of patients of different ages. *Ann Clin Res* 9:19, 1977.
37. Mougdil GC, Wade AG: Anaesthesia and immunocompetence. *Br J Anaesth* 48:31, 1976.
38. Krishnan EC, Mebust WK, Weigel JA, Jewell WF: Culture of peripheral monocytes in vitro in patients with renal cell carcinoma: a possible prognostic indicator. *J Urol* 130:597–601, 1983.
39. Nakano H, Nihira H, Toge T: Treatment of renal cancer by transcatheter embolization and its effect on lymphocyte proliferative responses. *J Urol* 130:24–27, 1983.
40. Ritchie AWS, James K, Micklem HS, Chrisholm GD: Lymphocyte subsets in renal carcinoma—a sequential study using monoclonal antibodies. *Br J Urol* 56:140–148, 1984.

12

Current Results of Infarction-Nephrectomy for Advanced Renal Adenocarcinoma

David A. Swanson, M.D.
Sidney Wallace, M.D.

Up to 57% of patients with primary adenocarcinoma of the kidney, or renal cell carcinoma, have been reported to have clinically apparent metastases at the time of initial diagnosis (1). Optimal treatment of such patients has long been vigorously debated, particularly with regard to whether nephrectomy should be performed (2, 3). Following preliminary reports from The University of Texas MD Anderson Hospital and Tumor Institute at Houston that embolic occlusion of the renal artery (angioinfarction) prior to nephrectomy might promote clinical regression of metastases and lengthen survival (4, 5), clinical management has become even more controversial. The authors' most recent analysis of 100 evaluable patients permits them to draw some tentative conclusions and to offer some guidelines regarding the role of infarction-nephrectomy in the management of stage IV renal cell carcinoma.

PATIENTS

One hundred patients with advanced untreated primary renal cell carcinoma presented to MD Anderson Hospital for evaluation and possible treatment between 1974 and 1981. All had clinically apparent metastatic disease. Parenchymal lung metastases were diagnosed in 64 patients, bone metastases in 36, metastases to hilar or mediastinal lymph nodes in 34, distant lymph node involvement in 7, malignant pleural effusion in 6, skin and liver metastases in 5 each, and metastases to other sites (brain, kidney, adrenal, breast, thyroid, pancreas, vagina, or other soft tissue) in 14. Eighty-four were men with a median age of 55 years (range 31 to 80), and 16 were women with a median age of 57 years (range 26 to 68).

Beginning in April, 1974, these patients were treated by angioinfarction (percutaneous arterial embolic occlusion of the renal circulation) of the primary tumor followed by radical nephrectomy. Parenteral medroxyprogesterone acetate, 400 mg twice weekly, was given to 88 of the 100 patients.

TREATMENT TECHNIQUE

The authors have used a variety of agents to occlude the renal circulation, all of them biologically inert. Most commonly, they used sterile gelatin sponge (Gelfoam), cut into 3 mm $\times$ 3 mm cubes or 5-mm strips, or particles of polyvinyl alcohol (Ivalon). Each of these agents was mixed with saline and contrast material, then injected slowly under fluoroscopic control into an angiographic catheter that had been advanced as far as possible into the renal artery in order to minimize the risk of escape of the embolic material.

The arterial flow carried the emboli passively to occlude the peripheral vasculature of the kidney and neoplasm. Once the peripheral vessels had been filled, one or more stainless steel coils were introduced through the catheter to occlude the main renal artery or arteries. The coil, which has multiple Dacron strands attached along its length to promote thrombus formation, is available in several different diameters. The combination of Gelfoam, Ivalon, and steel coils markedly reduces the blood supply to the tumor, although capsular and parasitic vessels prevent complete infarction (6). Microscopic examination of the infarcted kidney generally shows acute necrotizing arteritis and patchy hemorrhagic necrosis. Further details of the technique of angioinfarction have been reported elsewhere (7).

Although the interval between infarction and nephrectomy in these 100 patients ranged from several hours to 10 months, the median was 5 days, and three-quarters of all patients underwent nephrectomy 4 to 7 days after infarction. Radical nephrectomy was performed through a transabdominal incision in 98 patients and a subcostal flank incision in 2. Progesterone therapy generally was initiated 1 week postoperatively.

PATIENT RESPONSE

Eighty-five patients are known to be dead; one progressing patient was lost at 14 months and is presumed dead. The remaining 14 patients are alive and have been followed a minimum of 30 months.

Results were tabulated according to standard response criteria. Disappearance of all known metastatic disease constituted a complete response (CR). Decrease of greater than 50% in the product of the two maximum diameters of all lesions without any new lesions forming indicated a partial response (PR). A change of less than 25% in the product of the two maximum diameters of any lesion in the absence of any new lesions for a minimum of 12 months defined stabilization (5). Any new metastatic lesion or an increase greater than 25% in the product of the two maximum diameters of any lesion indicated progression, or nonresponse. Responding patients achieved a complete or partial response or stabilization.

Seven of the 100 patients achieved a CR. One of these remains alive without clinical evidence of recurrent disease 90 months after nephrectomy, whereas 6 developed new metastatic lesions after intervals of 7 to 31 months (median 13 months) and died of the disease (Table 12.1). Survival times ranged from 14 to 40 months; the median survival for the 7 complete responders was 19 months.

Eight patients exhibited a PR. Two remain alive at 30 and 36 months, the latter still without progression (Table 12.1). In 7, disease progressed after initially regressing more than 50% in 5 to 29 months (median 11 months) after nephrectomy. Survival times ranged from 12 to 64 months, and the median for all 8 was 21 months.

Disease in 13 of the 100 patients stabilized for longer than 1 year. It progressed subsequently in 8 patients 13 to 28 months after nephrectomy (median 18 months), but the other 5 patients remain stable (and alive) 31 to 70 months postnephrectomy (Table 12.1). In all, 7 patients remain alive at 31 to 70 months, while 6 have died at 17 to 62 months postnephrectomy (overall median survival 36 months). Five patients at or below the median survival time remain alive.

ANALYSIS

Among all 100 patients, 28 achieved some form of response (CR, PR, S). When the survival rate for the 28 responders is compared to that of the 72 nonresponders, the difference between the two curves is highly significant ($p = 0.000003$) (Fig. 12.1). The expected median survival for responding patients was 39.1 months, and 38% have survived 5 years.

Table 12.1
Recurrence, Progression, and Survival Data for 28 Responders

Complete Response (7 Patients)		Partial Response (8 Patients)		Stabilization (13 Patients)	
Months to Recurrence	Months Survival	Months to Progression	Months Survival	Months to Progression	Months Survival
9	14	5	12	15	17
14	17	8	12	15	22
7	19	5	17	No progression	31[a]
15	19	11	18	No progression	33[a]
12	30	16	24	21	34[a]
31	40	26	30[a]	No progression	36[a]
No recurrence	90[a]	No progression	36[a]	No progression	36[a]
		29	64	13	38
				15	39
				23	50
				28	55[a]
				28	62
				No progression	70[a]

[a] Alive.

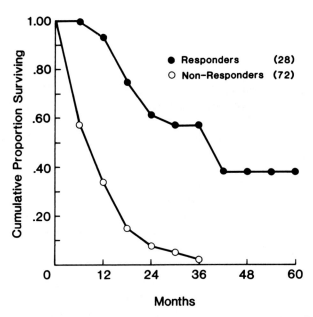

Figure 12.1. Survival curves of responders and nonresponders ($p = 0.000003$).

Table 12.2
Survival Rates for 60 Patients with Only Pulmonary Metastases

	Survival Rate (%)	
Years	Nephrectomy (18)	Infarction-Nephrectomy (42)
1	17	55
2	10	26
3		21
4		18
5		18
Median (months)	7.0	16.5

Nonresponding patients had an expected median survival of 8.4 months; only 5% survived 3 years, and none was alive at 5 years.

A comparison between the series of 100 patients treated by angioinfarction and nephrectomy and 43 patients treated by nephrectomy without prior infarction at MD Anderson Hospital in the early 1970s shows the survival rate of the angioinfarcted patients to be slightly, but not significantly, better ($p = 0.115$). However, if one compares those patients in the two groups whose metastases are only pulmonary, the difference in survival rates for 42 treated by infarction-nephrectomy and 18 similar patients treated by nephrectomy alone, the difference becomes significant ($p = 0.017$) (Table 12.2). The difference in expected median survival was 9½ months.

However, if patients with lung metastases are stratified into those with parenchymal metastases only and those with advanced lung disease, defined by either hilar or mediastinal adenopathy or malignant pleural effusion, with or without parenchymal lesions, one can see that among the patients treated by infarction-nephrectomy those with only paren-

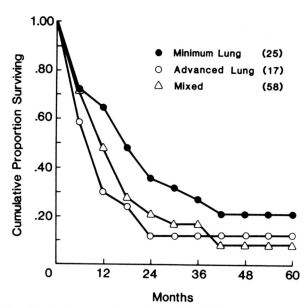

Figure 12.2. Survival curves for patients with different clinical presentations, all treated by angioinfarction plus radical nephrectomy ($p = 0.194$).

chymal lung metastases have a better apparent survival rate than those who also have adenopathy or effusion (advanced lung), although this difference is not significant ($p = 0.113$) (Fig. 12.2). Expected median survival times were 18.5 months and 9.25 months, respectively. In fact, patients with advanced lung disease have a survival time very similar to that of patients who have nonlung metastases or lung plus nonlung (mixed) metastases, whose expected median survival is 12.5 months ($p = 0.476$) (Fig. 12.2).

Although the 25 patients with only parenchymal lung disease appear to have the best survival rate, when they are compared to all others who underwent infarction-nephrectomy (75 patients with advanced lung and mixed metastases), the difference only approaches statistical significance ($p = 0.092$) (Fig. 12.3).

Finally, among the 83 patients from both groups who have mixed metastases (i.e., nonlung or lung plus nonlung), the survival rates for those undergoing nephrectomy alone and for those undergoing angioinfarction plus nephrectomy are virtually the same ($p = 0.980$) (Table 12.3). For these patients the authors cannot demonstrate that angioinfarction before nephrectomy confers any survival advantage.

Not only the survival rates, but also the response rates (objective clinical regression or stabilization of metastases), differ according to this breakdown of clinical presentation, i.e., lung parenchyma, advanced lung, or mixed metastases. Among patients who presented with parenchymal pulmonary metastases only, 5 achieved a CR, 2 a PR, and 4 were stable, for an overall response rate of 44% (Table 12.4). Among patients with advanced lung disease, there were 3 PRs and 2 stabilizations, for a 29% response rate. Finally, of patients with mixed metastases, 2 were CRs, 3 PRs, and 7 were stable, for a 21% response rate. Once again, although patients with only parenchymal lung disease had the

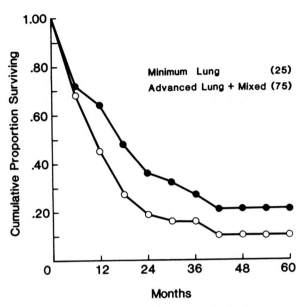

Figure 12.3. Survival curves for patients with either minimal lung metastases or more advanced clinical presentations, all treated by angioinfarction plus radical nephrectomy ($p = 0.092$).

Table 12.3
Survival Rates for 75 Patients with Mixed Metastases

Years	Survival Rate (%)	
	Nephrectomy (25)	Infarction-Nephrectomy (50)
1	48	48
2	25	21
3	25	17
4	25	08
5		08
Median (months)	11.5	12.5

Table 12.4
Correlation of Response to Clinical Presentation

Location of Metastases	No. of Patients	Response				
		CR	PR	S	Total	Rate
Lung parenchyma	25	5	2	4	11	44%
Advanced lung	17	0	3	2	5	29%
Mixed	58	2	3	7	12	21%
Total	100	7	8	13	28	28%

highest rate of clinical regression of metastases (11 of 25; 44%), when this response rate was compared to the response rate for all other patients (17 of 75; 23%) the difference was not statistically significant ($p = 0.076$).

COMMENT

In 1973 Almgard and his colleagues reported that 3 patients with pulmonary metastases were alive 12, 13, and 20 months after infarction (with autologous muscle) followed by radical nephrectomy, and that in only 1 the metastases had shown "some progress" (8). In view of the absence of effective therapy for patients with stage IV renal cell carcinoma, this observation fostered an early interest in the possible role of angioinfarction in the management of these patients. The authors' early experience at MD Anderson Hospital with this therapeutic combination, to which we added parenteral progestational therapy, led to 2 frank clinical regressions and increased survival times (4). An analysis of the first 50 patients with metastatic renal cell carcinoma treated by infarction, nephrectomy, and medroxyprogesterone acetate appeared to confirm the clinical benefit for selected patients (5), but the present analysis of 100 patients followed for a minimum of 30 months or until death demonstrates that the benefit is, indeed, for a highly selected group of patients.

The present analysis confirms the earlier observation that patients with only pulmonary metastases who undergo infarction followed by nephrectomy have an apparent survival advantage over similar patients treated by nephrectomy without prior infarction at the authors' institution several years earlier. Median survival duration was more than doubled in the infarction-nephrectomy patients, and the difference is statistically significant ($p = 0.017$). However, optimal survival time among patients treated by infarction-nephrectomy seemed to accrue primarily to patients with no mediastinal or hilar adenopathy, with no malignant pleural effusion, and no metastases outside the lungs. When patients have metastases outside the lung (with or without concomitant lung metastases), angioinfarction prior to nephrectomy produced no demonstrable improvement in survival rates.

It should not be surprising that patients with pulmonary parenchymal metastases secondary to renal carcinoma have the best survival rate, since the best results reported for any protocol generally occur in this group of patients. Most of the reported spontaneous regressions have been in the lung (9). DeKernion and associates noted a significantly better survival rate 1 year after nephrectomy among the subgroup of patients whose metastases were confined to the lung, although they make no mention of whether these patients had adenopathy or effusions (3). Hormone therapy has been most effective for pulmonary lesions (10), as has partially purified human leukocyte (α) interferon (11). Finally, Tykka and associates found that most objective tumor regressions in their patients occurred in lung metastases (12).

Although the overall response rate for the authors' initial 50 patients with metastatic renal cell carcinoma treated by angioinfarction and subsequent radical nephrectomy was 36% (5), it was only 20% for the next 50 patients, yielding a composite response rate of 28% for the complete series of 100 patients (Table 12.5). The difference in the response rate among the first 50 patients and that for the next 50 is not statistically significant ($p < 0.10$) and may represent only an apparent decrease, but the authors cannot explain the absence of any new complete responders (13). A difference in patient presentation is not the answer, since distribution of metastases in the two groups of 50 patients

Table 12.5
Responses among 100 Evaluable Patients

Response	Patients		
	Nos. 1–50	Nos. 51–100	Total
Complete	7	0	7
Partial	5	3	8
Stable	6	7	13
Total	18	10	28

Table 12.6
Comparison of Clinical Presentations among 100 Evaluable Patients

Location of Metastases	Patients	
	First 50	Last 50
Lung parenchyma	14	11
Advanced lung	8	9
Mixed	28	30

is fairly comparable (Table 12.6). Further experience must be accumulated before this and other questions regarding the most effective application of this protocol can be answered.

CONCLUSIONS

It is very risky to draw firm conclusions from a retrospective analysis of such a few patients, especially when comparisons include historical controls. Nonetheless, the combined response rate of 0.8% derived from multiple published reports totaling 571 patients has confirmed the unlikelihood of metastatic lesions regressing after radical nephrectomy not preceded by angioinfarction (14). The difference is highly significant between this 0.8% rate and the 15% objective response rate observed among the 100 patients in the present series. Furthermore, experience has shown that survival rates for patients with metastatic renal carcinoma who undergo radical nephrectomy without infarction are poor, as typified by the 38% 1-year survival rate reported by deKernion et al (3). In the present series, the comparable 1-year survival figures are 50% for all 100 patients and 64% for those 25 who had only parenchymal pulmonary metastases. That such a difference in survival rate exists demonstrates how critically important it is to stratify patients by site and volume of disease when reporting and comparing the results of treatment for patients with metastatic renal cell carcinoma. Despite the absence of stratification, however, the reported lack of response to nephrectomy alone seems valid because the large number of patients (571) is likely to surmount any bias secondary to clinical presentation.

The authors' current policy is to recommend angioinfarction plus delayed radical nephrectomy and medroxyprogesterone acetate to patients who present with parenchymal pulmonary metastases. Although analysis of their data may have done no more than identify this group of patients as being highly likely to do well clinically, the fact is that there are no published reports that document better results. At the other extreme, patients with nonpulmonary metastases (with or without concomitant lung lesions) have not demonstrated clinical regression of metastases or improved survival time after radical nephrectomy, even if preceded by angioinfarction; the authors routinely offer them an experimental protocol or only palliative therapy.

The meager number of patients with advanced lung disease retrospectively analyzed does not permit the authors to make a firm recommendation for them with any confidence. Although the expectation is that these patients are not as likely to respond as they would had they only parenchymal lesions, nonetheless the authors have seen 3 partial responses and 2 patients with prolonged stabilization among the 17 with advanced lung disease. In fact, 2 stable patients with biopsy-confirmed mediastinal adenopathy remain alive 50 and 70 months after nephrectomy, the latter patient still without evidence of any progression. In the absence of any demonstrably better therapeutic approach, it is the authors' opinion that some of these patients should be offered infarction-nephrectomy, although the data do not support its routine use in this group of patients.

The apparent clinical benefit for some patients may be easy to explain once the mechanism underlying this combination therapy is understood. It is not known how or why angioinfarction plus nephrectomy is associated with a good response in some patients; the observation is empiric. Clearly, more data are needed to resolve some of the questions raised. Ideally, a prospective randomized study would generate the most reliable answers. However, the slow rate of accrual (only 25 patients with parenchymal pulmonary metastases in over 7 years), the repeated demonstration that nephrectomy plus standard chemohormonal therapy does not promote regression of metastases or improve survival time, and the absence of any effective nonsurgical therapy for patients who progress make construction of such a trial difficult, if not unethical. Until better therapeutic strategies are reported, it seems reasonable to continue to employ angioinfarction and radical nephrectomy to treat carefully selected patients with metastatic renal cell carcinoma.

REFERENCES

1. Lokich JJ, Harrison JH: Renal cell carcinoma: natural history and chemotherapeutic experience. *J Urol* 114:371, 1975.
2. Johnson DE, Kaesler KE, Samuels ML: Is nephrectomy justified in patients with metastatic renal carcinoma? *J Urol* 114:27, 1975.
3. deKernion JB, Ramming KP, Smith RB: The natural history of metastatic renal cell carcinoma: a computer analysis. *J Urol* 120:148, 1978.
4. Bracken RB, Johnson DE, Goldstein HM, Wallace, S, Ayala AG: Percutaneous transfemoral renal artery occlusion in patients with renal carcinoma. Preliminary report. *Urology* 6:6, 1975.
5. Swanson DA, Wallace S, Johnson DE: The role of embolization and nephrectomy in the treatment of metastatic renal carcinoma. *Urol Clin North Am* 7:719, 1980.
6. McIvor J, Kaisary AV, Williams G, Grant RW: Tumour infarction after pre-operative embolisation of renal carcinoma. *Clin Radiol* 35:59, 1984.
7. Wallace S, Chuang VP, Swanson D, Bracken B, Hersh EM, Ayala A, Johnson D: Embolization of renal carcinoma. Experience with 100 patients. *Radiology* 138:563, 1981.

8. Almgard LE, Fernstrom I, Haverling M, Ljungqvist A: Treatment of renal adenocarcinoma by embolic occlusion of the renal circulation. *Br J Urol,* 45:474, 1973.
9. Freed SZ, Halperin JP, Gordon M: Idiopathic regression of metastases from renal cell carcinoma. *J Urol* 118:538, 1977.
10. Raghavaiah NV: Hormone treatment of advanced renal cell carcinoma. *Urology* 19:123, 1982.
11. Quesada JR, Trindade A, Swanson DA, Gutterman JU: Renal cell carcinoma: antitumor effects of leukocyte interferon. *Cancer Res* 43:940, 1983.
12. Tykka H, Oravisto KJ, Lehtonen T, Sarna S, Tallberg T: Active specific immunotherapy of advanced renal-cell carcinoma. *Eur Urol* 4:250, 1978.
13. Swanson DA, Johnson DE, von Eschenbach AC, Chuang VP, Wallace S: Angioinfarction plus nephrectomy for metastatic renal cell carcinoma: an update. *J Urol* 130:449, 1983.
14. deKernion JB, Berry D: The diagnosis and treatment of renal cell carcinoma. *Cancer* 45 (suppl):1947, 1980.

13

Metastatic Renal Adenocarcinoma

Saad Khoury, M.D.
A. Saul, M.B., B.S.

INTRODUCTION

Renal cell carcinoma is the third most common urologic cancer, accounting for about 7000 deaths/year in the United States. It is 3 times more common in males than in females. Thirty percent of patients with renal cell carcinoma have metastases at the time of diagnosis, and 95% have metastases at autopsy (1). Although some of these patients may have a relatively long survival (approximately 10% of patients will survive for more than 3 years (2)), the average survival is only 6 to 9 months. Secondary metastases appearing after removal of the primary neoplasm have a better prognosis than metastases present at the time of diagnosis (3).

Metastases occur in relatively young patients, with a mean age of 56 years. These lesions are often associated with pain and other symptoms that frequently require treatment, even if it is only palliative. The distribution of metastases in renal cell carcinoma is shown in Tables 13.1 and 13.2.

TREATMENT

Various methods have been used to treat metastatic renal cell carcinoma, with varying success. The essential problems raised by the management of this disease can be summarized by two questions: (*a*) Should routine radical nephrectomy be performed when metastases are present? (*b*) What is the therapeutic approach to the metastatic sites?

Radical Nephrectomy in Metastatic Renal Cell Carcinoma

For several decades, palliative nephrectomy has been the treatment of choice for metastatic renal cell carcinoma based on the assumption that: (*a*) the metastases may regress spontaneously after the removal of the primary tumor; (*b*) the removal of a large symptomatic tumor may

Table 13.1
Number of Metastases and Number of Organs Involved

	At Diagnosis (%)	At Autopsy (%)
Metastases		
Multiple	97	
Solitary	3	
Number of organs involved		
Limited to one organ	70	9
More than one organ	30	81

Table 13.2
Sites and Frequency of Metastases from Renal Cell Carcinoma

Site	At Diagnosis (%)	At Autopsy (%)
Lung and mediastinum	50	67
Bone	49	39
Skin	11	13
Liver	8	39
Brain	3	6

have an important palliative effect; (c) palliative nephrectomy may improve the survival. Experience has shown that these assumptions are a poor basis for routine nephrectomy in patients with metastatic renal cell carcinoma.

Spontaneous regression of metastases occurs very rarely after nephrectomy (in less than 0.5% of cases (4)), and often this regression is only transient. In addition, Freed et al (5) noted that three of the reported cases of spontaneous regression occurred in the absence of surgical intervention; thus, surgery is not a necessary concomitant of spontaneous regression. Furthermore, palliative nephrectomy is associated with an operative mortality of 2 to 10%, depending on the criteria of patient selection. Recent reports (6–8) suggesting a response of metastases after angiographic infarction of the primary tumor followed by nephrectomy need to be confirmed before such a procedure can be recommended as standard treatment.

Relief of symptoms is rarely a major concern in patients with metastases. The primary tumor is rarely associated with severe or significant symptoms, and patients with multiple metastases (97% of patients) have a poor prognosis; 50% will die within 6 months. In some cases, particularly in high risk patients, the indication for palliative nephrectomy in symptomatic patients can be replaced by angiographic infarction.

There is little evidence to suggest that patient *survival* is increased after adjunctive radical nephrectomy in patients with distant metastases. DeKernion and Lindner (9), Chatelain (10), and others have demonstrated that patients undergoing adjunctive nephrectomy have the same survival as the general population of patients with metastatic renal cell carcinoma.

Although routine adjunctive nephrectomy cannot be recommended in every case of metastatic renal cell carcinoma, this procedure may be beneficial in some patients:

1. In cases with severe symptoms caused by the primary tumor, such as bleeding or pain, in patients who have reasonable life expectancy of at least 5 months. Angiographic infarction should be reserved for poor risk patients, though serial infarction of segmental vessels to large tumors may provide a viable alternative to surgery.
2. In cases with solitary metastases (3% of all cases). Two-thirds of these patients will survive for more than 2 years. Therefore, resection of the solitary metastasis together with nephrectomy seems to be a reasonable approach.
3. As a means of psychologic support in patients in good condition who wish to have the tumor removed, other indications for adjunctive nephrectomy are more controversial. Maldazys and deKernion (11) studied the survival of a large number of renal carcinoma patients and identified favorable prognostic factors: a good performance status, a completely resectable primary tumor, limited tumor burden, and metastases limited to the lungs. The 3-year survival after adjunctive nephrectomy in this select group was over 30%. Perhaps the same survival would have been achieved without nephrectomy, but quality of life would probably have been compromised. Those authors currently offer patients in this group adjunctive nephrectomy followed by treatment on experimental protocols.

TREATMENT OF METASTATIC LOCALIZATIONS

Treatment Modalities

SURGICAL EXCISION OF METASTASES

Local excision is an effective form of treatment in patients with solitary metastasis (1 to 3% of all cases). Surgery is not indicated in cases with multiple metastases because of the poor survival. The indications and the techniques for the excision of metastases vary according to the site of the metastasis.

Lung metastases are the most frequent metastatic site and are usually treated surgically by wedge resection, rarely by lobectomy, and exceptionally by pneumonectomy. Survival after removal of solitary pulmonary metastases varies according to whether the lesion is concomitant (mean survival of 18 months) or secondary to radical nephrectomy (mean survival of 3 years).

However, because of the relative rarity of these lesions, a number of other diagnoses should also be considered. Sarcoidosis, tuberculosis, and certain collagen and fungal diseases can produce lesions on the chest X-ray that mimic lung metastases. These non-neoplastic lesions may regress spontaneously or in response to medical treatment. Whenever there is a doubt about the diagnosis, a period of observation may be justified. Although the best indication for surgery is solitary metastasis, multiple metastases can be excised when they are unilateral.

Bone metastases rank second in clinical frequency. Surgery has a place in the treatment of large lytic lesions in weight-bearing bones (especially the femur) with the aim of relieving pain and preventing pathologic fractures. In patients with a life expectancy of at least 3 or 4 months, an orthopaedic fixation can be performed, possibly associated with curettage of the lesions with or without local cryotherapy with liquid nitrogen (12). In some cases, a more aggressive attitude has been followed (12) with total replacement of the affected bone. The results are favorable in selected cases of solitary metastases, but the survival is poor in patients with multiple metastases.

Brain metastases are usually associated with significant clinical symptoms. In some cases, they may be the first sign of the disease. Surgery is the treatment of choice for solitary brain metastases. The selection of patients for surgery has been improved by the computerized tomography scan. The metastases can usually be "shelled" out, as they often have a plane of cleavage from normal brain tissue. The mean survival in patients with untreated solitary brain metastases is about 3 months, whereas in patients undergoing surgical resection of solitary brain metastases, the mean survival is about 7 months (13).

Liver metastases are much more frequent at autopsy than at diagnosis. They occur late in the course of the disease and are an index of poor prognosis. Solitary metastases can be treated by partial hepatectomy. The survival in these cases is generally very poor.

RADIOTHERAPY

Renal cell carcinoma is considered relatively radioresistant. Halpern and Harisiadis (14) treated 35 patients with 36 sites of bone pain and 14 obstructive or palpable masses and 10 sites of CNS metastasis. They compared treatment courses which differed in terms of time (T), total dose (D) and number of fractions (7). Bone pain responded in 77% of cases with TDF equivalent doses of 45 to 65. Eighty-six percent of these responses lasted for the remainder of the patient's life. In weight-bearing bones like the femur, a TDF equivalent dose of 75 to 86 may be required. The same authors found that brain metastases and spinal cord compression did not respond well to radiation. They concluded that painful bone metastases constitute the major indication for radiotherapy.

Attempts have been made to treat painful bone metastases with radioactive strontium. Despite promising results in some trials, the authors obtained no significant palliative effects in seven patients treated at the Hôpital de la Pitié in Paris. In view of the harmful environmental effects associated with strontium, they do not recommend the use of this treatment in clinical practice.

Systemic Treatment

HORMONE THERAPY

The use of hormones in renal cell carcinoma (Table 13.3) has a rational basis in animal model systems. Estrogens induce renal tumors in Syrian hamsters and some other species. Bloom and Wallace were the first to use hormones to treat patients with renal cell carcinoma. In 1971, Bloom reported a series of 80 patients and reviewed the literature.

Table 13.3
Trials of Hormone Therapy

Drug	Researchers	No. of Patients	CR	PR
Medroxyprogesterone acetate	Pizzocaro et al (30), Tirelli et al (31), Stolbach et al (18), Talley (32)	116	7	4
Testosterone	Talley (32), Tirelli et al (31)	48	0	0
Tamoxifen	Al-Sarraf (33), Glick et al (34), Mulder and Alexieva-Figusch (35), Ferrazzi et al (36), Weiselberg (21)	106	0	2
Nafoxidine	Feun et al (17), Stolbach et al (18)	39	2	2
Estramustine	Swanson and Johnson (37)	16	0	0
Flutamide	Ahmed (38)	25	0	1

He obtained an objective response in about 15% of cases. The criteria of response in this series and in the series which he reviewed were variable, and some of them would not be acceptable in modern clinical trials.

Since 1973, a number of trials have shown a very poor response to progestational agents. Hrushesky reported a series of 415 patients treated with hormones between 1971 and 1976 with a response rate of only 2% (15). More recently, there has been a loss of interest in progestagens in most centers. In a review of 110 patients at the University of California, Los Angeles, no patients were found to have an objective response to progestational agents (2). In a prospective, randomized study at this same center, no objective benefit was observed with progesterone or testosterone, compared with a placebo (16).

Although there have not been any good studies comparing the relative advantages of various doses and routes of administration (oral or intramuscular), the poor response to progesterone is unlikely to be due to inadequate doses (the average daily oral dose was 160 mg of diethylprogesterone).

Despite the limited data available, the authors can make a number of generalizations about hormone therapy: (a) Most responses appear to occur within 6 to 8 weeks of starting hormone treatment, so it is not useful to continue hormone therapy beyond this period in the case of nonresponse. (b) The response rate seems to be higher in men than in women, and progestational agents seem to be more effective than androgens. Antiestrogens have been reported to be active in renal cell carcinoma. Nafoxidine and tamoxifen have also been used with limited effectiveness (17–21).

Hormone receptor assays, which have been useful in predicting response in breast cancer, have also been studied in renal cell carcinoma. Concolino et al (19) demonstrated that some patients with positive progesterone receptors responded to therapy, while those with no receptors did not respond at all.

More recently, Nakano et al (22) studied the hormone receptors in the cytosol of 41 specimens of renal cell carcinoma. No significant correlation was observed between histopathologic findings and the hormone receptors. Seventeen patients with advanced disease were treated with medroxyprogesterone acetate, and although there was no regression in tumor size, the survival of patients with one or more receptors was significantly higher than in patients with negative receptors.

Hormone receptors are unable to predict accurately which patients are likely to respond to the commonly used hormonal agents. In any case, this new approach could hardly improve the overall response rate, which still remains minimal.

The major impetus for the continued use of progestational agents is the lack of effective chemotherapeutic agents and the relative paucity of side effects from hormone therapy. A beneficial trophic action may be observed. Patients occasionally experience nausea, vomiting, edema, breast tenderness, and uterine bleeding, but these symptoms are rarely severe. Detailed results of various trials of hormonal treatment for renal cell are reviewed by Torti (23). In Chapter 14 Bono presents a detailed analysis of all data related to hormone therapy and receptors.

CHEMOTHERAPY

There is a general consensus that renal cell carcinoma is one of the few solid tumors which has remained almost totally refractory to standard chemotherapy. Occasional reports suggesting a beneficial effect of a particular chemotherapy regimen are usually not confirmed by follow-up trials.

Single agents. Table 13.4 summarizes the literature concerning results of single-agent chemotherapy. Although the response criteria were not

Table 13.4
Single-Agent Chemotherapy Trials

Drug[a]	Researchers	No. of Patients	Complete Response	Partial Response
AMSA	Schneider et al (39), Van Echo et al (40)	37	0	1
Baker's antifol	Bukowski et al (41)	17	1	0
Methotrexate	Baumgartner et al (42)	20	0	2
Ifosfamide	Fossa and Table (43)	15	0	1
CTX (high dose)	Wajsman et al (44)	12	0	0
Methyl-GAG	Todd et al (45), Callahan and Knight (26)	76	1	6
CCNU	Merrin et al (46)	23	0	4
5-Fluorouracil	Talley (32)	12	0	0
Hydroxyurea	Stolbach et al (18), Talley (32)	24	0	1
Velban	Talley (32)	15	0	2
Actinomycin D	Hahn et al (47), Talley (32)	65	0	1
Triazimate	Hahn et al (47)	59	1	2
cis-Platinum	Rodriguez and Johnson (48)	32	0	0
NMHE	Amiel et al (27)	22	1	2

[a] AMSA, 4'-(g-acridinylamino)methanesulfon-*m*-anisidide; CTX, cyclophosphamide; NMHE, *N*-methyl-hydroxy-elliptinium.

uniform and the drug dosage schedules varied, there was an obvious lack of therapeutic effectiveness. The rare cases of complete response may correspond to the manifestation of the natural history of the disease, as this tumor can occasionally regress spontaneously without any treatment (5).

The agent most commonly used is vinblastine. Hrushesky and Murphy (24) recently made a retrospective review of 35 chemotherapeutic agents. He reported a 25% objective response rate following treatment with vinblastine, which surpassed the activity of any other single agents or combinations. As shown in Table 13.4, a number of partial responses have been attributed to vinblastine. DeKernion and Lindner (9) treated 16 patients with vinblastine and noted stabilization of metastases in 3 patients for 3 months or longer and partial regression in 1 patient. No patients had complete regression of metastases.

The other drug which is frequently recommended is CCNU (Table 13.4). Occasional responses have been reported, but the authors' experience of 11 cases has been disappointing, with no objective responses.

There was initial optimism following the report of several cases of partial regression with methyl-GAG (25). However, the toxicity was severe and subsequent reports indicated only 3 partial responses in a group of 51 evaluable patients (26).

N-Methyl-hydroxy-elliptinium acetate has been used by Amiel et al (27) in 22 evaluable patients; there were 2 partial responses, 7 cases of stabilization, and 1 complete, lasting remission. This protocol also appeared to have low toxicity.

In conclusion, the maximal objective response rate which one can expect from a single chemotherapeutic agent is approximately 15% (10). In the light of the natural history of this tumor, this low level of activity is probably not clinically significant. However, in patients with severe pain, even a low level of symptomatic activity may justify a trial of chemotherapy. Vinblastine, CCNU, and methyl-GAG appear to be the most appropriate choices.

Combination chemotherapy. In view of the poor response rate of metastatic renal cell carcinoma to single agents, the selection of agents for combination therapy has often been based on criteria of toxicity and patient tolerance rather than antitumor effect. Experience with combination chemotherapy is reviewed in Table 13.5.

Combination chemotherapy has not been shown to have any significant benefit over single-agent therapy. Randomized studies have not shown any advantage, but occasional studies appear to have higher partial response rates than when a single agent is used. However, the number of cases reported is often very small, and the toxicity of these combinations is usually significant. Complete responses are rare, and the duration of response is often limited.

The increased toxicity associated with combination chemotherapy must be weighed against the expected response rate. At the present time, the use of these combinations is only justified in well structured, rigorously conducted therapeutic trials in well informed patients.

Table 13.5
Combination Chemotherapy Trials

Drug[a]	Researchers	No. of Patients	Complete Response	Partial Response
VLB + CCNU	Davis and Munalo (49), Hahn et al (47), Merrin et al (46), Tirelli et al (31)	95	3	9
VLB + methyl CCNU	Merrin et al (46)	15	0	1
VLB + MTX + bleomycin	Levi et al (50), Bell et al (51)	34	0	10
VLB + MTX + bleomycin + tamoxifen	Levi et al (50), Bell et al (51)	34	0	10
VLB + CTX + 5-FU	Halpern et al (52)	10	0	0
VLB + CTX + 5-FU + hydroxyurea + MPA + prednisone	Talley et al (53)	45	1	6
CTX + 5-FU + vincristine + MTX	van der Werf-Messing and Mulder (54)	18	0	0
VLB + CTX + adriamycin + bleomycin + BCG	Dana and Alberts (55)	14	0	3

[a] VLB, vinblastine; CTX, cyclophosphamide; MTX, methotrexate; MPA, medroxyprogesterone acetate.

THE ROLE OF IN VITRO CHEMOTHERAPEUTIC TESTS

The response to chemotherapy has been studied in implanted renal cell carcinomas in athymic mice (28) and in clonogenic assays in vitro (29). In vitro sensitivity to chemotherapy was detected in five of the seven tumors, but no correlation was observed with the clinical results. The most extensive experience with the clonogenic assay for renal carcinoma is that of Michael Lieber at Mayo Clinic. The role of in vitro tests in predicting clinical response of human tumors has not yet been established, and in view of the lack of activity of cytotoxic agents in renal cell carcinoma, its predictive role in this cancer is very uncertain.

MANAGEMENT

Multiple Metastases

The only specific treatment of multiple metastases consists of radiotherapy to bone metastases for pain relief. A trial of hormone therapy may be administered but should be stopped after 2 months if there is no sign of response. High dose steroids may occasionally provide symptomatic relief in end-stage disease. Chemotherapy is only indicated for patients with intractable pain or as part of rigorous, controlled trials. Immunotherapy and interferon are still purely experimental.

Solitary Metastases

Solitary metastases may be more amenable to treatment. The prognosis of these lesions depends on the time of appearance of the metastases. Solitary lesions present at the time of diagnosis have a poorer prognosis than those appearing after radical nephrectomy.

Surgical excision of metastases present at the time of diagnosis is probably of little value. In the comparative study conducted at La Pitié Hospital in Paris (13), the 15 treated patients had the same survival as the untreated group. However, it should be attempted, whenever it is technically possible, as a complement to radical nephrectomy, especially in patients with a specific clinical problem, such as brain metastases or other symptomatic lesions.

Secondary solitary metastases appearing after nephrectomy should be excised whenever technically possible, as it seems to improve survival (13), but it is difficult to know whether this improvement is due to the treatment itself or to the fact that these lesions have a slow growth rate.

REFERENCES

1. Tolia BM, Whitmore WF: Solitary metastases from renal cell carcinoma. *J Urol* 114:836, 1975.
2. deKernion JB, Ramming KP, Smith RB: Natural history of metastatic renal cell carcinoma: computer analysis. *J Urol* 120:148, 1978.
3. O'Dea MJ, Zincke H, Utz DC, Bernatz PE: The treatment of renal cell carcinoma with solitary metastasis. *J Urol* 120:540–542, 1978.
4. Monti JE, Stewart BH, Straffon RA, Bunowsky LHW, Hewitt CB, Montague OK: The role of adjunctive nephrectomy in patients with metastic renal cell carcinoma. *J Urol* 117:272, 1977.
5. Freed SZ, Halperin JP, Gordon M: Idiopathic regression of metastases from renal cell carcinoma. *J Urol* 118:538–541, 1977.
6. Wallace S, Chuang VP, Swanson DA, Bracken B, Hersh EM, Ayala A, Johnson D: Embolization of renal carcinoma. *Radiology* 138:563, 1981.
7. Swanson DA, Wallace S, Johnson DE: The role of embolization and nephrectomy in the treatment of metastatic renal cell carcinoma. *Urol Clin North Am* 7:719, 1980.
8. Giuliani L, Carmignani G, Belgrano A, Puppo P, Quattrini S: Usefulness of preoperative transcatheter embolization of kidney tumors. *Urology* 17:431, 1981.
9. deKernion JB, Lindner A: Treatment of advanced renal cell carcinoma. In Kuss R, Khoury S, Murphy GP, Karr JP (eds): *Renal Tumors: Proceedings of the First International Symposium on Kidney Tumors.* New York, Alan R Liss, 1982.
10. Chatelain C: Is radical nephrectomy useful when metastases are present? In Kuss R, Khoury S, Murphy GP, Karr JP (eds): *Renal Tumors: Proceedings of the First International Symposium on Kidney Tumors.* New York, Alan R Liss, 1982.
11. Maldazys J, deKernion JB: Prognostic factors in metastatic and renal carcinoma. *J Urol* in press.
12. Marcove BC, Sadrieh J, Huvos AG, Grabstald H: Cryosurgery in the treatment of solitary or multiple bone metastases from renal cell carcinoma. *J Urol* 108:540, 1972.
13. Khoury S: The treatment of metastasis from renal cell carcinoma. In Kuss R, Khoury S, Murphy GP, Karr JP (eds): *Renal Tumors: Proceedings of the First International Symposium of Kidney Tumors.* New York, Alan R Liss, 1982.
14. Halpern EC, Harisiadis L: The role of radiation therapy in the management of metastatic renal cell carcinoma. *Cancer* 51:614–617, 1983.
15. Hrushesky WJ: Abstract: what's old and new in advanced renal cell carcinoma. Proc. AACR ASCO 18:318, 1977.
16. Cox C: Personal communication cited by de Kernion JB, Lindner A: Treatment of advanced renal cell carcinoma. In Kuss R, Khoury S, Murphy GP, Karr JP (eds): *Renal Tumors: Proceedings of the First International Symposium on Kidney Tumors.* New York Alan R Liss, 1982.
17. Feun LG, Drelichman A, Singhakowinte C, Vaitkevicius VK: Phase II study of nafoxidine in the therapy for advanced renal carcinoma. *Cancer Treat Rep* 63:149–150, 1979.

18. Stolbach LL, Begg CB, Hall T, Horton J: Treatment of renal carcinoma: a phase III randomized trial of oral medroxyprogesterone (Provera), hydroxyurea and nafoxidine. *Cancer Treat Rep* 65:689–692, 1981.
19. Concolino G, Marocchi A, Conti C, Tenaglia R, Silverio F, Brace U: Human renal cell carcinoma as a hormone-dependent tumor. *Cancer Res* 38:4340–4344, 1978.
20. Al-Sarraf M, Eyre H, Bonnett J, Saiki J, Gagliano R, Pugh R, Lehane D, Dixon D, Bottomly R: Study of tamoxifen in metastatic renal cell carcinoma and the influence of certain prognostic factors: a Southwest Oncology Group study. *Cancer Treat Rep* 65:447–451, 1981.
21. Weiselberg L, Budman D, Vinciguerra V, Schulman P, Degnan TJ: Tamoxifen in unresectable hypernephroma: a phase II trial and review of the literature. *Cancer Clin Trials* 4:195–198, 1981.
22. Nakano E, Tada Y, Fujioka H, Matsuda M, Osafune M, Kotake T, Sato B, Takaha M, Sonoda T: Hormone receptor in renal cell carcinoma and correlation with clinical response to endocrine therapy. *J Urol* 132:240–245, 1984.
23. Torti FM: Treatment of metastatic renal cell carcinoma. *Recent Results Cancer Res* 85:123–142, 1983.
24. Hrushesky WJ, Murphy GP: Current status of the therapy of advanced renal carcinoma. *J Surg Oncol* 9:277–288, 1977.
25. Knight WA III, Livinston RB, Fabian C, Costanzi J: Methyl-glyoxal bis-guanylhydrazone (methyl GAG, MGBG) in advanced human malignancy. *Proc Am Soc Clin Oncol* 20:319, 1979.
26. Callahan SK, Knight WA III: A phase II trials of methyl-glyoxal bisguanylhydrazone (MGBG methyl-GAG) in renal carcinoma. *Proc Am Soc Clin Oncol* 22:164, 1981.
27. Amiel JL, Rouesse J, Droz JP, Caille P, Travagli JP, Theodore C, Le Chevalier T, Ducret JP, Bidart M, Garnier HS: Traitement des cancers du rein metastases de l'adulte par l'acetate d'elliptinium. *Presse Med* 13:1555–1557, 1984.
28. Day JW, Sharivastav L, Lin G, Bonar RA, Paulson DF: In vitro chemotherapeutic testing of urologic tumors. *J Urol* 125:490, 1981.
29. Salmon SE, Hamburger AW, Soehnlen B, Durie BGM, Alberts DS, Moon TE: Quantitation of differential sensitivity of human tumor stem cells to anticancer drugs. *N Engl J Med* 298:1321, 1978.
30. Pizzocaro G, Valente M, Cataldo I, Vezzoni P, DiFronzo G: Estrogen receptors and MPA treatment in metastatic renal carcinoma. A preliminary report. *Tumori* 66:739, 1980.
31. Tirelli S, Frustaci S, Galligioni E, Veronesi A, Trovo MG, Magri DM, Crivellari D, Roncadin M, Tumulo S, Grigoletto E: Medical treatment of metastatic renal cell carcinoma. *Tumori* 66:235, 1980.
32. Talley RW: Chemotherapy of adenocarcinoma of the kidney. *Cancer* 32:1062, 1973.
33. Al-Sarraf M: The clinical trial of tamoxifen in patients with advanced renal cell cancer. A Southwest Oncology Group study. And vinblastine. *Proc Am Soc Clin Oncol* 20:378, 1979.
34. Glick J, Wein A, Nesendank W, Harris D, Brodovsky H, Padavic K, Torri S: Tamoxifen in metastatic prostate and renal cancer. *Proc Am Assoc Cancer Res.* 20:311, 1979.
35. Mulder JH, Alexieva-Figusch I: Tamoxifen in metastatic renal cell carcinoma. *Cancer Treat Rep* 63:1222, 1979.
36. Ferrazzi E, Salvango L, Fornasiero A, Gartei G, Fiorentino M: Tamoxifen treatment for advanced renal cell cancer. *Tumori* 66:601, 1980.
37. Swanson DA, Johnson DE: Estramustine phosphate (Emcyt) as treatment for metastatic renal carcinoma. *Urology* 17:344, 1981.
38. Ahmed T, Benedetto P, Yagoda A, Watson RC, Scher HI, Herr HW, Sogani PC, Whitmore WF, Pertschuk L: Estrogen, progesterone and androgen-binding sites in renal cell carcinoma. Observations obtained in phase II trial of flutamide. *Cancer* 54:477–481, 1984.
39. Schneider RG, Woodcock TM, Yagoda A: Phase II trial of 4′(g-acridinylamino) methanesulfon-*m*-anisidide (AMSA) in patients with metastatic hypernephroma. *Cancer Treat Rep* 64:183, 1980.
40. Van Echo DA, Marcus S, Aisner J, Wiernik PH: Phase II trial of 4′-(g-acridinylamino)

methanesulfon-*m*-anisidide (AMSA) in patients with metastatic renal cell carcinoma. *Cancer Treat Rep* 64:1009, 1980.

41. Bukowski RM, LuBuglio A, McCracken J, Pugh R: Phase II trial of Baker's antifol in metastatic renal cell carcinoma. *Proc Am Soc Clin Oncol* 20:402, 1980.
42. Baumgartner G, Heinz R, Arbes H, Lenzhofer R, Pridun N, Schuller J: Methotrexate-citrovorum factor used alone and in combination chemotherapy for advanced hypernephromas. *Cancer Treat Rep* 64:41, 1980.
43. Fossa SD, Table K: Treatment of metastatic renal cancer with ifosfamide and mesnum with and without irradiation. *Cancer Treat. Rep.* 64:1103, 1980.
44. Wajsman Z, Beckley S, Madajewicz S, Dragone N: High dose cyclophosphamide in metastatic renal cell carcinoma. *Proc Am Assoc Cancer Res* 21:423, 1980.
45. Todd RF, Granick MB, Canellos GP, Richie JP, Gittes RF, Mayer RJ, Skarin AT: Phase I-II trial of methyl-GAG in the treatment of patients with metastatic renal adenocarcinoma. *Cancer Treat Rep* 65:17, 1981.
46. Merrin C, Mittelman A, Famous N, Wajsman Z, Murphy GP: Chemotherapy of advanced renal cell carcinoma with vincristine and CCNU. *J Urol* 113:21, 1975.
47. Hahn RG, Begg CB, David T: Phase II study of vincristine-CCNU, triazinate and dactinomycin in advanced renal cell cancer. *Cancer Treat Rep* 65:711, 1981.
48. Rodriguez LH, Johnson DE: Clinical trial of cis-platinum (NSC 119875) in metastatic renal cell carcinoma. *Urology* 11:344, 1978.
49. Davis TE, Munalo FB: Combination chemotherapy of advanced renal cell carcinoma with CCNU and vinblastine. *Proc Am Assoc Cancer Res* 19:316, 1978.
50. Levi JA, Dalley D, Aroney R: A comparative trial of the combination vinblastine, methotrexate and bleomycin with and without tamoxifen for metastatic renal cell carcinoma. *Proc Am Assoc Cancer Res* 21:426, 1980.
51. Bell DR, Aroney RS, Fisher RJ, Levi JA: High-dose methotrexate with leucovorin rescue, vinblastine and bleomycin with or without tamoxifen in metastatic renal cell carcinoma. *Cancer Treat Rep* 68:587–590, 1984.
52. Halpern J, Brufman G, Shnider B, Biran S: Vinblastine, cyclophosphamide and 5-fluorouracil combination chemotherapy for metastatic hypernephroma. *Oncology* 38:193, 1981.
53. Talley RW, Oberhauser NA, Brownlee RW, O'Bryan RM: Chemotherapy of metastatic renal adenocarcinoma with five drug regimen. *Henry Ford Hosp Med J* 27:110, 1979.
54. van der Werf-Messing B, Mulder J: Metastatic kidney cancer treated with multiple drug therapy at the Rotterdam Radiotherapy Institute. *Br J Cancer* 29:491, 1974.
55. Dana BW, Alberts DS: Combination chemoimmunotherapy for advanced renal cell cancer with adriamycin, bleomycin, vincristine, cyclophosphamide plus BCG. *Cancer Clin Trials* 4:205, 1981.

14

Steroid Hormones and Hormonal Treatment in Renal Cell Carcinoma

Aldo V. Bono

INTRODUCTION

No treatment of renal cell carcinoma (RCC), except surgery, has proved to be effective so far. Hormonal therapy in metastatic patients has been advocated on the basis of a certain amount of experimental work. However, the correlations between the endocrine system and, in particular, between the male and female gonads and renal cancer are far from being fully investigated.

Some activities of steroid hormones on renal parenchyma in experimental animals have been well demonstrated. For instance, androgen administration has been known for four decades to induce renal parenchymal hypertrophy (1), whereas estrogens may cause degenerative changes and reverse androgen-induced hypertrophy (2).

Estrogen activity seems to be antagonized by progesterone, which increases renal volume previously reduced by estrogen administration (3). Further laboratory observations proved that prolonged estrogen treatment is able to induce renal adenomatoid tumors in golden Syrian hamsters (4). This requires more clinical investigation.

The results deriving from a number of clinical experiences using hormonal manipulation in human RCC cannot yet be considered conclusive. In fact, early reports showing a relevant percentage of favorable results obtained by hormonal therapy in human RCC were usually based on uncontrolled clinical trials. In contrast, in more recent controlled series, favorable responses induced by hormonal therapy in patients affected by RCC are relatively infrequent.

The matter becomes even more complex when the reports concerning steroid receptors in normal kidney and in human RCC are taken into account. The presence of hormonal receptors in renal parenchyma or in RCC is not universally accepted, and the significance, both in the concentration and in the threshold, is not agreed upon. Moreover, even if steroid receptors are found in noticeable concentration, the responsiveness of a given RCC to hormonal therapy cannot be taken for granted.

Finally, according to some observations, preoperative hormonal treatment might stimulate the formation of receptors. It is hoped that further investigations will be made so that this point can be fully elucidated. The aim of this chapter is to summarize the data and information related to the controversial issue of hormone dependence of human RCC.

GENERAL OBSERVATIONS

RCC is sometimes described as "hormone-dependent neoplasia" (5) and its responsiveness to the hormonal treatment is often emphasized (6). The basic observations supporting the previous statements are both experimental (tumor induction by estrogens and inhibition by estrogen antagonists) and clinical (the finding of specific hormonal receptors in renal normal tissue and in RCC, metastasis regression under hormonal manipulation, and longer survival in hormone-treated patients).

General factors, such as sex and age, have been postulated as demonstrative of the hormonal dependence of RCC. Many reports show that a variety of factors could be equally involved in RCC etiology. It may be worth recalling some of the most significant ones.

Notes on Epidemiology

It is well known that there is a substantial male predominance in sex distribution of incidence of RCC, which may indicate that human RCC is "under some sort of hormonal influence" (7). In various series, about twice as many RCCs are observed in males (8) as in females. Furthermore the age-adjusted rates usually show that the real incidence of renal cancer is perhaps almost 3 times greater in males than in females (9). According to some reports (10) the maximum predominance of RCC in males corresponds to the childbearing period in women and drops to a ratio of 2:1 in subjects above 40 years of age. This observation may suggest that "hormone changes in pregnancy act as a protective factor for women against RCC" and may thereby confirm the alleged "endocrine sensitivity" of RCC (11).

However, in contrast with the previous observations, incidence and mortality curves by sex for RCC and the comparison between the male-female age-specific death rates did not show any statistical difference within each age group in either Los Angeles County (12) nor in the district of Varese (13). Consequently, the interpretation of any sexual difference in the incidence of RCC is still open to question.

Even if the epidemiology of RCC has not been extensively studied, a certain number of observations probably indicate that factors different from sex and hormones are involved in the etiology of RCC:

1. *Age.* Prior to 35 years of age RCC is rare even if recent observations show a trend towards younger age group (14).

2. *Urbanization.* The incidence of RCC is statistically higher in urban and industrialized areas (15).
3. *Socioeconomic class.* Incidence and death rate are slightly but significantly associated with higher social classes (13).
4. *Environmental influence.* The age-adjusted incidence rates for RCC are almost 5 times higher in Scandinavian countries than in such low risk areas as Japan and Italy. It is interesting to note that Scandinavian people who migrate to low or medium risk countries, such as the U.S.A., show a lower incidence rate than in their native countries (12, 16).

Association of RCC with Endocrine Pathologic Condition

RCC has been correlated with a few endocrinopathies. There have been isolated reports of increased frequency of RCC in diabetes mellitus, adrenal cortical hyperfunction, and obesity.

A positive correlation between RCC and obesity was found by Wynder et al (17) in a case-control study, but this was only applicable to postmenopausal obese women. The interpretation of this observation could lie in the fact that the adipose tissues are rich in enzymes converting androstenediose into estrone, producing large amounts of circulating estrogens. The same report failed to demonstrate any correlation between excess body weight and RCC in males.

EXPERIMENTAL DATA

The first experimental observations relating estrogens to renal cancer were those of Matthews et al (4), who obtained adenomatoid renal tumors in male golden Syrian hamsters through prolonged estrogen administration. Subsequent studies (18) showed that the administration of diethylstilbestrol (DES) over a long period of time could induce bilateral renal tumors in 75% of the treated animals. Hormonal dependence of these tumors was partly confirmed by the observation that transplantation of the DES-induced tumors was possible, but only when estrogen was simultaneously administered to the recipient hamsters (19). The presence of estrogens is also required to allow in vitro growth of renal cancer cells (20). Moreover the transplantation of the DES-induced tumor required estrogen treatment of the recipient hamsters. It was not successful if antiandrogenic drugs were given at the same time (19, 21). Serial transplantation, however, gradually released neoplastic tissue from hormone dependence.

Administration of testosterone and progesterone simultaneously with DES prevented the transplant from being accepted (22, 23). Other hormones or related substances, such as corticosteroids (19) and bromoergocriptine (24), had an inhibitory effect on the DES-induced tumor (22).

Extirpation of endocrine glands in experimental animals was extensively studied in order to clarify the effects of estrogen administration, but the results are still controversial and poorly understood.

Adrenalectomy in a hamster bearing a well developed RCC transplant reduced the growth rate of the transplanted tumor (25). In other words, corticosteroid suppression, reached through bilateral adrenalectomy, seems to have an inhibitory effect similar to that produced by corticosteroid administration. Kirkman and Bacon (18) pointed out that the maximum incidence of estrogen-induced tumors could be observed in the male hamster after castration. Yet orchidectomy seemed to depress the development of tumors as well as the growth of well established transplants (19). Even in animals in which RCC had been obtained in spite of previous adrenalectomy, orchidectomy produced some regression of the tumor (25).

It is well known that in female Syrian hamsters estrogen treatment can induce renal tumors only before sexual maturity or after it has come to an end. Ovariectomy during the fertile period allows the development of experimental tumors, perhaps because of the suppression of the source of natural progestagens (22). However, ovariectomy also abolished the most important sources of natural estrogens. Therefore, it is not clear why a sharp reduction of natural estrogens should facilitate the development of RCC through exogenous estrogens.

The pituitary gland plays an important role in DES induction of RCC in hamsters. In castrated and hypophysectomized golden Syrian hamsters, estrogen administration by itself cannot induce renal tumors or allow the survival of subcapsular RCC grafts. From these observations Lin et al. (26) came to the conclusion that the hypophysis might produce a promoting substance which is essential to tumor induction. This hypothesis is also supported by the fact that simultaneous administration of luteinizing, hormone, follicle-stimulating hormone, and prolactin does not restore the possibility to produce RCCs from estrogen administration in hypophysectomized hamsters.

On the basis of the findings concerning tumor inhibition obtained by progesterone associated with cortisone (27), and taking into account some data from the observation of experimental ablative endocrine surgery, progestational therapy has been proposed for humans (27). So far, however, experimental studies have not completely elucidated the complex problem of tumorigenesis in experimental animals. The greatest uncertainty is derived from the fact that the golden Syrian hamster is actually the only animal species in which estrogen administration causes renal tumors. Even if other reports (28) suggest that the European hamster may also be prone to DES-induced RCC, it seems unlikely that these particular experimental observations might be entirely transferred to human pathology.

Finally it is also important to point out that other information concerning a nonhormonal etiology of RCC is available: (a) Naturally occurring RCC seems to be a relatively rare tumor in lower animals, and, in particular, there are no reports of spontaneous renal tumors in hamsters (29). (b) In animals RCC can also be produced through viral infection. The early observation of the viral origin of leopard frog RCC (30) is well known. More recently, in birds and rodents, many viruses have been recognized as etiologic factors of RCC (31). (c) In spontaneous animal tumor models, results which are in contrast with the hypothesis of estrogen induction of RCC have been observed. In 1973 Soloway and

Myers (32) in an extensive study on spontaneous RCC in mice, reported that tumor growth inhibition could be registered in both sexes with either DES or testosterone administration, whereas cortisone and medroxyprogesterone acetate (MPA) did not show any inhibitory effect.

In 1982 Murphy (33) studied an RCC in an inbred line of BALB mice. Administration of MPA did not affect the tumor developmental patterns at all. Testosterone induced a more extensive spread of metastases and shorter survival periods if compared with controls. As in the previous model DES administration reduced the survival time and enhanced metastasization.

STEROID RECEPTORS IN NORMAL KIDNEY AND IN RENAL CELL CARCINOMA

Introduction

Recent laboratory investigations tend to demonstrate the presence of cytoplasmic and nuclear hormone receptors in tissues that are not usually considered to be targets for the hormones. For example, there are few investigations demonstrating a significant amount of androgen receptors in the epithelium of the larynx in both sexes (34). In the female, the bladder trigone has been found to be rich in estrogen receptors (35). In clinical oncology, estrogen and progesterone receptors have been hypothesized since 1976 in human malignant melanoma (36). The presence of hormone receptors in these normal tissues and in tumors whose hormone dependence is unclear suggested the possibility that steroid receptors might exist in tissues that are not manifestly under the hormonal action, and thereby that tumors arising from them could be hormonally dependent. Human RCC, owing to the above mentioned experimental and epidemiologic premises, may fall into this class of hormone-dependent or hormone-related neoplasias (37). The reported activity of progestagens against human RCC might be explained if a significant amount of progesterone receptors could be demonstrated in cancer tissues of responsive patients.

Outline of Receptor Assays

Laboratory assays for the determination of steroid receptors in tissue are complex and numerous. Each method offers disadvantages and limitations. A complete survey of such methods is beyond the scope of this chapter, but some remarks will be useful for the purpose of understanding the problem.

Usually the tissue specimens are quickly frozen with liquid nitrogen after removal and after the dissection of necrotic areas. At the moment of the assay the frozen tissue is pulverized with an automatic device and the powder so obtained is thawed to 0 to 4°C, buffered, homogenated, and centrifuged (from 30,000 to 200,000 g). At the end of the centrifugation, the layer of floating lipids is removed and the protein-containing supernatant (usually called cytosol) is recovered. The protein content of cytosol is estimated by spectophotometry and then diluted to a concentration of 4 to 10 mg/ml.

Two parallel methods of receptor assays are frequently used at this stage: (*a*) the dextran-coated charcoal assay and (*b*) the sucrose-gradient centrifugation.

For method *a*, aliquots of cytosol are added to a parallel series of tubes containing H3-steroid hormone solutions in increasing concentration in either the presence or the absence of a 100- to 500-fold excess of unlabeled steroid. The reagents commonly used are: DES and R 2858 for estrogen receptors (ER); R5020 synthetic progestin or H3-progesterone 2, 4, 6, 7 or H3-*d*-norgestrel for progesterone receptors (PGR); dexamethasone for corticosteroids; R1881 for androgens (AR). Cytosols are then incubated for a long period of time (15 to 18 hours), the free hormone is usually removed with activated dextran-coated charcoal (38), the samples are centrifuged, and the supernatant radioactivity is measured. The binding capacity and affinity are finally analyzed by Scatchard's method (39).

In addition to the previous assay, other methods use gel filtration in buffered Sephadex LH20 columns for the incubated cytosols (40), agar gel electrophoresis (41), or precipitation in protamine sulfate (42).

For method *b*, aliquots of buffered cytosols are allowed to react with tritiated or unlabeled hormones and then are treated in the same way as in the charcoal assay. The supernatant fluids are assayed for receptor activity by layering over linear 50 to 200 gr/liter sucrose gradients. After centrifugation the bottoms of the tubes are pierced and a few drops of the fractions are collected for the measurement of radioactivity.

Recently new techniques for simultaneous determination of ER and PGR (43) and new approaches for the ERs using fluorescent ligands have been proposed (44). The addition of dexamethasone to the incubating cytosols is advocated in PGR determination to ensure that R5020 does not bind to glucocorticoid receptors (45). Some laboratories, however, do not perform this step.

It is therefore not surprising that modifications in the methods performed by various institutions may occur—differences in rate of centrifugation, dilution of cytosols, entity of the excess steroids, choice of radioligands, time of incubation, etc. This results in the final measurement being affected due to the incidence of variable factors. It is also clear that the threshold beyond which the presence of the receptors has to be considered positive may become questionable and can vary when specific methods are used. For example, the threshold of positivity is usually considered to be the binding capacity of 5 fmoles/mg of protein with a K_d of 0.5 to 6.5×10^{-9} M for ER and of 10 fmoles/mg of protein with a K_d of 2 to 10×10^{-9} M for PGR. Table 14.1, modified from Karr et al (45), summarizes the values of receptors for the human kidney as determined in various laboratories.

Hormonal Receptors in Kidneys of Experimental Animals

The presence of steroid receptors in the normal kidney of experimental animals has been reported by many investigators. Estrogen receptors have been found in rats (46), in guinea pigs (47), and in golden Syrian hamsters (48). Androgen receptors have been detected in mice (49) and

Table 14.1
Cytosol Receptors in Human Kidney and RCC[a]

	Normal Kidney		RCC	
	Fmoles/mg of Cytosol Protein	K_d	Fmoles/mg of Cytosol Protein	K_d
Androgen	1–12	$1–5 \times 10^{-9}$ M	1–27	$1 \times 10^{-9}/50 \times 10^{-10}$ M
Estrogens	0–60	$2–7 \times 10^{-9}$ M	1–10	$1–9 \times 10^{-9}$ M
Progestin	8–40	$2–64 \times 10^{-9}$ M	0–50	$3 \times 10^{-8}/9 \times 10^{-9}$ M
Glucocorticoid	4.2–18	$4.3–10 \times 10^{-9}$ M	7–118.5	$0.4 \times 10^{-8}/9.5 \times 10^{-9}$ M
Aldosterone	1–110	$3 \times 10^{-7}/3 \times 10^{-9}$ M	1–7	1×10^{-8} M

[a] From data of Bojar et al (107), Chen et al (65), Concolino et al (108), Di Fronzo et al (64), Hemstreet et al (63), Karr et al (45), Rafestin-Obin et al (52), Robustelli Della Cuna et al (83), Tobin et al (71).

in Syrian hamsters (50); mineralocorticoid receptors (51) and a glucocorticoid receptor (52) have been found in rats. Low levels of progesterone receptors are reported in Syrian hamster kidney (53).

However, the presence of steroid receptors in normal kidneys is not correlated to their susceptibility to spontaneous or DES-induced RCC (45). It is remarkable to note that the normal kidney of the rat shows ER concentrations almost double those of the intact Syrian hamster kidney (54).

In the estrogen-treated hamster the concentration of renal steroid receptors usually increases in a very significant way. The administration of 17β-estradiol, estrone, or DES induces the appearance of high quantities of PGRs, while the withdrawal of estrogens rapidly decreases their concentration (55). Estrogen treatment is followed by an increase of ER concentration even before the occurrence of RCC (54). The RCC hamster model is characterized by the significant presence of cytosolic receptors for progesterone, estradiol, dihydrotestosterone, dexamethasone, and aldosterone (45) mentioned in their order of concentration: these receptor findings persist even after some intraperitoneal passages (56). In the murine spontaneous tumor model (57), receptor determinations showed a measurable presence of ER, whereas PGRs were absent and ARs were present in traces (45). This tumor, however, was unaffected by medroxyprogesterone acetate (inhibiting Syrian hamster DES-induced tumor) and showed an enhancement in growth under testosterone administration.

Hormonal Receptors: Experience in Humans

In this chapter we previously reported that hormonal therapy for human RCC has been introduced on the basis of a somewhat empirical rationale (58). As some responses in advanced cases had been registered, the research of steroid receptors (SR) was widely performed by urologic oncologists in an attempt to assess the possibility of some hormone responsiveness, as in the case of breast cancer.

Many institutions systematically undertake receptor profiles in RCC patients, and the presence of high affinity/low capacity binding sites for steroid hormones is frequently reported (Table 14.1). However, the value of receptor concentrations often ranges between very low and very

STEROID HORMONES AND HORMONAL TREATMENT   211

high figures, which makes the results look clearly conflicting. For example, in human kidney progesterone receptors were found in significant concentrations (from 11.22 to 45.26 fmoles/mg of protein), as were estrogen receptors (ER = 30.04 to 53.23 fmoles/mg of protein). These results were reported by Concolino et al (59, 60), which lead the authors to define the kidney as a "target tissue" for steroid hormones. But the concentrations of ER and PGR determined in the oncologic division laboratory of the Fondazione Clinica del Lavoro, (Pavia, Italy) on 76 specimens—half normal and half neoplastic kidney, including specimens of both normal renal tissue and the tumor*—ranged from 0.001 to 9.57 fmoles for the ER and from 0 to 12.12 fmoles for the PGR. The previous quotations represent striking extremes of the data which are reported in the literature and are summarized below.

ESTROGEN RECEPTORS

ERs were first described in renal tissue by Fanestil et al (61) and by Bojar et al (62) with a binding capacity ranging from 20 to 60 fmoles/mg of cytosol protein. In 1976 the above mentioned results by Concolino et al were published, and a mean of 24 fmoles/mg of protein was reported in 1980 by Hemstreet et al (63) in normal kidney and RCC. However, the results shown in other studies were not in agreement with these findings. Di Fronzo et al (64) found that only 3 of 31 specimens of normal kidneys had a concentration of ER greater than 5 fmoles and only two RCCs were positive. It is interesting to note that in a single case of RCC reported by Di Fronzo et al with undectable ER in primary tumor, 13 fmoles of ER were found in lymph node metastases.

Chen et al (65) and the author's group (66) found ER only in traces. Karr et al (45) reported 3 cases of positive ER (ranging from 14.2 to 24.2 fmoles) in 18 tumorous kidneys examined, whereas only 2 normal tissue specimens were positive for ER. The CNR group (67, 68) found ER in significant concentration in 5 of 27 (18.5%) M_0 RCCs and in 4 of 23 (17.4%) M_1 RCCs with means of 4.2 fmoles and of 3.2 fmoles/mg of protein, respectively.

PROGESTERONE RECEPTORS

The literature offers similar discrepancies concerning the concentration of PGR. Usually the same authors reporting high concentration of ER tend to confirm the presence of PGR in large amounts. Bojar et al (69, 70) analyzed 88 cases of RCC, but the PGR concentrations were low, as a rule under 5 fmoles. These results appear to be in agreement with those of other laboratories (71, 72). The same authors made an attempt to induce higher levels of PGR by preoperative estrogen priming in 24 patients. No specimen of the low dose treated cases ($n = 8$) and only 2 of the 16 treated with high dose estrogen showed PGR in concentrations above the level of 5 fmoles. The presence of progestin binding inhibitors was eventually excluded in a subsequent study (73).

A very interesting experience has recently been reported by Bracci et

---

* The specimens were harvested at the Urological Department of the Regional Hospital of Varese, Italy.

al (74), who treated patients affected by RCC for 7 days before nephrectomy with an antiestrogen (tamoxifen, 20 mg/day). The PGR concentrations in both normal renal tissue and in RCC from ablated kidney were always very high compared with the untreated patients (femtomoles of PGR in untreated patients: normal tissue = 2.96 − RCC = 4.09 ± 2.81; femtomoles of PGR in tamoxifen-treated patients: normal tissue = 66.13 − RCC = 16.43 ± 4.05.

ANDROGEN RECEPTORS AND GLUCOCORTICOID RECEPTORS

The assay of androgen receptors is not as frequently performed as ER and PGR determinations. In 10 tumor specimens Chen et al (65) found significant amounts of AR (from 1.4 to 26.7 fmoles with a mean of 13.5 ± 8.4), and these findings were confirmed by Concolino et al (6), who reported positive findings for nuclear AR (assayed by the methods of Anderson et al (75) and of Walters and Clark (76) in 8 of 14 RCC specimens.

However, Karr et al (45) could not confirm these results in a series of 12 cases, as they found only very low values of AR (1 to 4.5 fmoles). The above mentioned CNR group reported positivity for AR in only 6 of 68 (8.8%) specimens of RCC with a mean of 6.3 fmoles/mg of protein.

On the contrary, glucocorticoid receptors were almost always detected in normal kidneys and in RCC (45, 52, 65, 69, 70, 73, 77).

MINERALOCORTICOID RECEPTORS

According to Pasqualini et al (78) mineralocorticoid receptors are present in normal kidney tissue, but in RCC they appear in lower concentrations (6 to 7 times less). An explanation for this may be the well known fact that RCC originates from proximal tubule cells (52, 79).

From all of the data obtained by steroid receptor determinations, it may be assumed that the response of some patients to progestational therapy could be mediated at the intracellular level.

Medroxyprogesterone acetate inhibits more than 80% of specific binding in the tumor tissue (69, 70, 73, 77), thus reducing the growth-facilitating action of glucocorticoids on neoplastic cells.

In conclusion, the preceding review suggests that receptor analysis of renal specimens may be useful for the further elucidation of the biochemical behavior of RCC. It may even be useful for diagnostic purposes, provided there proves to be a correlation between steroid receptors and responsiveness of the tumor to hormonal treatment.

HORMONAL TREATMENT IN RENAL CELL CARCINOMA

Hormonal Treatment in Advanced Cases

Hormonal therapy of RCC was introduced soon after the observations on estrogen induction of renal cancer in hamsters. Bloom (27) started treating advanced human RCC with MPA and testosterone and reported a 20% partial response rate. Since then many clinical experiences have been published with MPA, megestrol acetate, progesterone caproate, testosterone, and tamoxifen. Table 14.2 shows the results of hormonal treatment of the first generation of clinical trials—after the first 5 years, favorable results of hormonal therapy have progressively decreased. Table 14.3 summarizes the percentages of positive responses registered in the past decade. Only few authors report favorable results during this period, and the extensive review of Luderer et al (80) demonstrates that a bare 8% response rate can be expected from progestational therapy, whenever strict criteria of evaluation of objective response are used (i.e., bidimensional measurability of indicator lesions). Table 14.4 takes into account the favorable results from hormonal therapy in advanced cases, grouped over periods of 5 years. The number of patients treated with single hormonal agent tends to decrease, and the response percentage is usually very low. In most clinical trials the hormone dosage used and the administration schedules vary considerably. The oral route is employed as well as the parenteral one, and both are often used together. Early progesterone therapy was usually administered intramuscularly (100 to 250 mg) two to three times/week or given orally (150 to 300 mg/day). The poor response to MPA (Table 14.4) might indeed be due to the insufficient dosage of the drug administered (81).

Recently, plasma levels of 100 ng/ml have been considered to be optimum to achieve a therapeutic effect in advanced breast cancer (82). These plasma concentrations can be reached by using a dose of 1000 mg/day administered orally or 500 mg/day administered intramuscularly. For practical therapeutic purposes, combination of the two routes

Table 14.2
Summary of Early Results of Hormonal Treatment in Metastatic Disease (1964 to 1973)

Author	Hormone[a]	No. of Patients	Responses	%
Bloom (27)	P	20	4/20	20
Melander et al (90)	P + A	20	4/20	20
Jenkin (109)	A	15	1/15	7
Woodruff et al (110)	P	27	5/27	18
Samuels et al (111)	P/A	23	4/23	17
Papac (112)	P/A	12	4/12	33
Paine et al (113)	P	15	3/15	20
Bloom (114)	P/A	80	13/80	16
Wagle and Murphy (115)	P/A	43	8/43	19
Van der Werf Messing and Gilse (116)	P	31	2/31	6
	A	2	0/2	0
Talley (117)	P	61	7/61	11
	A	37	0/37	0
Alberto and Senn (118)	A	23	0/23	0
	P	17	0/17	0
	A + P	20	0/20	0
Bloom (89)	A/P	60	13/60	21
		496	68/496 (13.7%)	

[a] P, progestagens; A, androgens.

Table 14.3
Summary of More Recent Results of Hormonal Treatment in Metastatic Disease (1974 to 1983)

Author	Hormone[a]	No. of Patients	Responses	%
Morales et al (119)	P	18	0/18	0
	A	20	1/20	5
Lokich and Harrison (120)	P/A	73	0/73	0
Hahn and Brodovsky (121)	P	166	0/166	0
Papac et al (122)	P/A	21	5/21	23
Bloom and Hendry (123)	P/A	60	9/60	16
Bracci and Di Silverio (34)	P	17	3/17	17
Concolino et al (124)	P	2	0/2	0
Luderer et al (80) (review)	P	356	30/356	8
	A	188	5/188	3
DeKernion et al (125)	P	110	0/110	0
Pannuti et al (86)[b]	P	20	2/20	10
Bono et al (100)	P	11	0/11	0
Pizzocaro et al (126)	P	10	0/10	0[c]
Takesue and Ueda (127)	P	16	0/16	0
Pearson et al (128)	P	10	0/10	0
Nakano et al (129)	P/A	32	3/32	9.3
Stolbach et al (130)	P	20	0/20	0
Pizzocaro and CNR	P	24	0/24[d]	0
cooperative group (67)	A	9	0/9[d]	0
Wicklund (85)[b]	P	12	3/12	25

[a] P, progestagens; A, androgens.
[b] High dose MPA.
[c] Stable disease in two cases.
[d] Stable disease in 33%.

Table 14.4
Favorable Response to Hormonal Therapy in Patients Affected by Metastatic RCC Resulting from Reports Published in Different Periods

Years	No. of Patients	No. of Responses	%
1964–1968	105	22	20.9
1969–1973	328	31	9.45
1974–1978	497	20	4
1979–1983	260	6	2.3

of administration can be considered. A loading period with 500 mg/day by intramuscular injection and a maintenance period with a dose of 1000 mg/day orally has been recommended (83–85).

Increased understanding of the kinetics of MPA, the most widely used drug in human RCC, has led to the adoption of higher therapeutic doses. This has led to some useful responses in a few studies (86, 87) but not in others (68).

Androgens have also been used in the treatment of advanced RCC, often in patients nonresponsive to progestagens or when progression occurred after MPA therapy. In some trials the combination of progestagens and androgens was administered from the very beginning. The sequential therapy (progestagens-androgens) was chiefly adopted by the British group (21, 88, 89). It apparently obtained the best response rate

(Tables 14.2 and 14.3: 50 of 364 cases = 13.7%) with significant prolongation of survival. On the contrary, the androgens, as single agents, have not yielded really favorable results, as partial responses of only 3% have been reported (80). The progestagen-androgen combination yielded comparably low responses, with the only exception being the series by Melander et al (90), who registered a 20% response rate in 20 cases.

Antiestrogen Therapy in Metastatic Patients

The logical consequence of work on experimental renal tumors in hamsters was the attempt at therapeutic trials with antiestrogenic drugs. The most used drug is tamoxifen (TAM) (Table 14.5), which is a nonsteroidal compound that binds to ER in target tissue: for this reason it is widely employed in advanced breast cancer (83, 84).

Dosages of TAM differ in the published series, ranging from 10 to 100 mg/day. From a survey of the known data, the mean objective response rate is very low (4.72%). However, in a small series of 10 patients (8 male, 2 female), Paladrine et al (91) recorded 3 partial responses, all in males, with MPA treatment. As the disease progressed further, nafoxidine treatment was initiated and again a partial response was observed in all 3 patients. They showed an additional partial response when megestrol acetate was administered upon disease progression, thus suggesting, as in breast cancer, a priming effect of antiestrogens. It may therefore be assumed that sequential administration of antiestrogen therapy could be of some value in patients responding to progestagens.

Combination Chemohormonal Therapy

The report that hormonotherapy with MPA yielded a 15% response rate in advanced RCC (88, 89) suggested a number of tentative trials

Table 14.5
Antiestrogen Therapy in Advanced RCC

Author	No. of Patients	No. of Responses	%
Giuliani et al (131)[a]	3	2/3 (+)[d]	0
Feun and Oïshi (132)[a]	21	4/21	5
Al Sarraf (133)[a]	49	2/49	15
Mulder and Alexieva-Figusch (134)[a]	23	0/23	0
Paladrine et al (91)[b]	10	3/10	33
Ferrazzi et al (135)[a]	12	0/12	0
Glick et al (136)[a]	15	0/15	0
Papac et al (137)[a]	3	0/3	0
Weiselberg et al (138)[a]	10	0/10	0
Al Sarraf et al (139)[a]	79	5/79	6.3
Stolbach et al (130)[a]	19	3/19	15.8
Lanteri et al (140)[a]	15	2/15	13
Fuks et al (141)[c]	14	0/14	0

[a] Tamoxifen.
[b] Nafoxidine.
[c] Tamoxifen + MPA.
[d] (+), Only bone metastases.

combining MPA with chemotherapeutic agents (Table 14.6). The mean response rate was 12.8%, similar to the response rate obtained from MPA alone and not superior to the response to vinblastine alone (92). However, in three reports concerning small series of patients, very high response percentages were recorded. The addition of bacille Calmette-Guérin (BCG) to a chemohormonal regimen (MPA, vincristine, adriamycin) yielded one complete response and four long lasting partial responses (93). Since then these results have not been confirmed by other series: the writer's experience in 12 cases treated by a similar regimen, without BCG, was negative. It is possible that the combination of immunotherapy with chemohormonal therapy may have synergistic effects, as BCG treatment by itself in some trials either prolonged survival (31) or reduced measurable metastases (94, 95).

Katakkar and Franks (96), in a small series of eight patients with lung metastases, obtained four partial remissions and one complete response, but of very short duration. The treatment consisted of a three-drug regimen with additional MPA (Table 14.5). Finally, by adding TAM to a combination of anticancer drugs, Levi et al (97) obtained a good response rate (35%). Such a regimen might thus be considered for further trials.

Adjuvant Hormonal Therapy in Operable Disease

Following Bloom's first report of clinical activity of progestagens, some institutions began to use MPA as an adjuvant therapy after nephrectomy in every stage of the disease.

The most extensive study has been carried out by the Rome University group (34). From 1967 to 1976, 168 patients entered the study and were

Table 14.6
Chemohormonal Therapy in Advanced RCC

Author	Regimen[a]	Responders	%
Alberto and Senn (118)	MPA/Test. + VLB/5FU	0/20	0
Ishmael et al (93)	MPA + VCR + ADM + BCG	5/14	35.7
Hahn and Brodovsky (121)	MPA + VLB + 5FU	0/20	0
Katakkar and Frans (96)	MPA + ADM + VLB + HDU	5/8	62
Hahn et al (142)	MPA + MeCCNU	4/38	10.5
	MPA + VLB	3/38	7.9
Talley (117)	MPA + VLB + CTX + HDU + Prednisone	7/45	15
Levi et al (97)	TAM + VLB + MTX + BLM	5/14	35
Swenson (143)	Estramustine	0/16	0
Bono (65)[b]	MPA + VLB + ADM	0/12	0
Engelhom et al (144)	MPA + VLB	4/24	16.6
Altman et al (145)	MPA + Yoshi 864	2/30	7
		35/279	
		(12.5%)	

[a] ADM, adriamycin (Doxorubicin); BCG, bacille bilié de Calmette-Guérin; BLM, bleomycin; CTX, cyclophosphamide; 5FU, 5-fluorouracil; HDU, hydroxyurea; MeCCNU, lomustine; MPA, medroxyprogesterone acetate; MTX, methotrexate; TAM, tamoxifen; Test., testosterone; VCR, vincristine; VLB, vinblastine.

[b] Unpublished data, 1982.

divided into two unbalanced, nonrandomized groups: group 1° = nephrectomy alone (52 patients) and group 2° = nephrectomy plus MPA (116 patients) without any stratification for N− and N+ cases. (The dosage schedule was as follows: 250 mg/day intramuscularly for a month; 250 mg three times a week for the second month; 250 mg a week for the third month; 250 mg every 10 days or 100 mg orally daily from the fourth to the twelfth months; and in the second and third years, 250 mg intramuscularly every 2 weeks.)

The occurrence of metastases (13 of 52 in the first group and 8 of 116 in the second group) and the 6-year actuarial survival rate (29% *versus* 61%)—analyzed in 1983 on 82 evaluable patients (74)—showed results strikingly in favor of the MPA group. However, the lack of randomization is likely to arouse some criticism, as is the lack of stratification for N− and N+ cases, because lymph node involvement worsens the prognosis (98, 99) (Table 14.7).

The same group carried out another study on 50 consecutive patients all treated with MPA after nephrectomy. Thirty-four patients were pT2 (of which 12 were N+ = 35%) and 16 pT3 (of which 5 were N+ = 35%). The 5 year survival rate was surprisingly high, and the probability of survival appeared to be especially favorable in ER-positive cases. The Varese group, on the other hand (100), in a retrospective study comparing 46 hormone-treated patients with 42 nontreated patients after nephrectomy, could not demonstrate any difference in long term survival rates. The patient groups were homogeneous for age, sex and pathologic stage. The incidence of metastases and the disease-free interval seemed unaffected by the therapy. In the majority of cases, however, the treatment lasted only for an average of 3 months and consisted of 750 mg of progestans a week.

A cooperative group from Yokohama University and related hospitals studied 80 patients collected from 1968 to 1978. After radical nephrectomy, 35 were treated with MPA at a low oral dosage (40 mg for 2 months) and 45 were left untreated (101). The treated group showed a 26% incidence of metastases (9 of 35) against a 44% incidence (20 of 45) in the control group. The authors came to the conclusion that there was a beneficial effect which could be attributed to the MPA adjuvant treatment. Some criticism can also be made about this report, again because the patients were not randomized and only cases coming from hospitals outside the university were allocated in the control group. Finally, the statistical analysis made on the reported figures (chi-square test) do not show any significant difference in the incidence of metastases in both groups.

Recently the CNR cooperative group (68) has published a preliminary

Table 14.7
RCC Series of Varese Regional Hospital—Lymph Node Involvement—5-Year Survival

	No. of Patients (%)	Dead (%)	Mean Survival (Months)
N− (pN0) pT3	24 (65)	8/24 (33)	33.5
N+ (pN1–4) pT3	13 (35)	11/13 (84)	16.6

report on a prospective randomized trial carried out on a series of 70 evaluable patients affected by M_0 category RCC. After radical nephrectomy, 32 patients received MPA as adjunctive treatment (500 mg three times a week for 1 year, given orally after 2 months) and 38 received no further therapy. No difference in relapse rates between the treated and control groups, even stratifying by sex and pathologic stage, could be detected. The group concluded that these preliminary data did not support any evidence of a protective activity of MPA adjunctive therapy. Moreover, in an unpublished subsequent analysis of the results of the study (113 patients; December 1983), the group has found a trend toward a higher percentage of relapses in MPA-treated female patients in comparison with controls.

CONCLUSIONS

As the correlations between human RCC and hormonal status have not yet been completely assessed, conclusions are certainly not easy to reach. However, some facts stand out and need to be emphasized.

Estrogen-induced RCC in the male hamster is a suitable model for laboratory studies on tumor kinetics, biochemical properties of cells, etc. These interesting experiments, however, do not warrant the speculative generalization that renal cancer spontaneously occurring in other species is necessarily hormone dependent. It should rather be stressed that the hamster is actually the only animal prone to estrogen-induced renal cancer.

As far as man is concerned there are two arguments against the hormonal etiology of RCC (102): (a) the rare occurrence in both men and women of bilateral tumors and (b) the age of maximum incidence of the neoplasia at the age when hormone production declines. Even the reason why there is a predominant incidence of RCC in males has not been clarified. The supposed "protection" exerted by progesterone in women during the fertile period is in contrast with the obvious remark that the amount of circulating estrogens is high for most of a woman's life and yet females are less subject to RCC than males. Another observation which may deny the possible role of estrogens in the etiology of human RCC is that estrogen therapy in male subjects does not usually increase the incidence of renal tumors. As has been well known since the first report of Higgins (103), a great number of men affected by prostate cancer have been treated over very long periods of time with high dose estrogens (usually DES). Moreover, a great number of them were castrated before the therapy was started. Nevertheless, the literature reports only three cases of RCC in patients treated with estrogens for 3 to 7 years (104, 105).

The conflicting figures reported for steroid receptor concentrations in normal kidney and in RCC make it uncertain whether this assay should be considered useful in clinical practice. The need for standardization of techniques in various laboratories is urgent to compare and interpret results correctly. The clinical significance of the relatively high concentrations of glucocorticoid and mineralocorticoid receptors often found in neoplastic tissue has not been completely elucidated. The hypothesized blockade of glucocorticoid receptors by high dose MPA administration could be of primary clinical relevance. Indeed, it has been observed that glucocorticoids show an in vitro stimulatory effect on the growth kinetics of human RCC cells (106). MPA might therefore compete with the growth-promoting effect of glucocorticoids through saturation of glucocorticoid receptors. Unfortunately, repeated determinations in different tumor areas demonstrate that human RCC very frequently consists of irregularly distributed, "biochemically heterogeneous cell subpopulations" (77) and that receptor molecules are "restricted to a subpopulation" of cells. It is possible that the favorable action of MPA may be limited to the scattered cells endowed with receptors.

On the whole, this point of view is consistent with the data produced by controlled clinical trials and by a few other statistically evaluable series. Objective responses to progestagens or to antiestrogenic treatment in metastatic patients are rare and too frequently of short duration. These poor results could be accounted for by activity exerted upon the few sensitive cellular subpopulations. The results of hormonal therapy in advanced RCC, which average a 15% response rate only in the most favorable series (34, 88, 89), should be considered as disappointing when realistically examined. Moreover even though chemotherapeutic agents are ineffective and hormone therapy has few side effects, in the author's opinion, chemohormonal therapy is not justified as adjuvant treatment after radical nephrectomy. The use of a drug as adjunctive therapy which has not yielded at least a 50% objective response in advanced cases would be against the basic rules of oncology.

The author believes, however, that the most important observation emerging from the data concerning receptor profiles and hormonal therapy trials in RCC is that antiestrogenic priming can induce the formation of high quantities of PGR, as is the case for breast cancer (74). This interesting phenomenon deserves further investigations and will probably open the way to new therapeutic approaches for the treatment of RCC. The pharmacologic induction of high concentrations of PGR in tumor tissue may cause most tumorous cell populations to become sensitive to treatment with progestational agents.

Acknowledgment. The receptor assays for these studies were performed at the laboratory of the Oncologic Division of Fondazione Clinica del Lavoro (Pavia, Italy) by C Zibera under the supervision of Professor G Robustelli Della Cuna. The author wishes to thank them both for their highly qualified work and, in particular, is grateful to Professor Robustelli Della Cuna for his invaluable advice. Grateful thanks are extended to Mrs. Luisa Golzi for her help with the revision of the English text.

REFERENCES

1. Lattimer JK: The action of testosterone propionate upon the kidneys of rats, dogs and men. *J Urol* 48:778–784, 1942.
2. Kirkman H, Bacon RL: Malignant renal tumors in male hamsters (*Cricetus auratus*) treated with estrogens. *Cancer Res* 10:122–124, 1950.
3. Selye H: Toxic effect of estrogens as influenced by progesterone. *Can Med Assoc J* 42:188–197, 1940.

4. Matthews VS, Kirkman H, Bacon RL: Kidney damage in the golden hamster following chronic administration of diethylstilbestrol and sesame oil. *Proc Soc Exp Biol Med* 66:195–196, 1947.

5. Concolino G, Marocchi A, Conti C, Tenaglia R, Di Silverio F, Bracci U: Human renal carcinoma as a hormone dependent tumor. *Cancer Res* 38:4340–4344, 1978.

6. Concolino G, Marocchi A, Toscano V, Di Silverio F: Nuclear androgen receptor as marker of responsiveness to medroxyprogesterone acetate in human renal cell carcinoma. *J Steroid Biochem* 15:397–402, 1981.

7. Pavone-Macaluso M: Aetiology of renal cancer. In Kuss R, Murphy GP, Khoury S, Karr JP (eds): *Renal tumors: Proceedings of the First International Symposium on Kidney Tumors.* New York, Alan R Liss, 1982, pp 255–271.

8. Bennington JL, Beckwith JB: Renal adenocarcinoma. In Bennington JL, Beckwith JB (eds): *Tumors of the Kidney, Renal Pelvis, and Ureter.* Washington, DC, Armed Forces Institute of Pathology, 1975, pp 93–199.

9. Bennington JL, Kradijan RH: *Renal Carcinoma.* Philadelphia, WB Saunders, 1967, pp 38–42, 180–196.

10. Finger-Cantor AL, Meigs JW, Heston JF, Flannery JT: Epidemiology of renal cell carcinoma in Connecticut 1935–1973. *J Natl Cancer Inst* 57:495–500, 1976.

11. Concolino G: Renal cancer: steroid receptors as a biochemical basis for endocrine therapy. In Thompson EB, Lippman ME (eds): *Steroid Receptors and the Management of Cancer.* Boca Raton, FL, CRC Press, 1979, vol 1, pp 174–197.

12. Paganini-Hill A, Ross RK, Henderson BE: Epidemiology of kidney cancer. In Skinner DG (ed): *Urological Cancer.* New York, Grune and Stratton, 1983, pp 383–407.

13. Berrino F: Epidemiologia e patogenesi del carcinoma renale. In Veronesi U, Lasio E, Emanuelli H, Pizzoccaro G, De Lena I (eds): *I Tumori Urologici.* Milan, CEA, 1982, pp 3–7.

14. Bono AV: New perspectives in nephrocarcinoma. *Urologia* 49:3–14, 1982.

15. Blot WJ, Fraumeni JF Jr: Geographic patterns of renal cancer in the United States. *J Natl Cancer Inst* 2:363–366, 1979.

16. Waterhouse J, Muir C, Shanmugaratam P: *Cancer Incidence in Five Continents.* Lyon, IARC Scientific Publications, 1982, vol 4.

17. Wynder EL, Mabuchi K, Whitmore W: Epidemiology of adenocarcinoma of the kidney. *J Natl Cancer Inst* 53:1619–1634, 1974.

18. Kirkman H, Bacon RL: Estrogen induced tumors of the kidney. I. Incidence of renal tumors in intact and gonadectomized male golden hamster treated with diethylstilbestrol. *J Natl Cancer Inst* 13:745–765, 1952.

19. Bloom HJG, Dukes CE, Mitchley BCV: Hormone dependent tumours of the kidney. I. The oestrogen-induced renal tumour of the Syrian hamster: hormone treatment and possible relationship to the carcinoma of the kidney in man. *Br J Cancer* 17:611–645, 1963.

20. Algard FT: Hormone induced tumors: hamster flank organ and kidney tumors in vitro. *J Natl Cancer Inst* 25:557–572, 1960.

21. Bloom HJG, Hendry WF: Special oncology: kidney. Influence of hormones. In Chisholm GD, Williams DI (eds): *Scientific Foundations of Urology.* London, Heinemann, 1982, pp 684–689.

22. Kirkman H: Estrogen-induced tumors of the kidney. *Natl Cancer Inst Mongr* 1:1–59, 1959.

23. Horning ES: Endocrine factors involved in induction, prevention and transplantation of kidney tumors in the male golden hamsters. *Z. Krebsforsch.* 61:1–21, 1956.

24. Hamilton JM, Flaks A, Saluja PG, Maguire S: Hormonally induced renal neoplasia in the male golden Syrian hamster and the inhibitory effect of 3-bromo-alpha-ergocriptine methansulphonate. *J Natl Cancer Inst* 54:1385–1400, 1975.

25. Bloom HJG, Baker WH, Dukes CE, Mitchley BCV: Hormone dependent tumors of the kidney. II. Effect of endocrine ablation procedure on the transplanted oestrogen-induced renal tumour of the Syrian hamster. *Br J Cancer* 17:646–656, 1963.

26. Lin YC, Loring JM, Villee CA: Permissive role of the pituitary in the induction and growth of estrogen-dependent renal tumors. *Cancer Res* 42:1015–1019, 1982.

27. Bloom HJG: Hormone treatment of renal tumors. Experimental and clinical obser-

vations. In Riches EW (ed): *Tumor of the Kidney and Ureter.* Baltimore, Williams
& Wilkins, 1964, pp 311–320.

28. Reznick G, Schuller H: Carcinogenic effect of diethylstilbestrol in male Syrian golden
hamster and European hamster. *J Natl Cancer Inst* 62:1083–1088, 1979.

29. Guérin M, Chouroulinkov I, Rivière MR: Experimental kidney tumors. In Rouiller
C, Muller AF (eds): *The Kidney. Morphology, Biochemistry, Physiology.* New York:
Academic Press, 1969, vol 2, pp 199–268.

30. Lucké B: Kidney carcinoma in the leopard frog: a virus tumor. *Ann NY Acad Sci*
54:1093–1109, 1952.

31. Brosman S: Non specific immunotherapy in genito-urinary cancer. In *Proceedings
of the Clinical Symposium of Chicago.* Chicago, Franklin Institute Press, 1977, pp
97–99.

32. Soloway MS, Myers GM Jr: The effect of hormonal therapy on a transplantable
renal cortical adenocarcinoma in the syngeneic mice. *J Urol* 109:356–361, 1973.

33. Murphy GM: Murine renal cell carcinoma: a suitable human model. In Kuss R,
Murphy GP, Khoury S, Karr JP (eds): *Renal Tumors: Proceedings of the First
International Symposium on Kidney Tumors.* New York: Alan R Liss, 1982, pp
175–206.

34. Bracci U, Di Silverio F: Ormonodipendenza. *Atti Soc Ital Urol* 44:167–194, 1976.

35. Saez S, Martin PR: Evidence of estrogen receptors in the trigone area of human
urinary bladder. *Biochemistry* 15:317–319, 1981.

36. Fisher RI, Neifeld JP, Lippman ME: Oestrogen receptors in human malignant
melanoma. *Lancet* 2:337–342, 1976.

37. Van Maillot K, Hermanek P, Geutsch HH: Steroid receptors in tumors of tissues
generally considered to be hormone-independent. *J Cancer Res* 93:77–84, 1979.

38. McGuire WL: Quantitation of estrogen receptor in mammary carcinoma. *Methods
Enzymol* 36:248–254, 1975.

39. Scatchard G: The attraction of protein for small molecules and ions. *Ann NY Acad
Sci* 51:660–672, 1949.

40. Ginsburg M, Greebstein BD, MacLusky NJ, Morris ID, Thomas PJ: An improved
method for the study of high affinity steroid binding. *Steroids* 23:773–792, 1974.

41. Wagner RK: Characterization and assay of steroid hormone receptors and steroid
binding serum proteins by agar gel electrophoresis. *Zentralbl Physiol Chem*
352:1235–1245, 1972.

42. Chamness GC, McGuire WL: Scatchard plots: common errors in correction and
interpretations. *Steroids* 26:538–542, 1975.

43. Pollow K: New assays: development in assay procedures. A new assay system for
aestrogen and progesterone receptors: double labeling (125-I) oestradiol and (3,4)-
R5020 as radioligand. In Cavalli F, McGuire WL, Pannuti F, Pellegrini A, Robustelli
Della Cuna G (eds): *Proceedings of the International Symposium on MPA.* Amsterdam, Excerpta Medica, 1982, pp 555–556.

44. Martin PM, Magdalena THP, Benyahia B, Rigaud O, Katzenellbogen JA: New
approach for visualizing estrogen receptors in target cells using inherently fluorescent
ligands and image intensification. *Cancer Res* 43:4956–4965, 1983.

45. Karr JP, Schneider S, Rosenthal H, Sandberg AA, Murphy GP: Receptor profiles in
renal cell carcinoma. In Küss R, Murphy GP, Khoury S, Karr JP (eds): *Renal
Tumors: Proceedings of the First International Symposium on Kidney Tumors.* New
York, Alan R Liss, 1982, pp 211–244.

46. Murono EP, Kirdani RY, Sandberg AA: Specific estradiol 17-binding component in
adult rat kidney. *J Steroid Biochem* 11:1347–1351, 1979.

47. Pasqualini LR, Sumida C, Gelly C: Steroid hormone receptors in fetal guinea pig
kidney. *J Steroid Biochem* 5:977–985, 1974.

48. Li JJ, Villee CA: Estrogen binding sites in Syrian hamster kidney cytosol and
comparison with binding component in other tissues. In *Proceedings of the Fifth
International Congress on Pharmacology,* San Francisco, 1972, pp 140–141.

49. Bullock PL, Bardin CW: The presence of estrogen receptor in kidney from normal
and androgen insensitive tfm/y mice. *Endocrinology* 97:1106–1111, 1975.

50. Li JJ, Li SA: Translocation of specific steroid hormone receptors into purified nuclei
in Syrian hamster tissues and estrogen dependent renal tumors. In Vermeulen A,

Junglbut P, Klopper A, Sciarra F (eds): *Research on Steroids*. Amsterdam, Elsevier, 1977, pp 837–853.

51. Fanestil DD, Edelman IS: Characteristics of renal nuclear receptors for aldosterone. *Proc Natl Acad Sci USA* 56:872–879, 1966.

52. Rafestin-Obin ME, Roth-Meyer C, Claire M, Michand A, Baviera E, Brisset JM, Carsol P: Are mineralocorticoids present in human renal adenocarcinoma? *Clin Sci* 57:421–425, 1979.

53. Li JJ, Li SA: Specific progesterone binding in the estrogen dependent renal adenocarcinoma of the Golden hamster. *Proc Endocr Soc NYC* 18:20, 1975.

54. Anderson NS, David Y, Fanestil DD: Estrogen receptor in hamster kidney during estrogen induced renal tumorigenesis. *J Steroid Biochem* 10:123–128, 1978.

55. Li JJ, Li SA: Estrogen induced progesterone receptor in Syrian hamster kidney. II. Modulation by synthetic progestins. *Endocrinology* 108:1751–1756, 1981.

56. Li JJ, Li SA: High yield of primary serially transplanted hamster renal carcinoma: steroid receptor and morphologic characteristics. *Eur J Cancer* 16:1119–1125, 1980.

57. Murphy GP, Hrushesky WJ: A murine renal cell carcinoma. *J Natl Cancer Inst* 50:1013–1025, 1973.

58. Spiers ASD: Cytotoxic drugs and hormonal manipulations in the management of carcinoma of the kidney. In Spiers ASD (ed): *Chemotherapy and Urological Malignancy*. Berlin, Springer-Verlag, 1982, pp 9–28.

59. Concolino G, Marocchi A, Concolino F, Sciarra F, Di Silverio F, Conti C: Human kidney steroid receptors. *J Steroid Biochem* 7:831–835, 1976.

60. Concolino G, Marocchi A, Di Silverio F, and Conti C: Progestational therapy in human renal carcinoma and steroid receptors. *J Steroid Biochem* 7:923–927, 1976.

61. Fanestil DD, Vaughn DA, Ludens JH: Steroid hormone receptors in human renal carcinoma. *J Steroid Biochem* 5:338,1974.

62. Bojar H, Dreyfürst R, Balzar K, Staib W: Östrogen Rezeptoren in menschlichen Nierencarzinomen. *J Chem Clin Biochem* 14:551–556, 1976.

63. Hemstreet GP, Wittliff JL, Sarrif AM, Hall ML, McRae LJ, Durant JR: Comparison of steroid receptor levels in renal cell carcinoma and autologous kidney. *Int J Cancer* 26:769–775, 1980.

64. Di Fronzo G, Ronchi E, Bertuzzi A, Vezzoni P, Pizzocaro G: Estrogen receptors in renal carcinoma. *Eur Urol* 6:307–311, 1980.

65. Chen L, Weiss FR, Chaichik S, Klydar I: Steroid receptors in human renal carcinoma. *Israel J Med Sci* 16:756–760, 1981.

66. Bono AV, Zibera C, Robustelli Della Cuna G, Gianneo E: Estradiol and progesterone cytoplasmic receptors in renal cell carcinoma and autologous normal kidney. In *Proceedings of the Fifth Congress of the European Society of Urology*. Vienna, 1982, p 370.

67. Pizzocaro G, Di Fronzo G, Cappelletti V, Piva L, Salvioni R, Ronchi E, Giongo A, Dormia E, Zanollo A, Giannoni R, Maffeis U, Lasio E: Hormone treatment and sex steroid receptors in metastatic renal cell carcinoma: report of a multicentric prospective study. *Tumori* 69:215–220, 1983.

68. Pizzocaro G, Di Fronzo G, Piva L, Salvioni R, Ronchi E, Cappelletti V, Giongo A, Mastrobernardino E, Cozzoli C, Dormia E, Minervini S, Zanollo A, Fontanella U, Giannoni R, Maggioni A, Lasio E: Adjunctive medroxyprogesterone acetate to radical nephrectomy in category M_0 renal cell carcinoma. *Eur Urol* 9:202–206, 1983.

69. Bojar H, Maar K, Staib W: The endocrine background of human renal cell carcinoma. I. Binding of the highly potent progestin R5020 by tumor cytosol. *Urol Int* 34:302–311, 1979.

70. Bojar H, Maar K, Staib W: The endocrine background of human renal cell carcinoma. II. Attempt to induce the R5020-binding component by oestrogens. *Urol Int* 34:312–319, 1979.

71. Tobin EH, Monhaddeb J, Bloom ND: Analysis of specific progesterone receptor proteins in human kidney and renal cell carcinoma. In Wittliff JL, Dapunt O (eds): *Steroid Receptors and Hormone-Dependent Neoplasia*. New York, Masson, 1980, pp 197–202.

72. Roth-Meyer C, Rafestin-Obin ME, Michand A, Claire M, Brisset JM, Corval P: Steroid receptors in normal and neoplastic human kidney. In Wittliff JL, Dapunt O

STEROID HORMONES AND HORMONAL TREATMENT   223

(eds): *Steroid Receptors and Hormone-Dependent Neoplasia.* New York, Masson, 1980, pp 171–173.

73. Bojar H, Maar K, Staib W: The endocrine background of human renal cell carcinoma. III. Role of inhibitors of R5020 binding in tumor cytosol. *Urol Int* 34:321–329, 1979.

74. Bracci U, Di Silverio F, Concolino G: Hormonal therapy of renal cell carcinoma. In Küss R, Murphy GP, Khoury S, Karr JP (eds): *Renal Tumors: Proceedings of the First International Symposium on Kidney Tumors.* New York, Alan R Liss, 1982, pp 623–640.

75. Anderson J, Clark JH, Peck EJ Jr: Oestrogen and nuclear binding sites. Determination of specific sites by H3-oestradiol exchange. *Biochem J* 126:561–567, 1972.

76. Walters MR, Clark JM: Cytosol and nuclear compartmentalization of progesterone receptors of the rat uterus. *Endocrinology* 103:601–609, 1978.

77. Bojar H, Maar K, Staib W: The endocrine background of human renal cell carcinoma. IV. Glucocorticoid receptors as possible mediators of progestagen action. *Urol Int* 24:330–338, 1979.

78. Pasqualini JR, Portois MC, Kuss R, Khoury S, Petit J, Degennes JL, Dairon F: Aldosterone and estradiol specific binding in normal and carcinoma human renal tissue. In *Proceedings of the Tenth European Congress of the International College of Surgeons,* Milan, 1977.

79. Oberling C, Rivière M, Haguenau F: Ultrastructure of the clear cells in renal carcinomas and its importance for the demonstration of their renal origin. *Nature* 186:402–403, 1960.

80. Luderer RC, Opipari MI, Perrotta AL: Treatment of metastatic renal cell carcinoma. Review of experience and world literature. *J Am Obstet Assoc* 77:590–603, 1978.

81. deKernion JB, Linder A: Treatment of advanced renal carcinoma. In Küss R, Murphy GP, Khoury S, Karr JP (eds): *Renal Tumors: Proceedings of the First International Symposium on Kidney Tumors.* New York, Alan R Liss, 1982, pp 641–659.

82. Tamassia V, Battaglia A, Ganzina F, Isetta AM, Sacchetti G, Cavalli F, Goldhirsh A, Kiser J, Bernardo G, Robustelli Della Cuna G: Pharmacokinetic approach to the selection of dose schedules of medroxyprogesterone acetate in clinical oncology. *Cancer Chem Pharmacol* 8:151–155, 1982.

83. Robustelli Della Cuna G, Bernardo-Strada MR, Ganzina F: High-dose medroxyprogesterone acetate in metastatic breast cancer. A critical review. In Cavalli F, McGuire WL, Pannuti F, Pellegrini A, Robustelli Della Cuna G, (eds): *Proceedings of the International Symposium on MPA.* Amsterdam, Excerpta Medica, 1982, pp 280–305.

84. Robustelli Della Cuna G, Pellegrini A, Ganzina F: Chemotherapy and hormone treatment of advanced breast cancer. Farmitalia S.P.A., Monographs, Milan, 1982, pp 77–100.

85. Pannuti F, Martoni A, Carnaggi CM, Strocchi E, Di Marco AR, Rossi AP, Tomasi L, Giovannini M, Cricca A, Frnet F, Lelli G, Gianibiasi ME, Canova N: High-dose MPA in oncology. History, clinical use and pharmacokinetics. In Cavalli F, McGuire WL, Pannuti F, Pellegrini A, Robustelli Della Cuna G (eds): *Proceedings of the International Symposium on MPA.* Amsterdam, Excerpta Medica, 1982, pp 5–46.

86. Pannuti F, Martoni A, Cricca A: Treatment of renal clear cell carcinoma by high doses of MPA: pilot study. *IRCS Med Sci* 6:177–180, 1978.

87. Wicklund H: High-dose medroxyprogesterone acetate in patients with advanced renal cell carcinoma. In Cavalli F, McGuire WL, Pannuti F, Pellegrini A, Robustelli Della Cuna G (eds): *Proceedings of the International Symposium on MPA.* Amsterdam, Excerpta Medica, 1982, pp 420–424.

88. Bloom HJG: Hormone-induced and spontaneous regression of metastatic renal cancer. *Cancer* 32:1066–1071, 1973.

89. Bloom HJG: Adjuvant therapy for adenocarcinoma of the kidney: present position and prospects. *Br J Urol* 45:237–257, 1973.

90. Melander O, Notter G, Von Schreeb T: Hormonbehanding av metastaserande renal cancer. *Nordisk Med* 78:1039–1044, 1967.

91. Paladrine W, Longacre D, Hemmings P, Harper G: Nafoxidine, an anti-estrogen in hypernephroma. *Proc Am Soc Clin Oncol* 20:293, 1979.

92. Hrushesky WJ, Murphy GP: Current status of the therapy of advanced renal carcinoma. *J Surg Oncol* 9:277–288, 1977.
93. Ishmael DR, Bottomley RH, Hoge A: Treatment of renal cell adenocarcinoma (hypernephroma) with Depo-Provera and combination chemoimmunotherapy. *Proc Am Soc Clin Oncol* 17:265, 1976.
94. Minton JP, Pennline K, Nowrocki JF: Immunotherapy of human kidney cancer. *Proc Am Soc Clin Oncol* 17:301, 1976.
95. Morales A, Eidinger D: Bacille Calmette-Guérin in the treatment of adenocarcinoma of the kidney. *J Urol* 115:377–380, 1976.
96. Katakkar SB, Franks CR: Chemohormonal therapy for metastatic renal cell carcinoma with adriamycin, hydroxyurea, vinblastine and medroxyprogesterone acetate. *Cancer Treat Rep* 62:1379–1380, 1978.
97. Levi JA, Dalley D, Aroney R: A comparative trial of the combination vinblastine, methotrexate and bleomycin with and without tamoxifen for metastatic renal cell carcinoma. *Proc Am Soc Clin Oncol* 21:426, 1980.
98. Holland JM: Cancer of the kidney. Natural history and staging. *Cancer* 32:1030–1042, 1973.
99. Robson CJ, Churchill BM, Anderson W: The results of radical nephrectomy for renal cell carcinoma. *J Urol* 101:287–301, 1969.
100. Bono AV, Benvenuti C, Gjanneo E, Comeri GC, Roggia A: Progestagens in renal cell carcinoma. *Eur Urol* 5:94–96, 1979.
101. Satomi Y, Takay S, Kondo I, Fukushima S, Furuhata A: Postoperative prophylactic use of progesterone in renal-cell carcinoma. *J Urol* 128:919–922, 1982.
102. Kantor AF: Current concepts in the epidemiology and etiology of primary renal cell carinoma. *J Urol* 117:415–417, 1977.
103. Huggins C, Hodges CV: Studies on prostatic cancer. I. The effect of castration, of estrogens and of androgens injection on serum phosphatase in metastatic carcinoma of the prostate. *Cancer Res* 1:293–297, 1941.
104. Bellet RE, Squiteri AP: Estrogen-induced hypernephroma. *J Urol* 112:160–161, 1974.
105. Nissenkorn I, Servadio C, Avider I: Oestrogen-induced renal carcinoma. *Br J Urol* 51:6–9, 1979.
106. Card DJ, Kohorn EJ, Lytton B: Effects of hormones on whole organ cultures of renal cell carcinoma. *Surg Forum* 21:523–533, 1970.
107. Bojar H, Wittliff JL, Balzer K, Dreyfürst R, Boeminghaus F, Staib W: Properties of specific estrogen binding components in human kidney and renal carcinoma. *Acta Endocrinol* 193:51, 1975.
108. Concolino G, Di Silverio F, Marocchi A, Tenaglia R, Bracci U: Steroid receptors in normal human kidney and in human renal cell adenocarcinoma. In *Proceedings of the Tenth European Congress of the International College of Surgeons.* Milan, 1977.
109. Jenkin RD: Androgens in metastatic renal adenocarcinoma. *Br Med J* 1:361, 1967.
110. Woodruff MW, Wagle D, Gailam SD, Jones R: The current status of chemotherapy for advanced renal carcinoma. *J Urol* 97:611–618, 1967.
111. Samuels ML, Sullivan P, Howe CD: Medroxyprogesterone acetate in the treatment of renal cell carcinoma (hypernephroma). *Cancer* 22:525–532, 1968.
112. Papac JR: Hormonal therapy of renal cancer. *Proc Am Soc Clin Oncol* 10:67, 1969.
113. Payne CH, Wright FW, Ellis F: The use of progestagen in the treatment of metastatic carcinoma of the kidney and uterine body. *Br J Cancer* 24:277–282, 1970.
114. Bloom HJG: Medroxyprogesterone acetate (Provera) in treatment of metastatic renal cancer. *Br J Cancer* 25:256–265, 1971.
115. Wagle DG, Murphy GP: Hormonal therapy in advanced renal cell carcinoma. *Cancer* 28:318–321, 1971.
116. Van Der Werf Messing B, Gilse HA: Hormonal treatment of metastatases of renal carcinoma. *Br J Cancer* 25:423–427, 1971.
117. Talley RW: Chemotherapy of adenocarcinoma of the kidney. *Cancer* 32:1062–1065, 1973.
118. Alberto P, Senn HJ: Hormonal therapy of renal carcinoma alone and in association with cytostatic drugs. *Cancer* 33:1226–1229, 1974.
119. Morales A, Kiruluta G, Lott J: Hormones in the treatment of metastatic renal cancer. *J Urol* 114:692–693, 1975.

120. Lokich JJ, Harrison JM: Renal cell carcinoma: natural history and chemotherapeutic experience. J Urol 114:371–374, 1975.
121. Hahn RG, Brodovsky H: MethylCCNU, Velban and Depo-Provera treatment trials in advanced renal cancer. Proc Am Soc Clin Oncol 17:246, 1976.
122. Papac JR, Ross SA, Levy A: Renal cell carcinoma, analysis of 31 cases with assessment of endocrine therapy. Am J Sci 274:281–290, 1977.
123. Bloom HJG: Renal cancer. In Stoll E (ed): Endocrine Therapy in Malignant Disease. Philadelphia, WB Saunders, 1972, pp 339–441.
124. Concolino G, Marocchi A, Tenaglia R, Di Silverio F, Sparano F: Specific progesterone receptor in human renal cancer. J Steroid Biochem 9:399–402, 1978.
125. deKernion JP, Ramming KP, Smith RB: Natural history of metastatic renal cell carcinoma: computer analysis. J Urol 120:148–152, 1978.
126. Pizzocaro G, Valente M, Cataldo I, Vezzoni P, Di Fronzo G: Estrogen receptors and MPA treatment in metastatic renal carcinoma. A preliminary report. Tumori 66:739–742, 1980.
127. Takesue F, Ueda T: Progesterone treatment of renal cancer. Nishinihon J Urol 43:252–256, 1981.
128. Pearson J, Friedman MA, Hoffman PG Jr: Hormone receptors in renal cell carcinoma. Their utility as predictors of responses to endocrine therapy. Cancer Chemother Pharmacol 6:151–154, 1981.
129. Nakamo E, Fujioka H, Matsuda M: Clinical evaluation of endocrine therapy of renal cell carcinoma. Nishinihon J Urol 43:695–701, 1981.
130. Stolbach LL, Begg CB, Hall T, Horton J: Treatment of renal carcinoma: a phase III randomized trial of oral medroxyprogesterone (Provera), hydroxyurea and nafoxidine. Cancer Treat Rep 65:689–692, 1981.
131. Giuliani L, Pescatore D, Giberti C, Martorana G: Usefulness and limitation of estrogen receptor protein (ERP) assay in human renal cell carcinoma. Eur Urol 4:342–347, 1978.
132. Feun LG, Oishi N: Phase II study of nafoxidine in the therapy for advanced renal carcinoma. Cancer Treat. Rep. 63:149–150, 1979.
133. Al Sarraf M: The clinical trial of tamoxifen in patients with advanced renal cancer. A Southwest Oncology Group Study. Proc Am Soc Clin Oncol 20:378, 1979.
134. Mulder JM, Alexieva-Figusch I: Tamoxifen in metastatic renal cell carcinoma. Cancer Treat Rep 63:1222–1224, 1979.
135. Ferrazzi E, Salvagno L, Fornasiero A, Gartei A, Fiorentino M: Tamoxifen treatment for advanced renal cell cancer. Tumori 66:601–605, 1980.
136. Glick JH, Wein A, Torri S, Alavi J, Harris D, Brodovsky H: Phase II tamoxifen in patients with advanced renal cell carcinoma. Cancer Treat Rep 64:343–344, 1980.
137. Papac R, Luikhart S, Kirkwood J: High-dose tamoxifen in patients with advanced renal cell carcinoma and malignant melanoma. Proc Am Soc Clin Oncol 21:358, 1980.
138. Weiselberg L, Budman D, Vinciguerra V, Schulman P, Degnan TJ: Tamoxifen in unresectable hypernephroma. A phase II trial and review of the literature. Cancer Clin Trials 4:195–198, 1981.
139. Al Sarraf M, Eyre H, Bonnet S, Saiki S, Gagliano R, Pugh R, Lehane D, Dixon D, Bottomley R: Study of tamoxifen in metastatic renal cell carcinoma and the influence of certain prognostic factors: a Southwest Oncology Group study. Cancer Treat Rep 65:447–451, 1981.
140. Lanteri VJ, Beckley S, Dragone H, Wajsman Z, Choudhury M, Pontes JE: High-dose tamoxifen in metastatic renal cell carcinoma. Urology 19:623–625, 1982.
141. Fuks JZ, Aisner J, Van Echo DA, Wiernik PH: Phase II study of medroxyprogesterone acetate with tamoxifen in advanced renal cell cancer. Cancer Treat Rep 66:1773–1774, 1982.
142. Hahn RG, Temkin NR, Savlov ED, Perlia C, Wampler GL, Horton J, Marsh J, Carbone PP: Phase II study of vinblastine, methyl-CCNU and medroxyprogesterone acetate in advanced renal cell cancer. Cancer Treat Rep 62:1093–1099, 1978.
143. Swanson DA, Johnson DE: Estramustine phosphate as treatment for metastatic renal carcinoma. Urology 17:344–346, 1981.
144. Engelholm, SA, Kjaer M, Walbom-Jörgensen S, Hansen HH: Combined chemotherapy and hormonal therapy in metastatic renal adenocarcinoma. A controlled

trial. In Cavalli F, McGuire WL, Pannuti F, Pellegrini A, Robustelli Della Cuna G (eds): *Proceedings of the International Symposium on MPA.* Amsterdam: Excerpta Medica, 1982, pp 425–431.

145. Altman SJ, Stephens RL, Bonnet JD: Yoshi plus medroxyprogesterone acetate in adenocarcinoma of the kidney: a Southwest Oncology Group Study. *Cancer Treat Rep* 66:1781–1782, 1982.

15

Experimental Chemotherapy of Renal Adenocarcinoma

Karl Heinz Kurth, M.D.
J. C. Romijn, M.D.
J. W. van Dongen, M.D.
Michael M. Lieber, M.D.
Fritz H. Schröder, M.D.

THE HUMAN KIDNEY CARCINOMA XENOGRAFT—A VALID MODEL IN EXPERIMENTAL CHEMOTHERAPY?

The treatment of metastatic renal adenocarcinoma is usually ineffective. Hormonal therapy inaugurated following experimental evidence for the hormonal control of renal tumor growth (1–4) yielded disappointing clinical results (5–7). The ability of vaccines of whole irradiated cells with or without adjuvants to produce tumor immunity has been demonstrated in animal models (8). Huben et al (9) reported the response to various immunotherapy schedules in a spontaneous murine renal cell carcinoma model. Tumor cells were implanted intrarenally. Specific immunotherapy with a crude membrane preparation of tumor cells plus complete Freund's adjuvant (CFA) led to a significant decrease in survival in an experimental model in which locally recurrent tumor was induced. In clinical trials specific immunotherapy afforded complete and partial remission of measurable kidney carcinoma metastases, but only 20 to 25% of the patients treated were responders (10–15). Spontaneously occurring, transplantable renal adenocarcinoma in a murine model has been used as a testing system for various chemotherapeutic agents (16, 17). Unfortunately, there is little evidence that the responsiveness to cytostatic drugs in these experimental models can be reproduced in human renal cancer. Since congenitally athymic nude mice have become available, many reports on the xenografting of human tumors into immune-deficient animals have appeared (18). It is clear that there are different rates of success in xenografting human tumors

(19) (Table 15.1). Successful transplantation of renal adenocarcinoma on nude mice has been reported (20–26). The extent to which a xenograft maintains the properties of the source tumor is crucial to the question as to which model is better: the xenografted human tumor on immunodeficient animals or the syngeneic mouse tumor. The human origin of xenografted tumor cells has been confirmed by karyotype studies (27, 28), immune fluorescence studies (29), and the production of lactate dehydrogenase-isoenzyme (30) and of tumor marker (26, 31).

The growth kinetics of xenografts, however, differs significantly from the relatively slow growth of many human tumors. It seems that those grafts that grow in mice are either selected for rapid growth or accelerate to more rapid growth (32). Cell proliferation in xenografts tends to be faster than would be expected of the source tumors. However, as shown by Bogden et al (33), even when histologic changes were observed in a mammary tumor xenografted on athymic mice, the sensitivity to melphalan was broadly maintained in the xenografts. The value of xenografts in experimental cancer therapy depends ultimately upon the extent to which they maintain the therapeutic sensitivity of the source tumor. There are few publications in which the authors report a therapeutic responsiveness of xenografted kidney carcinoma that is in line with clinical experience (34).

An important obstacle in xenograft research is the pharmacodynamic problem of comparing drug treatment in man and mouse. There is no secure basis for the judgment as to what dose in a mouse is equivalent to a clinical treatment. Another problem that limits the use of xenografts

Table 15.1
Take Rates of Human Cancers Xenografted in Nude Mice or T-Deprived Mice (44)

I. *Good take rate* (more than 50% of biopsy samples established as transplantable
 Colorectal carcinoma
 Metastatic melanoma
 Oat cell carcinoma (bronchus)
II. *Fair take rate* (20–50%)
 Bladder carcinoma
 Bronchial carcinoma (others)
 Gliomas
 Ovarian carcinoma
 Pancreatic carcinoma
 Renal carcinoma
 Sarcoma (most types)
 Uterine carcinoma
III. *Poor take rate* (occasionally)
 Acute myeloid leukemia
 Chronic carcinoma
 Prostatic carcinoma
 Breast carcinoma
 Gastric carcinoma
 Teratoma testis
IV. *No reported transplantable lines*
 Carcinoid
 Seminoma
 Mesothelioma

for predicting and selecting appropriate chemotherapy for individual patients is the time required to establish xenografts and subsequently to test drugs. The predictive screening to select drugs for an individual patient may exceed the survival of the patient. However, because there is good evidence that xenografted human tumors retain their morphologic characteristics (20, 21, 26, 31, 35) and functional activity (35, 36), their use in chemotherapeutic studies may be more appropriate than that of transplantable rodent tumors for chemotherapeutic studies. The major advantage of xenografts may be in the primary screening of new agents (37).

ASSAY EVALUABILITY OF DRUG TESTING SYSTEMS

The authors evaluated the take rate of human kidney carcinoma in nude mice in their laboratory and used the established tumor cell lines to investigate the assay evaluability of three different drug testing systems: the subrenal capsule assay, as described by Bogden et al (33), the in vitro assay with labeled DNA precursor (38), and the stem cell assay (39, 40). The discovery of the role of the thymus and thymus-derived lymphocytes in transplantation immunology (41) offered new methods for xenografting. The nude (nu/nu) mouse described by Flanagan (42) and Pantelouris (43) has been shown to be congenitally athymic and lacking in T cell-mediated immune responses. The animals have been shown to be receptive to a wide range of human tumor xenografts. It is difficult to piece together an overall picture of the proportion of human tumors that may be expected to grow as xenografts in nude mice or "T-deprived" mice. Selby (44) attempted to summarize the complex literature by dividing histologic types of tumor into categories according to the ease with which they had been established as transplantable xenograft lines (Table 15.1). Renal carcinoma has been evaluated as fairly transplantable (take rate 20 to 50%). It is unclear why some tumors grow well as xenograft and others fail to grow. The reasons may lie in the viability of the implanted tissue, its actual content of malignant cells, the ability to stimulate vascularization, or the residual immune response of the host.

Take Rate of Xenografted Kidney Carcinoma on Nude Mice

From March 1980 to February 1983 fresh surgical tissue specimens from 39 consecutive resected kidney carcinomas were subcutaneously inserted bilaterally on the back of female BALB-c nu/nu mice as described previously by Höhn and Schröder (20). Tumor fragments weighing 50 to 200 mg were transplanted into two to six animals. All animals were observed for possible tumor growth until they died or were killed because of weakness.

Observation periods ranged from 1 to 11 months, the average being 4.25 months. Fourteen transplanted tumors that grew in the animals to a measurable size were transplanted into a second generation of mice (Table 15.2). Five tumors showed growth in the second passage. Finally

Table 15.2
Transplantable Human Renal Cell Carcinoma Maintained on Nude Mice (BALB-c nu/nu)

Tumor Line	No. of Passages	Doubling Time (Days)	Maximum Volume (mm³)[a]
RC-2	43	11.0 ± 7	600
RC-8	40	11.0 ± 4.6	500
RC-21	49	3.2 ± 1.4	1600
RC-43	18	4.7 ± 1.4	1600

[a] Calculated 28 days after transplantation; to determine the total load of tumor carried by one mouse, the volume must be doubled.

Table 15.3
Immunohistochemical Staining of Renal Carcinoma Cell Lines with Monoclonal Antibodies

Moabs[a]	Localization of Staining	RC-2	RC-21	RC-43	RC-51	NC-65
RC-43	Tamm-Horsfall protein	−	−	−	−	−
RC-25	Glomeruli	−	−	−	−	−
RC-2	Proximal tubules and Henle's loop	−	−	−	−	−
RC-4		−	−	−	−	−
RC-3		−	−	−	−	−
RC-69	Proximal tubules	−	−	−	−	−
RC-154		−	−	−	−	−
RC-38	Glomeruli	−	−	−	(+)	−
RC-250	Kidney and other carcinomas	−	+	+	−	−
Antikeratin	Keratin protein	+	+	+	+	+
Antivimentine	Vimentine intermediate filaments	+	+	+	+	+
Anti-HLA-ABC	HLA-ABC	+	+	+	+	+

[a] Moabs isolated by E. Oosterwijk et al (75).

four tumors were maintained as serially transplantable human renal carcinoma on nude mice. Thus, the take rate (> five passages on nude mice) was 4 of 39 (10%). The tumor cell lines are listed in Table 15.3. One tumor cell line (NC-65), used for the assays described below, had already been established in 1977, and some of its characteristics have been published elsewhere (20, 26, 27). All transplantable tumor cell lines originated from patients who already had metastases at the time of diagnosis or developed metastatic disease soon after surgery. Comparison of the histologic features of the human neoplasms with their nude mouse counterparts revealed the tumors to be identical (Fig. 15.1*A*). Electron microscopy showed features characteristic of kidney carcinoma (Fig. 15.1*B*). Growth curves are shown in Figure 15.2. There was no evidence of progressive dedifferentiation of the transplanted tumor following repeated mouse passages. Monoclonal antibodies (Moabs) that react with the proximal tubules of the nephron did not

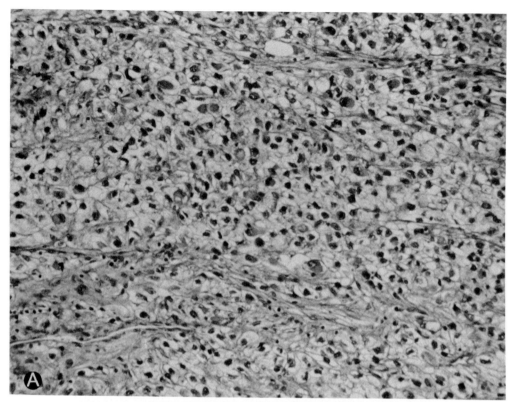

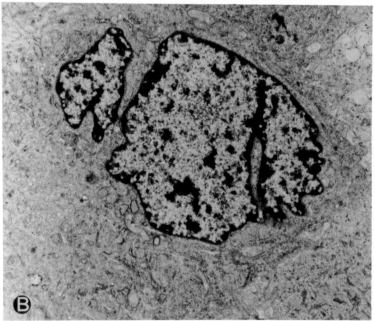

Figure 15.1. *A,* Human clear cell renal adenocarcinoma grown in a nude mouse (RC-8, eighth passage). ×200. *B,* Electron microscopy showing cytoarchitecture of a human renal adenocarcinoma supported by a nude mouse (NC-65, fiftieth passage). Indentation of the nucleus and clumped chromatin. Cytoplasma contains an abundance of glycogen and lipid. ×3400.

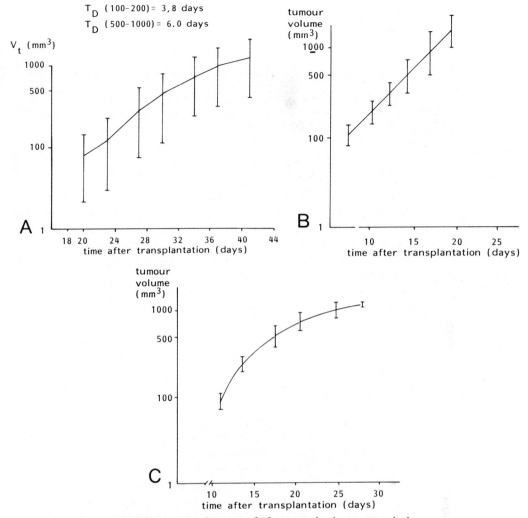

Figure 15.2. RCC-14. *A,* Mean growth curve of 12 tumors in the twenty-ninth mouse passage. After a lag phase of 20 days, the transplanted tumors became measurable and grew with a doubling time of 3.8 days until day 33. Thereafter they grew with a doubling time of 6.0 days. *B,* RCC-21. Mean growth curve of 16 RC-21 tumors in the ninth passage. The tumors becames palpable on day 7 after transplantation and grew with a doubling time of 3.2 days. The animals were sacrificed before the growth curve reached a plateau. *C,* Mean growth of 16 NC-65 tumors in the fifty-eighth mouse passage. Doubling time was 3.8 days.

stain the tumor lines histochemically, except for a weak staining by Moab RC-250, whereas Moabs reacting with human keratine protein and vimentine intermediate filaments stained all examined lines (Table 15.4). HLA-ABC was found to be present on the surface of nucleated cells. Thus the human origin of the established kidney carcinoma was proven in all lines. By the time that the human tumor had been successfully transplanted for serial passages, all of the patients who had delivered the source tumors had died. In no case could the subcutaneous assay be used for individual chemosensitivity testing.

Table 15.4
Human Renal Carcinoma Transplanted Directly from Surgical Specimens into Nude Mice

Transplants		Serial Passages	
Attempted	Successful	Attempted	Successful[a]
39	14 (35.9%)	13	4 (30.8%)

[a] Five or more successive passages in nude mice.

Evaluability of the Subrenal Capsule Assay

The subrenal capsule assay (SRC) provides an in vivo method for quickly determining the responsiveness of human tumor xenografts to chemotherapeutic agents in situ. Transplantation studies using both athymic nude mice and normal immunocompetent mice (NIC) as hosts for human tumor xenografts suggested that SRC assay methodology would permit the use of the NIC mouse instead of the athymic nude animal (45). By limiting the assay to 6 days it should be possible to avoid the complications of an immune response (46). By applying the SRC assay methodology in a 6-day time frame, it was demonstrated that tumor sensitivity to chemotherapeutic agents could be determined by using fresh surgical explants of human breast and colon tumors as first transplant generation xenografts in the normal immunocompetent mouse. Of 254 xenografts implanted under the renal capsule of NIC mice, 62% showed positive measurable growth, 18% showed no measurable change, and 20% showed some degree of partial regression. The average growth of xenografts in assays having a mean increase in tumor size (+ TS) was 1.5 ocular micrometer units (OMU) $\pm$ 1.1 SD, the range being 0.3 to 6.0. For untreated xenografts that exhibited a decrease in tumor size (− TS) following implantation, comparison of the average regression rates in ocular micrometer units per day, revealed that they regressed in nude mice and immunocompetent mice at similar rates averaging 0.2 OMU/day. Bogden et al (46) argued that, since a decrease in xenograft size is dependent upon the normal lytic and clearance mechanisms of the host, it would appear that these mechanisms at least are of similar effectiveness in athymic and immunocompetent mice. Increasing mean + TS values should reflect tumors with increasingly greater growth potential. Thus, by examining the mean TS control value for each assay, one could recognize an assay that might yield doubtful results (mean ΔTS < 0.5 OMU using tumor line, mean Δ TS < −0.5 OMU for primary tumor).

The authors examined the growth of fresh surgical explants from the established kidney carcinoma tumor lines after implantation under the renal capsule, using the method described by Bogden et al (33). Criteria for the evaluability of the assay were (a) growth of the tumor fragment transplanted under the renal capsule of immunocompetent BALB-c nu/+ mice and immunoincompetent BALB-c nu/nu mice (mean ΔTS (tumor size) > 0.5 OMU) and (b) histologically proven presence of tumor tissue.

METHODS AND MATERIALS—SRC ASSAY

Athymic female BALB-c nu/nu mice (AN), immunocompetent BALB-c nu/+ mice (NIC), and immunocompetent BALB-c nu/+ mice pretreated by whole body irradiation (IIC) with 5 Gy were used to receive explants of the established renal carcinoma cell lines. BALB-c mice were obtained from the breeding colony in the authors' laboratory. Preselected 1-mm³ fragments of tumor tissue were implanted under the renal capsule. Since the renal capsule of the mouse is transparent, measurements of the fresh tumor tissue fragments were made under magnification by means of a stereoscopic microscope fitted with an ocular micrometer. Two diameters were measured (length and width) and recorded in ocular micrometer units. Magnification was calibrated so that 10 OMU was equal to 1 mm. Tumor size (TS) was expressed as the average of the two diameters. Tumor size was measured on day 0 and day 11 in athymic mice, and on day 0 and day 6 in immunocompetent irradiated and nonirradiated mice. The change in tumor size was calculated for each animal, and the average TS values were computed for each tumor line. After the last measurements the kidney bearing the xenograft was excised and prepared for histologic examination. The following renal carcinoma tumor lines were used to investigate the SRC assay evaluability: NC-65, RC-2, RC-8, RC-21, RC-43, and RCC-14 (RCC-14 by courtesy of U Otto, Department of Urology, University of Hamburg, West Germany).

RESULTS OF THE SRC ASSAY EVALUABILITY

Three tumor lines were tested in BALB-c nu/nu mice. In all experiments tumor growth above the critical level of 0.5 OMU was observed (Table 15.5). The computed values represent the mean growth of the transplanted tumor fulfilling the first criterion of evaluability. Histologically, however, only small islands of tumor cells surrounded by fibroblasts and lymphocytes could be identified under the renal capsule at the end of the 6-day assay in immunocompetent BALB-c nu/+ mice (Fig. 15.3). In BALB-c nu/+ animals treated by total body irradiation 1 day prior to transplantation, on the other hand, tumor growth and viable tumor tissue was visible under the microscope (Fig. 15.3B). Tumor in situ at the end of the 6-day assay (A) and the tumor-bearing kidney (B) are shown in Figure 15.3.

Summarizing the experiments with the SRC assay in athymic, immunodeficient (irradiated), and immunocompetent mice, evaluable assays were obtained with athymic or immunodeficient mice. Immunocompetent mice fulfilled only one criterion of assay evaluability. Although measurements of the implants after 6 days delivered a mean growth of > 0.5 OMU, the histology of day 6 xenografts revealed varying degrees of host-versus-graft reaction ranging from incursion of host cells to total replacement of the implant by histiocytes with formation of a pseudotumor. If one were to rely merely on measurements of the transplanted tumor, no useful information could be obtained. AE Bogden (personal communication), using gynecologic xenografts, did not detect severe host reactions of this type in immunocompetent mice

Table 15.5
Subrenal Capsule Assay Evaluability

Tumor Line	Assay Duration (Days)	BALB-c nu/nu Athymic Mice[a]		BALB-c nu/+ Immunocompetent Mice		BALB-c nu/+ Irradiated Immunocompetent Mice	
		Tumor Size (OMU)	No. of Animals	Tumor Size (OMU)	No. of Animals	Tumor Size (OMU)	No. of Animals
NC-65	6	+5.6 (±1.7)	4	+5.2 (±3.8)	8	+5.4 (±3.1)	9
				+6.5 (4.5)	7		
	11	+3.9 (±6.2)	8				
RC-2	6					+3.1 (±4.1)	7
RC-8	6	NE[b]	8	+0.3 (±15.6)	6	NE[c]	8
	14	4.5 (±3.1)	5				
	35	+22.1 (±17.1)	4				
RC-21	6			+25.7 (±6)	6[a]	+8.8 (±4.6)	6
						+9.4 (±3.8)	6
RC-43	6					+12.0 (±2.6)	6
RCC-14	11	+5.8 (±3.6)	6				
	6					+7.9 (±1.6)	8
	6					+5.3 (±1.7)	6

[a] Swiss mice +/+.
[b] NE, not evaluated, intercurrent death in 4 of 8; in 2 of 8 total regression of the transplanted tissue was histologically proved.
[c] Intercurrent death in 1 of 8; total regression in 5 of 8.

at the end of the 6-day assay. Actual cell counts indicated that tumor cells comprised approximately 85% of the fragment mass at the end of the assay period. Host response may be greater to some types of tumor. Irradiation of immunocompetent mice prior to transplantation under the renal capsule can suppress host reaction, and NIC mice therefore should not be used without immune deprivation. Similar experience has been reported by others (47, 48). Edelstein et al (48) also pointed out that there is a discrepancy between macroscopic and histologic evaluation of human tumor response when normal mice are used for the SRC assay. To suppress an invasion by (mouse) host cells during the 6-day period of the assay, they pretreated by whole body irradiation with 4 or 6 Gy (24 hours prior to implantation) or 4.5 Gy (less than 4 hours before implantation), or cortisone acetate suspension 0.75 to 2.5 mg/mouse subcutaneously, or 2.5 mg/mouse of a colloidal suspension of silica intravenously. Combinations of cortisone acetate (0.75 mg) and whole body irradiation were also tested. Whole body irradiation best fulfilled the criteria for assay evaluability (tumor growth and high percentage of histologically viable tumor cells). In preirradiated normal mice, the percentage of tumor cells observed under the kidney capsule (per microscopic field) was generally higher for tumor line transplants than for transplants from primary tumors. Since a part of the heterogeneity seen in the histologic sections taken on day 6 was already present in the 1-mm³ tumor pieces, prior to implantation, Edelstein et al (49) suggested that the intrinsic heterogeneity of tumors is such that only a fraction of them demonstrate tumor growth after transplantation into preirradiated host, even though almost all of them fulfill the minimum requirements for bulk growth.

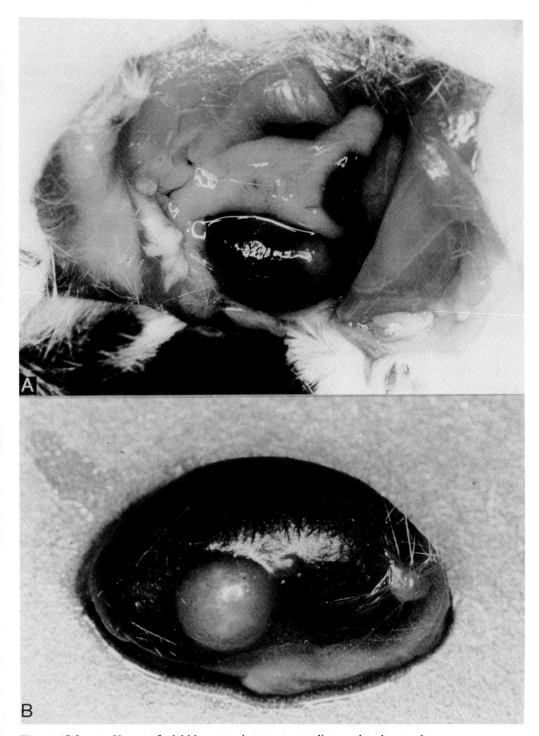

Figure 15.3. *A,* Xenografted kidney carcinoma tumor line under the renal capsule of a preirradiated BALB-c nu/+ mouse (day 6). *B,* Tumor-bearing kidney from preirradiated BALB-c nu/+ mouse (day 6).

In Vitro Assay with Labeled DNA Precursor

Several in vitro drug testing assays have been developed for solid tumor tissue. Morphologic changes in the tumor cells (50), the inhibition of cell population increases (39, 51, 52), inhibition of cellular respiration (53), and inhibition of the cell metabolism (54, 55) have all been used as a measure of drug activity. In 1980 Shrivastav and Paulson (38) developed an in vitro assay to measure the susceptibility to chemotherapeutic drugs of cells from human tumors, utilizing freshly isolated live cells. Cells were incubated in vitro, and the drug-induced inhibition of the incorporation of radiolabeled precursor into DNA, RNA, and protein was measured. The assay was sensitive to concentrations of chemotherapeutic drugs in the therapeutic range and was reproducible when tested with replicates of the same tumor cell population. For the assay, a live cell suspension containing 5 to 6×10^5 cells/ml was added to each of the 96 wells on a microtiter plate. The plates were incubated with drugs for 24, 48, and 72 hours. Tritiated thymidine (or uridine or an amino acid mixture) was then added, and incubation was continued for a further 12 hours. The authors used several of the established human kidney carcinoma lines xenografted on nude mice to determine the evaluability of the assay with labeled DNA precursor. The tumor cell lines NC-65, RC-21, and RCC-14 (by courtesy of U Otto, Hamburg, West Germany) were prepared for the assay immediately after surgical excision. NC-65 was also cultured in a medium until the sixth passage and then used for the assay. The assay (Fig. 15.4) was regarded as evaluable if (a) the [^{3}H]thymidine incorporation increased both with time and with increasing number of cells plated and (b) the inhibition of [^{3}H]thymidine incorporation in treated cells was dose dependent.

The assay system used in this investigation was a slight modification of that described by Shrivastav and Paulson (38). Fresh tumor tissue was dissected from nude mice, cut into 1 to 2-mm pieces with scissors, and incubated in Eagle's minimum essential medium (MEM) containing 200 units/ml of collagenase (type I) for 4 hours at 37°C in a humidified atmosphere of 5% CO_2 in air. After incubation, tissue fragments were aspirated in a pipette several times to complete dispersion.

The suspension was centrifuged at 1500 rpm. The supernatant was discarded and the pellet was washed with phosphate-buffered saline (PBS) by resuspension and centrifugation as many times as necessary. Finally the cells were suspended in MEM + 10% fetal calf serum (FCS). Single-cell suspension was obtained by sieving through a nylon gauze with a pore size of 40 μm. The number of viable cells was determined by the trypan blue exclusion test. After dilution, cells were seeded in 100 μl of MEM + 10% FCS into the wells, and 50 μl of extra medium—in some experiments containing cytostatic drug—were added. The microtiter plates were incubated for 24, 48, 72, or 144 hours in a humidified atmosphere of 5% CO_2 in air at 37°C. After this, 50 μl of a solution of [^{3}H]thymidine in MEM + 10% FCS were added, the final activity being 1.5 μCi/well (200 μl), and the plates were incubated overnight (16 hours). Incorporation was terminated by centrifuging the microtiter plates at 1500 rpm for 10 minutes. The supernatants were

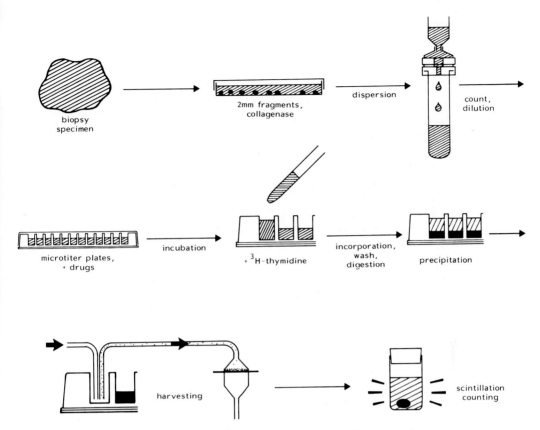

Figure 15.4. Method DNA precursor [³H]thymidine assay. For further explanations see the text (under "In Vitro Assay with Labeled DNA Precursor").

discarded, the cell plates were washed with PBS containing 0.5 mM unlabeled thymidine, and the plates were centrifuged for 5 minutes at 1500 rpm. After removal of the supernatant, the pellets were dissolved with the aid of 1 drop of 2.5% trypsin at 37°C for 7 to 10 minutes. One hundred microliters of cold 10% trichloroacetic acid were added to each well. The plates were allowed to stand overnight at 4°C, and the acid precipitable radioactivity was collected on Whatman glass filter paper using a precipitation cell harvester. The radioactive material was solubilized in 1 ml of Soluene 350 in a scintillation flask for 30 minutes. After the addition of 10 ml of Instagel scintillation fluid containing 10 ml of acetic acid and 1 g of butylated hydroxytoluene/liter, radioactivity was measured using a liquid scintillation counter.

RESULTS—EVALUABILITY OF THE DNA PRECURSOR ASSAY

With all of the cell lines tested, a high level of incorporation of radioactive thymidine was measured after a cultivation period of 24 to 144 hours. Figure 15.5 demonstrates that, with cells isolated from NC-65 tumors grown in the nude mouse, the amount of radioactivity incorporated was dependent on the initial cell number (i.e., the number

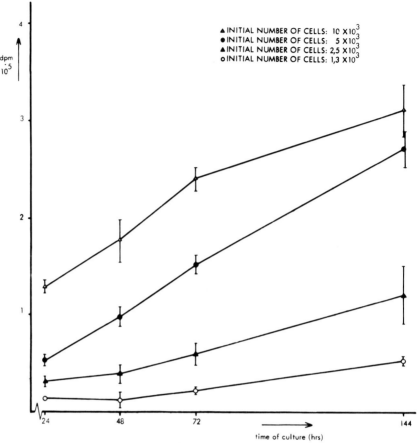

INITIAL NUMBER OF CELLS: 10×10^3
INITIAL NUMBER OF CELLS: 5×10^3
INITIAL NUMBER OF CELLS: $2,5 \times 10^3$
INITIAL NUMBER OF CELLS: $1,3 \times 10^3$

$\frac{dpm}{10^5}$

time of culture (hrs)

Figures 15.5 and 15.6. Cells isolated from tumor cell line NC-65. There is a good relationship between the number of cells plated and incorporation of [³H]thymidine until 72 hours. A linear relationship is found when 10×10^3 cells/well are plated (Fig. 15.5). Similar results were found for cultured cells from NC-65 tumor (Fig. 15.6).

of cells plated). A linear relationship between cell number and [³H]-thymidine incorporation was observed when the number of cells initially plated was in the range 1.3 to 10×10^3. The incorporation of radioactivity increased linearly when 10×10^3 or fewer NC-65 tumor cells were plated. In the same experiment the incorporation of thymidine by NC-65 cells that had been maintained in culture for five passages was studied (Fig. 15.6). A higher level of thymidine incorporation was noted with the cultured cells than with the freshly isolated tumor cells.

The same phenomenon was observed with the other tumor lines studied. The incorporation of radioactive thymidine by cells of the NC-65 tumor line, at various cell concentrations and after various times of cultivation, is shown in Figure 15.7. The incorporation decreased after preincubation of tumor cells exceeding 24 hours. Maximal incorporation occurred with 1×10^5 NC-65 cells. When 6×10^5 cells were plated, however, the incorporation of thymidine represented only a fraction of the maximal level. The importance of these findings becomes clear in

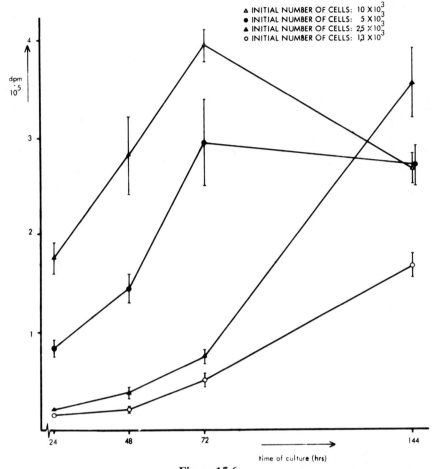

Figure 15.6.

the next experiment. The authors measured the inhibition of thymidine incorporation in the presence of drugs under various conditions. Figure 15.8 shows that [³H]thymidine incorporation by RCC-14 cells, plated at 1×10^4 cells/well, was increasingly inhibited by increasing doses of adriamycin. This dose-dependent effect was no longer demonstrable when 6×10^4 cells/well were plated.

Summarizing the experience in determining the evaluability of the in vitro assay with labeled DNA-precursor, the optimal level for [³H]-thymidine incorporation was reached after different culture times for different numbers of cells seeded. Consequently, the incorporation of radioactivity measured after longer periods in culture did not correctly reflect the number of cells originally plated. In the series of experiments, the number of live tumor cells in suspension was gradually increased. When larger numbers of tumor cells were plated up to 6×10^5 ml as recommended by Shrivastav and Paulson (38), the maximal level of incorporated [³H]thymidine was not reached, probably due to contact inhibition of growth, which may prevent incorporation of [³H]thymidine for DNA synthesis. Therefore, both the time of incubation and the number of cells plated appear to be of critical importance for the amount

EXPERIMENTAL CHEMOTHERAPY   241

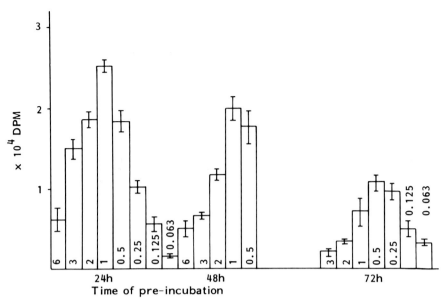

Figure 15.7. Cell isolated from tumor cell line NC-65. Maximal incorporation of [³H]thymidine occurred with 1×10^4 cells. The incorporation decreased after preincubation of tumor cells in medium for more than 24 hours.

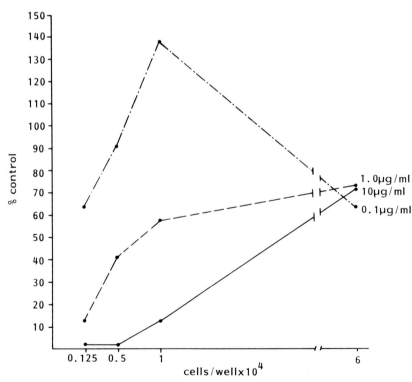

Figure 15.8. Cells isolated from tumor cell line RCC-14. The incorporation of [³H]thymidine is inhibited in a dose-dependent manner in the presence of adriamycin when 0.5×10^4 cells/well are plated. When 6×10^4 cells/well were plated, no dose-dependent effect was observed.

of radioactivity ultimately incorporated by the cells. A dose-dependent inhibition of [³H]thymidine incorporation after preincubation with cytostatic drugs was seen only when smaller numbers of tumor cells from tumor lines were plated (0.5 to 2×10^4 cells/well equal to 0.5 to 2×10^5 cells/ml). The authors regard the variation of the optimal condition for incorporation as a major disadvantage in the possible clinical application of this test system, since it is not feasible in such situations to determine in advance the best conditions for the test. The pattern of inhibition of thymidine incorporation by cytostatic drugs may be critically influenced by the experimental conditions, especially by the number of live tumor cells plated in vitro for the assay.

The question of the nature and origin of the cell prepared from kidney tumor lines may be of importance. In addition to the neoplastic epithelial cells, the tumors also contain supporting stroma, which in the nude mouse-supported tumor is of mouse origin (56). However, as demonstrated by Shrivastav and Paulson (38), cells attached to the microtiter wells were chiefly of epithelioid morphology. It was speculated that collagenase has some selective adverse effect on fibroblastic cells, since epithelial cell lines could easily be subcultured in 0.1% collagenase in culture medium, while the fibroblastic cells from a rhabdomyosarcoma could not (38). Thus, although it is not possible to establish beyond doubt the origin and nature of cells present in the cell fraction obtained of the collagenase-treated kidney tumor line, some findings suggest that these cells are mainly from epithelial origin.

Human Tumor Stem Cell Assay (Colony Formation Assay)*

The stem cell assay uses cells obtained directly from a tumor and attempts to predict the clinical response to various drugs in the laboratory. The system for solid tumors was developed by Hamburger and Salmon (40). Roper and Drewinko (57) evaluated several in vitro tests of antineoplastic agent activity, including measurements of labeling index, doubling time, ⁵¹Cr release, vital dye exclusion, and colony formation. They concluded that the colony-forming assay provides the most reliable dose-dependent index of drug-induced cell death. Evidence that colonies grown in agar were derived from the original tumor obtained from the patient was provided by injection of colonies into nude mice, where they produced histopathologically identical tumors. The cells in colonies grown in a two-layer system are referred to as stem cells. This term implies the capacity for self-renewal. In a population of tumor cells, the stem cells are those that regrow after subcurative therapy (58, 59). A number of reports of the application of the stem cell assay (or clonogenic assay) to human genitourinary tumors have appeared recently (60–65). Using fairly liberal criteria for growth, the probability of culturing a given renal cell carcinoma successfully is about 50% (63, 66, 67). To date, it has turned out that so-called "single-cell suspensions" from primary human solid tumors prepared by mechanical or enzymatic

---

*All experiments to determine the assay evaluability of the stem cell assay utilizing kidney carcinoma lines and chemosensitivity testing with the stem cell assay were performed by M Lieber and co-workers (Mayo Clinic, Rochester, MN).

techniques contain not only single tumor cells, but also many small aggregates of tumor cells. As reported by Agrez and co-workers (68), most of the cell colonies observed 1 to 2 weeks after culture initiation result from the proliferative enlargement of the small cell aggregates initially seeded. With this in mind, it is evident that cultures prepared from cell suspensions must be counted the day after seeding in order to identify the size and number of cell aggregates (68). Cultures which contain many cell aggregates greater than 60 μm in diameter must be discarded as nonevaluable. To distinguish whether the cells observed in the cell colonies are alive or dead when the cultures are assessed, vital staining with the tetrazolium dye, INT, can be used (69). When such cytotoxic control compounds as mercuric chloride, sodium azide, or chromomycin were used, it was found that the presumed "tumor cell colony proliferation," which should be inhibited by the presence of supercytotoxin in high concentrations, was not prevented. Therefore, assays of chemotherapy sensitivity depending on colony formation in soft agar can only be expected to yield worthwhile data if computerized "day 1" counting, a positive cytotoxic control compound, and vital staining are part of the assay (67).

METHODS AND MATERIALS—EVALUABILITY OF THE STEM CELL ASSAY

For the soft agar system, at least 2 g of grossly non-necrotic tumors obtained from the cell lines NC-65, RC-2, RC-21, and RCC-14 were minced mechanically into pieces of approximately 1 mm^3.

After storage at 4°C in complete cell culture medium, the minced tumor was incubated for disaggregation for 90 minutes in an enzyme mixture as described by Lieber and Kovach (61). Red blood cells were removed by exposure to lysing buffer. One volume of tumor cell pellet was suspended in 10 volumes of lysing buffer for 8 minutes at room temperature, centrifuged, and washed with complete medium. Tumor cells were then resuspended in complete medium and filtered through a 100-mesh stainless steel sieve (Cellector Tissue Sieve). Cell concentration was determined (1.5 × 10^7 cells/ml) and viability was scored by trypan blue (0.4%) exclusion.

For the soft agar stem cell assay, simplified culture media were used. Assays were performed in 35-mm Falcon plastic Petri dishes in 1 ml of Dulbecco modified Eagle's medium with 10% calf serum supplemented with 0.3% agar plated over 1 ml of the same medium containing 0.5% agar. Five × 10^5 viable tumor cells were seeded/plate. Plates were maintained in a humidified incubator in 95% air/5% CO$_2$ at 37°C for 3 weeks. Colony counting of six plates for each tumor specimen was performed on day 1 after plating. Mean day 1 counts were subtracted from those obtained later for each set of six plates. Significant colony formation was defined as an increase of 50 or more in the mean colony count for the six plates of 50 or greater as assessed 7 to 21 days after plating. Counting was performed electronically by an FAS-II Image Analysis Scanner (Bausch & Lomb). The criterion for the evaluability of the assay in this study was growth of at least 50 colonies/plate after

Table 15.6
Growth of Human Kidney Carcinoma Cell Lines in the Colony Formation Assay (Stem Cell Assay) after Seeding of 5×10^5 Viable Tumor Cells/Plate

Tumor Line	Mean No. of Colonies on 6 Plates (±SD)	
NC-65	98.5	(±10)
	110	(±15)
	212	(±35)
	875	(±18)
	202	(±87)
	181	(±68)
RC-2	64	(±15)
	109	(±68)
	121	(±32)
RC-21	157	(±69)
	191	(±24)
	309	(±40)
	345	(±47)
	788	(±61)
RCC-14	173	(±15)
	311	(±51)
	704	(±12)
	797	(±160)
	985	(±71)

500,000 trypan blue excluding nucleated cells had been seeded on each plate.

All tumor cell lines cultured in soft agar grew sufficiently to reach the critical limit of more than 50 colonies/plate (Table 15.6). Enough material was gained from the surgical specimens to perform chemosensitivity testing. Summarizing the experience obtained with kidney carcinoma cell lines in the stem cell assay, one can conclude that with the excellent growth observed they may be useful for pharmacologic studies of drug interaction.

Von Hoff (70) and Selby et al (71) recently discussed the possible value of the "human tumor stem cell assay." Both authors emphasized—as others have done—the major advantage in the study of human tumor biology which has been brought about by the ability to generate colonies in culture from cells of human tumors. But they also stated, however, that the use of this assay in the routine selection of anticancer drugs is premature. It should be stressed that at present only 50% or fewer of solid tumors coming to the laboratory can be successfully propagated in vitro (67). Regardless of any possible value of drug testing systems for predicting chemosensitivity, one requires that an assay should be evaluable in a high percentage of cases. This goal is not yet achieved when donor patients' tumors are worked up for the stem cell assay.

CHEMOTHERAPY STUDIES IN VIVO AND IN VITRO

Subcutaneous Assay

The tumors used for these experiments were obtained by hetero-transplanting human kidney carcinoma directly from the patient to nude mice. BALB-c nu/nu mice, bred and maintained in the authors' laboratory, were employed. The chemosensitivity of the serially transplantable tumor lines NC-65, RC-21, and RCC-14 (by courtesy of U Otto, University of Hamburg, West Germany) was examined. Tumor pieces weighing between 50 and 200 mg were subcutaneously transplanted into both shoulders (Fig. 15.9). When the tumor had become palpable, after a lag phase of 6 (RC-21), 10 (NC-65), or 20 days (RCC-14), respectively, the mice were divided into groups of six to eight animals and injected with anticancer drugs. Control animals received on injection of saline. The tumor diameters were measured twice a week, and the volume of the tumor was calculated from the formula V_t $= \frac{\pi}{6} (d1 \times d2)^{1.5}$. The criterion for drug activity was a significant reduction in tumor growth compared to controls. Drugs, treatment schedule, and route of injection are listed in Table 15.7.

RESULTS OF DRUG TESTING IN THE SUBCUTANEOUS ASSAY

In tumor line NC-65 one of the 11 drugs tested, DFMO/MGBG (difluoromethylornithine/methylglyoxal bis[guanylhydrazon]) reduced tumor growth significantly (DFMO was a generous gift from the Centre de Research, Merrel International). In tumor line RC-21 (Table 15.7, Fig. 15.10), two of the seven drugs tested reduced tumor growth (vin-

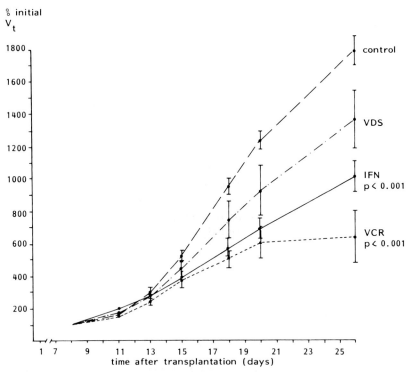

Figure 15.9. Effect of treatment on subcutaneously growing RC-21 tumor line with vindesine, vincristine, and α-interferon. Growth is expressed as the mean percentage of the initial tumor volume ± SEM at day 8.

Table 15.7
Activity of Drugs against Subcutaneously Implanted Human Kidney Carcinoma Xenografts in Nude Mice and Comparison of Final Tumor Volume in Controls and Treated Animals (Results Expressed as Percentage of Control)

Compound	Dose Level (mg/kg/week)	Route	Tumor Growth in Renal Carcinoma Lines as Percentage of Control (Range of Tumor Volume in cm^3)		
			NC-65 (0.7–2.5)	RC-21 (1.3–1.8)	RCC-14 (0.7–1.2)
Adriamycin	0.5/3×/3 wks	i.p.	92		
	2.0/1×/3 wks	i.p.	83		
	5.0/1×/2 wks	i.v.	71		
	10.0/1×/2 wks	i.v.	100	61	107
Vinblastine	1.0/1×/3 wks	i.p.	76		
	2.5/1×/3 wks	i.v.			66^b
	3.3/3× in 12 days	i.p.		81	
Methyl-GAG	100/1×/3 wks	i.p.	60		
DFMO^a/methyl-GAG	2%/100 (1×/2 wks)	p.o./i.p.	40^b	56	33^b
Vindesine	0.8/1×/3 wks	i.p.	75	87	
Vincristine	0.15/1×/3 wks	i.p.	92	38^b	
Methotrexate	1.0/1×/3 wks	i.p.	84		
Epi-adriamycin	10.0/1×/3 wks	i.v.	60	60	
Mitoxantrone	5/3× in 12 days	i.p.		87	
Cis-platinum	5/1×/3 wks	i.p.	90	80	110
α-Interferon	2 × 10^5 units/daily 21 days	s.c.		55^b	50^b

^{a} DFMO, difluoromethylornithine.
^{b} Wilcoxon test $p < 0.05$.

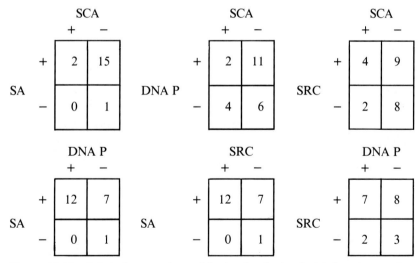

Figure 15.10. Mutual comparison of the results obtained with four drug testing systems in tumor lines NC-65, RC-21, and RCC-14. SCA, subcutaneous assay; SA, stem cell assay; SRC, subrenal capsule assay; DNA P DNA precursor [^{3}H]-thymidine assay; +/+ tumor sensitive in both assays; −/−, tumor resistant in both assays.

cristine, human α-interferon (Ropheron)), and in tumor line RCC-14, three of the five drugs tested (vinblastine, DFMO/MGBG, α-interferon) did as well (Table 15.6). Assay duration for tumor line RC-21 ranged from 20 to 31 days, for NC-65 from 22 to 33 days, and for RCC-14 from 40 to 41 days. The mean doubling times for the three tumor lines were 3.2 days, 3.6 days, and 3.8 days, respectively. In none of the animals could tumor growth be completely suppressed. The reduction achieved could be described as partial remission in four experiments and as minimal remission in two experiments.

Subrenal Capsule Assay

Immunocompetent BALB-c nu/+ mice, pretreated with whole body irradiation (5 Gy, 24 hours prior to transplantation), were selected to receive fresh surgical explants of the kidney carcinoma lines NC-65, RCC-14, RC-2, RC-21, and RC-43. Preselected 1-mm^3 fragments of tumor tissue were implanted under the renal capsule and measured under magnification by means of a stereoscopic microscope. Two diameters were measured, and the average of the two diameters was recorded in ocular micrometer units. The animals were divided into groups of six mice and injected with anticancer drugs from day 1 to day 5. Animals were sacrificed on day 6, and final measurements were performed. The change in tumor size was calculated for each animal and the average tumor size volumes were computed for each tumor line. The criterion for drug activity was either significant reduction in tumor growth compared to controls or tumor regression.

RESULTS OF SUBRENAL CAPSULE 6-DAY ASSAY

Tumor growth was significantly reduced by 5 of the 10 drugs tested in tumor line NC-65, 3 of the 6 drugs tested in RC-2, 5 of the 9 drugs tested in RC-21, and 1 of the 6 drugs tested in tumor line RC-43 (Table 15.8). Vindesine, mitoxantrone, and adriamycin caused tumor regression in tumor lines NC-65, vincristine in tumor line RC-2, and vinblastine in tumor line RC-21.

Table 15.8
Activity of Drugs against Human Kidney Carcinoma Xenografts Transplanted under the Renal Capsule of Irradiated Mice (BALB-c nu/+)[a]

Compound	Dose Level (mg/kg/injection)	Route	ΔTS Tumor Line				
			NC-65	RCC-14	RC-2	RC-21	RC-43
	Control		5.4/5.9	7.9	5.9	8.8/9.4	12.0
Vincristine	1.0	s.c.	2.8		−0.8[b]	1.2[b]	1.2[b]
Vinblastine	1.0	s.c.	1.1[b]	5.4[b]	1.1[b]	−3.0[b]	6.9
Vindesine	1.0	s.c.	−0.4[b]		0.0[b]	4.2	
DFMO[c]/methyl-GAG	2%/100	p.o./s.c.	0.8[b]	5.7		0.4[b]	10.3
Methotrexate	4.0	s.c.	4.5				
Mitoxantrone	5.0	s.c.	−0.7[b]			4.3	
Adriamycin	4.0	i.v.	−0.13[b]	1.6	1.9	5.0	11.0
Epi-adriamycin	4.0	i.v.	3.6			1.5[b]	
Cis-platinum	2.0	s.c.	4.2	6.0	4.8	6.6	12.9
Mitomycin-C	0.7	s.c.					12.2
α-Interferon	10^5 U	s.c.	4.1	6.1		1.9[b]	

[a] ΔTS expressed in ocular micrometer units (10 OMU = 1.0 mm). Six-day assay; injections on days 1 to 5.
[b] Wilcoxon-test p < 0.05.
[c] DFMO, difluoromethylornithine.

DNA Precursor [³H]Thymidine Assay

Cell suspensions were prepared from solid tumors of the tumor lines NC-65, RC-2, RC-8, RC-21, and RCC-14. Cells were seeded in microtiter wells in the presence of various drugs. Optimal cell concentration was determined for each tumor line prior to the experiments with drugs. After 48 hours' incubation in 100 μl of MEM + 10% FCS and drugs in 50 μl of MEM, 50 μl of [³H]thymidine solution were added (the final activity being 1.5 μCi/well) and the cells in suspension were incubated overnight (16 hours). Radioactivity was then measured using a liquid scintillation counter.

RESULTS—DNA PRECURSOR [³H]THYMIDINE ASSAY

If the results of the in vitro cytostatic testing are evaluated at a dose level comparable with the peak plasma concentration obtainable in vivo ($\pm$ 1μg/ml), then at this concentration six of the nine drugs reduced [³H]thymidine incorporation to 30% or below controls in tumor line NC-65; one of the five drugs in line RC-2; one of the five drugs in line RC-8; eight of the nine drugs in line RC-21; and zero of the five drugs in line RCC-14 (Table 15.9).

Stem Cell Assay

Minced tumor tissue was worked up for the stem cell assay as described above. Chemosensitivity of the tumor lines NC-65, RC-2, RCC-14, and RC-21 was tested with the drugs used for the subcutaneous assay, the SRC assay, and the DNA precursor assay.

RESULTS—STEM CELL ASSAY

All tumor lines showed significant colony formation in vitro and allowed drug testing to be successfully carried out. In 54 of the 68 assays performed in triplicate with peak plasma concentrations, more than 70% inhibition of colony formation (> 60 μm) compared to controls was observed (Table 15.10). Methotrexate was the only drug showing no activity against the tumor lines. Thus, the in vitro sensitivity data gathered with maximally achievable plasma concentrations and continuous drug exposure do not correspond with what is known of the drug activity in the clinic.

Comparison of the in Vivo and in Vitro Assay

In vivo and in vitro chemosensitivity tests have been applied to kidney carcinoma. The tumor cells were first grown as xenografts in athymic mice. The serially transplantable tumors were implanted subcutaneously, and the animals were treated with cytostatic drugs as soon as the tumor became measurable (subcutaneous assay). The results of this in vivo assay with precise measurements of the sensitivity are compared with the results obtained with the subrenal capsule assay, the DNA precursor [³H]thymidine assay, and the stem cell assay, utilizing the same tumor line for all assays.

Table 15.9
Drug Testing in Vitro: Inhibition of Thymidine Incorporation in Cells of Human Kidney Carcinoma Lines Established on Nude Mice (Results Expressed as Percentage of Control)

Compound	Dose (μg/ml)	NC-65 (1×10^5)	RC-2 (2×10^5)	RC-8 (2×10^5)	RC-21 (1×10^5)	RCC-14 (1×10^5)
		— % [³H]Thymidine Incorporation in Tumor Lines (Cells/ml)				
Vinblastine	0.1	32	42	57	22	94
	1.0	30	42	52	26	79
	10.0	31	30	38	13	57
Vincristine	0.1	27	42	55	36	
	1.0	27	34	61	34	
	10.0	27	30	65	25	
Vindesine	0.1	28	33	81	34	
	1.0	32	42	56	28	
	10.0	32	25	48	20	
Adriamycin	0.1	30	63	20	13	138
	1.0	8	12	14	<1	60
	10.0	<1	2	6	<1	13
Cis-platinum	0.1	72	105	86	42	125
	1.0	17	100	83	15	91
	10.0	2	88	67	1	31
Mitoxantrone	0.1	112			11	
	1.0	91			1.4	
	10.0	87			0	
Epi-adriamycin	0.1	44			51	
	1.0	2			3	
	10.0	1			1	
DFMO[a]/methyl-GAG	1 mM/1 μM	27			9	56
α-Interferon	7×10^5 U/ml	57			8	59
Methotrexate	0.1	45				
	1.0	40				
	10.0	45				

[a] DFMO, difluoromethylornithine.

Table 15.10
Stem Cell Assay of Xenografted Kidney Carcinoma Lines[a]

Drug	Concentration (μg/ml)	RC-2	RC-14	RC-21	NC-65	Total
Cis-platinum	1.5	2/2	2/2	2/2	1/1	7/7
Methotrexate	2.75	0/2	0/2	0/3	0/1	0/8
Methyl-GAG	5.0	0/2	0/2	1/2	1/1	2/7
Mitoxantrone	0.25	2/2	2/2	2/2	2/2	8/3
Adriamycin	0.6	2/2	2/2	2/2	2/2	8/8
Epi-adriamycin	0.6	2/2	2/2	3/3	2/2	9/9
Vincristine	0.8	2/2	1/1	2/2	1/1	6/6
Vindesine	0.6	1/2	2/2	3/3	2/2	8/9
Vinblastine	0.05	1/1	1/1	1/1	3/3	6/6

[a] Drug testing by continuous exposure with maximally achievable plasma concentrations in vivo (peak plasma concentration). Frequency of drug which was shown to be active (>70% inhibition of colony formation)/number of assays performed.

Comparison showed a higher rate of resistant tumors in the in vivo assays than in the in vitro assays when the tumors were exposed to the same drugs (Fig. 15.11). If the results of the subrenal capsule assay, the stem cell assay, and the DNA precursor [³H]thymidine assay are compared with the results obtained with the source tumor (kidney tumor lines NC-65, RC-21, and RCC-14), then the best correlation is found with the SRC assay and the [³H]thymidine assay (Fig. 15.11). At least for the tumor lines both of these assays had the highest predictive value. Griffin et al (72) reported on a retrospective and prospective clinical trial performed to determine the usefulness of the 6-day SRC assay. The overall predictive accuracy retrospectively evaluated in 55 patients with a variety of solid malignancies was 85%. Of 37 patients with chemotherapy-refractory cancers treated in a prospective trial with single-agent chemotherapy selected on the basis of the assay, 14 patients (38%) responded. Thus the SRC assay showed potential value as a rapid predictive test for chemotherapeutic selection on an individual patient basis.

Comparing the SRC assay with the stem cell assay, Bogden and Von Hoff (8) found a greater number of evaluable assays with the in vivo

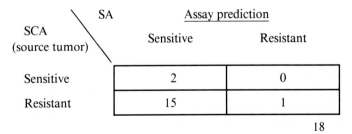

Figure 15.11. Comparison of the subcutaneous assay (SCA, source tumor) with the subrenal capsule assay (SRC), the stem cell assay (SA), and the DNA precursor assay (DNA P). Comparison of the results in tumor lines NC-65, RC-21, and RCC-14.

method, suggesting that the subcapsular site, for a limited period of 6 days, is a more favorable medium for solid human tumor explants. The SRC assay was predictive of clinical sensitivity for three of three drugs tested, while there was no correlation for sensitivity between the clinical response. However, the stem cell assay was predictive of clinical resistance for 10 of 10 drugs tested, and the SRC assay showed prediction for 16 of 20 drugs tested.

In the authors' tumor lines, the SRC assay and the [^{3}H]thymidine assay predicted both the sensitivity and the resistance better than the stem cell assay. Of course, the relative resistance of kidney carcinoma to cytostatic treatment means that this type of tumor is not ideal for drug testing. On the other hand, as shown, evaluable SRC assays can nearly always be obtained with kidney carcinoma explants, and therefore this method may be used to test the effectiveness of new drugs against kidney carcinoma. The [^{3}H]thymidine assay seems to be less ideal for clinical study because of the need to determine optimal assay conditions. To demonstrate that the SRC assay or any other given assay technique is more effective in predicting clinical response to drug treatment than a medical oncologist's empirical techniques, further randomized prospective clinical trials are needed (73).

CONCLUSION

New drugs that are not in clinical use are initially selected for secondary screening on the basis of experimental results obtained with transplanted tumors in mice. It may be doubted whether these models are indeed capable of predicting the response of human cancers, especially since apparently similar human cancers do not respond in a uniform manner to drugs. Differences in the host and other still unrecognized factors must be responsible. The relatively poor correlation between drug activity in human and animal cancers may be due to the following reasons, which have been formulated by Atassi (74):

1. There is no common etiology between experimental animal tumors and human tumors.
2. There are few unequivocal data establishing that the biochemical pathways in tumor cells are different from those in normal human or animal cells.
3. The failure of animal models to predict drug responsiveness of human tumors may be due to differences in the burden of tumor cells.
4. Criteria for anticancer activity differ from those in the clinic and are not comparable.
5. The growth rate of transplantable tumors is accelerated, and they are less differentiated than human cancers.
6. The dose administration used in animal models cannot be used in humans.

It should be possible to make a meaningful comparison between experimental and human anticancer activity by giving more attention to points 3 to 6. Experimentally, treatment of a transplantable tumor should be started when the tumor is measurable (i.e., the body burden of tumor cells is higher than 10^8). Thus, the tumor should be treated when the disease is diagnosed (visible), as in a clinical situation, and not at an early, undetectable stage. Instead of an increase in life span or a reduction of tumor growth, a significant regression of the tumor mass should be used for a positive correlation between animal model and human tumor.

Furthermore, cell proliferation should be close to that observed in human cancers. Human tumor xenografts implanted subcutaneously in nude athymic mice are expected to provide better information than the murine tumor. However, after several passages in nude mice, growth kinetics are no longer comparable with those of the original tumor. The use of fresh surgical xenografts implanted under the renal capsule of irradiated immunocompetent mice as a first transplant generation allows rapid determination of the sensitivity to chemotherapeutic agents (46). In contrast to an established tumor line, originating from a donor who may have been either sensitive or resistant to chemotherapy and thus showing a homogeneous response, fresh surgical xenografts from several patient donors with the same type of tumor may show heterogeneous responses to a treatment.

The human tumor cloning assay and the assay with labeled DNA or RNA precursors (thymidine or uridine) measure the response of a single cell population in vitro after the microarchitecture of the tumor has been destroyed. Results obtained by measurements in vivo and in vitro may be complementary. More notice should be taken of the dose aspect in experimental models. It is desirable that reduction in tumor growth should be achieved by nontoxic doses. Optimal doses equal to or exceeding the LD-10 may indicate chemosensitivity in the model, but are meaningless because the equivalent of the optimal dose can never be used by clinicians.

Finally, the parameters used in the clinic—i.e., partial or complete tumor regression, disease-free intervals, and cures—should be demonstrable in the experimental model.

At present the authors cannot claim to know the best experimental model for in vivo or in vitro screening of new anticancer agents. Efforts need to be continued to find the most suitable and reliable tumor model for examining the drug sensitivity of human cancer.

Acknowledgment. This research was supported in part by a grant from the Nierstichting, The Netherlands.

REFERENCES

1. Bloom HJG: Treatment of renal cell carcinoma with steroid hormones: observations with transplanted tumors in the hamster and incurable cancer in man. In King JS (ed): *Renal Neoplasia.* Boston, Little, Brown, and Co, 1967, p 605.
2. Bloom HJG: Medroxyprogesterone (Provera) in treatment of metastatic renal cancer. *Br J Cancer* 25:250–265, 1971.
3. Soloway MS, Meyers GH Jr: The effect of hormonal therapy on a transplantable renal cortical adenocarcinoma in syngeneic mice. *J Urol* 109:356–361, 1973.
4. Horning E: Endocrine factors involved in the induction, prevention and transplantation of kidney tumors in the male golden hamster. *Z Krebsforsch* 61:1, 1956.

5. van der Werf-Messing BJ, van Gilse H: Hormonal treatment of renal carcinoma. *Br J Cancer* 25:423–427, 1973.
6. Laucius JF, Patel YA, Lusch CJ, Koons LS, Bellet RE, Mastrangelo MJ: A phase-II evaluation of Bacille Calmette-Guérin plus megestrol acetate in patients with metastatic renal adenocarcinoma. *Med Pediatr Oncol* 3:237–242, 1977.
7. Neidhart JA, Gagen M, Young D, Wise H: A randomized study of polymerized tumor antigen admixed with adjuvant (PTA) for therapy of renal cancer. In Proceedings of the American Society of Clinical Oncology, San Diego, 1983, abstract C-189.
8. Bogden AE, Von Hoff DD: Comparison of the human tumor cloning and subrenal capsule assays. *Cancer Res.* 44:1087–1090, 1984.
9. Huben RP, Conelly R, Goldrosen MH, Murphy GP, Pontes EJ: Immunotherapy of a murine renal cancer. *J Urol* 129:1075–1078, 1983.
10. Tykkä H, Oravisto KJ, Lehtonen T, Sarna S, Tallberg T: Active specific immunotherapy of advanced renal cell carcinoma. *Eur Urol* 4:250–258, 1978.
11. Neidhart JA, Murphy SG, Hennick LA, Wise HA: Active specific immunotherapy of stage IV renal carcinoma with aggregated tumor antigen adjuvant. *Cancer* 46:1128–1134, 1980.
12. Klippel FF, Jacobi GH, Schulte-Wisserman H: Immunotherapie beim metastasierenden Hypernephrom. *Akt Urol* 12:161–165, 1981.
13. Kurth KH, Marquet R, Warnaar SD, Zwartendijk J, Schröder FH, Jonas U: Active specific immunotherapy with autologous tumor cells admixed with Corynebacterium parvum in patients with metastatic renal cell carcinoma. In Bracci U, Di Silverio F (eds): *Advances in Urological Oncology and Endocrinology.* Acta Medica, 1984, pp 269–283.
14. McCune CS, Shapira DV, Henshaw EC: Specific immunotherapy of advanced renal carcinoma: evidence for the polyclonality of metastases. *Cancer* 47:1984–1987, 1981.
15. Schärfe T, Becht E, Klippel KF, Jacobi GH, Hohenfellner R: Active immunotherapy of stage IV renal cell cancer using autologous tumor cells. In Klippel KF (ed): *Immunotherapie in der Urologie,* Band 9, Klin. und. Exp. Urologie. München, W Zuckschwerdt Verlag, 1984, pp 59–66.
16. DeVere White R, Olsson CA: Renal adenocarcinoma in the rat. *Invest Urol* 17:405–412, 1980.
17. Murphy GP: Murine renal cell carcinoma: a suitable human model. In Küss R, et al (eds): *Renal Tumors: Proceedings of the First International Symposium on Kidney Tumors.* New York, Alan R Liss, 1982, pp 175–206.
18. Rygaard J, Povlsen CO: *Proceedings of the First International Workshop on Nude Mice.* Stuttgart, Gustav Fischer Verlag, 1974.
19. Steel GG: The growth and therapeutic response of human tumors in immune-deficient mice. *Bull Cancer* 65:465–472, 1978.
20. Höhn W, Schröder FH: Renal cell carcinoma: 2 new cell lines and a serially transplantable nude mouse tumor (NC-65). *Invest Urol* 16:106–112, 1978.
21. Otto U, Klöppel G, Baisch H: Transplantation of human renal cell carcinoma into NMRI nu/nu mice: reliability of an experimental tumor model. *J Urol* 131:130–133, 1984.
22. Katsuoka Y, Baba S, Hata M, Tazaki H: Transplantation of human renal cell carcinoma to the nude mice: as an intermediate of in vivo and in vitro studies. *J Urol* 115:373–376, 1976.
23. Shrivastav S, Yarief Y, Day JW, Reich CF, Bonar RA: Establishment and characterization of a human renal carcinoma cell line (SS 78). *In Vitro* 17:1117–1124, 1981.
24. Williams RD, Strewler GJ, Nissenson RA: Human renal cancer model with associated hypercalcemia in nude mice. In Proceedings of the American Urological Association, Las Vegas, 1983, abstract 78, p 111.
25. Tamaoki N, Hata J, Izumi S, Ueyama Y, Toyama K: Systemic effects of human renal cell carcinoma on nude mice: polycythemia, anemia, hypervolemia and hepatomegaly. In Nomura T, Ohsawa N, Tamaoki N, Fujiwara K (eds): *Proceedings of the Second International Workshop on Nude Mice.* Tokyo, University of Tokyo Press, 1977, pp 417–426.
26. Kurth KH, Weissglas GM, Romijn JC, Schröder FH, van Dongen JW: In vitro and in vivo chemotherapeutic testing of human renal carcinoma in the nude mouse. *Akt Urol* 14:223–229, 1983.

27. Hagemeijer A, Höhn W, Smit EME: Cytogenetic analysis of human renal carcinoma cell lines of common origin (NC-65). *Cancer Res* 39:4662–4667, 1979.

28. Reeves BR, Houghton JA: Serial cytogenetic studies of human colonic tumor xenograft. *Br J Cancer* 37:612, 1978.

29. Warenius HM: Identification and separation of murine and human components of heterotransplanted human tumors. In *Symposium on Immuno-deficient Animals in Cancer Research*. London, Macmillan, 1980.

30. Pesce AJ, Bubel HC, DiPersio L, Michael JG: Human lactic dehydrogenase as a marker for human tumor cells growth in athymic mice. *Cancer Res* 37:1998, 1977.

31. Wirth M, Inglin B, Romen W, Ackermann R: Human embryonal cell carcinoma in nude mice. *Cancer Res* 43:5526–5532, 1983.

32. Lamerton LF, Steel GG: Growth kinetics of human large bowel cancer growing in immune-deprived mice and some chemotherapeutic observations. *Cancer* 36:2431, 1975.

33. Bogden AE, Kelton DE, Cobb WR, Gulkin TA, Johnson RK: Effects of serial passage in nude athymic mice on the growth characteristics and chemotherapy responsiveness of 13762 and R323OAC mammary tumor xenografts. *Cancer Res* 38:59, 1978.

34. Otto U, Huland H,: Baisch H, Klöppel G: Transplantation of human renal cell carcinoma into NMRI nu/nu mice. Evaluation of response to vinblastine sulfate monotherapy. *J Urol* 131:134–138, 1984.

35. van Steenbrugge GJ, Groen M, Romijn JC, Schröder FH: Biological effects on hormonal treatment regimen on a transplantable human prostatic tumor line (PC-82). *J Urol* 131:812–817, 1984.

36. Houghton JA, Taylor DM: Growth characteristics of human colorectal tumors during serial passage in immune-deprived mice. *Br J Cancer* 37:213, 1978.

37. Giovanella BC, Stehlin JS, Shepard RC, Williams LJ: Correlation between response to chemotherapy of human tumors in patients and in nude mice. *Cancer* 52:1146–1152, 1983.

38. Shrivastav S, Paulson DF: In vitro chemotherapy testing of transitional cell carcinoma. *Invest Urol* 17:395–400, 1980.

39. Salmon SE, Hamburger AW, Soehnlen B, Durie BGM, Alberts DS, Moon TE: Quantification of differential sensitivity of human tumor stem cells to anticancer drugs. *N Engl J Med* 298:1321–1327, 1978.

40. Hamburger AW, Salmon SE: Primary bio-assay of human tumor stem cells. *Science* 197:461–463, 1977.

41. Miller JFAP: The thymus and transplantation immunity. *Br Med Bull* 21:111–117, 1965.

42. Flanagan SP: Nude, a new hairless gene with pleiotropic effects in the mouse. *Genet Res (Camb)* 8:295–309, 1966.

43. Pantelouris EM: Absence of thymus in a mouse mutant. *Nature* 217:370–371, 1968.

44. Selby PJ: Human tumor xenografts in cancer research. *Cancer Topics* 2:9, 1979.

45. Bogden AE, Haskell PM, lePage DJ, Kelton DE, Cobb WR, Esber HJ: Growth of human tumor xenografts implanted under the renal capsule of normal immunocompetent mice. *Exp Cell Biol* 47:281–293, 1979.

46. Bogden AE, Cobb WR, LePage PM, Haskell PM, Gulkin TA, Ward A, Kelton DE, Esber HJ: Chemotherapy responsiveness of human tumors as first transplant generation xenografts in the normal mouse: six-day subrenal capsule assay. *Cancer* 48:10–20, 1981.

47. Bennett JA, Nguyen M, Pilon V, MacDowell RT: Histopathological changes induced by human colon cancer xenografts implanted under the kidney capsule of immunocompetent and immunosuppressed mice. *Proc Am Assoc Cancer Res* 25:372, 1984.

48. Edelstein MB, Fiebig HH, Smink T, van Putten LM, Schuchhardt C: Comparison between macroscopic and microscopic evaluation of tumor responsiveness using the subrenal capsule assay. *Eur J Cancer Clin Oncol* 19:995–1009, 1983.

49. Edelstein MB, Smink T, Ruiter DJ, Visser W, van Putten LM: Improvements and limitations of the subrenal capsule assay for determining tumor sensitivity to cytostatic drugs. *Eur J Cancer Clin Oncol* 20:1549–1556, 1984.

50. Wright JC, Walker D: A predictive test for the selection of cancer chemotherapeutic agents for the treatment of human cancer. *J Surg Oncol* 7:381–392, 1975.

51. Hamburger AW, Salmon SE, Kim MB, Trent JM, Soehnlen BJ, Alberts DS, Schmidt

HJ: Direct cloning of human ovarian carcinoma cells in agar. *Cancer Res* 38:3438–3444, 1978.

52. Holmes HL, Little JM: Tissue culture microtest for predicting response of human cancer to chemotherapy. *Lancet* 2:985–987, 1974.

53. Buskirk HH, Crim JA, Van Giessen GH, Petering GHG: Rapid in vitro method for determining cytotoxicity of antitumor agents. *J Natl Cancer Inst* 51:135–138, 1973.

54. Knock FE, Galt RM, Oester YT, Sylvester R: In vitro estimate of sensitivity of individual human tumors to antitumor agents. *Oncology* 30:1–22, 1974.

55. Phillips BJA: A simple, small scale cytotoxicity test, and its uses in drug metabolism studies. *Biochem Pharmacol* 23:131–138, 1974.

56. Mickey DD, Stone KR, Wunderli H, Mickey GH, Vollmer RT, Paulson DF: Heterotransplantation of human prostate adenocarcinoma cell line in nude mice. *Cancer Res* 37:4049, 1977.

57. Roper PR, Drewinko B: Comparison of in vitro methods to determine drug-induced cell lethality. *Cancer Res* 36:2182–2188, 1976.

58. Johnson PA, Rossof AH: The role of the human tumor stem cell assay in medical oncology. *Arch Intern Med* 143:111–114, 1983.

59. Buik RN, Mac Killop WJ: Measurements of self-renewal in culture of clonogenic cells from human ovarian carcinoma. *Br J Cancer* 44:349–355, 1981.

60. Stanisic TH, Buick RN: An in vitro clonal assay for bladder cancer: clinical correlation with the status of the urothelium in 33 patients. *J Urol* 124:30–33, 1980.

61. Lieber MM, Kovach JS: Soft agar clonogeneic assay for primary renal cell carcinoma: in vitro chemotherapy drug sensitivity testing. *Invest Urol* 19:111–114, 1981.

62. Dow LW, Bhakta M, Wilimas J: Clonogenic assay for Wilms' tumor: improved technique for obtaining single cell suspensions and evidence for tumor cell specificity. *Cancer Res* 42:5262, 1982.

63. Sarosdy MF, Lamm DL, Radwin HM, von Hoff DD: Clonogenic assay and in vitro chemosensitivity testing of human urologic malignancies. *Cancer* 50:1332–1338, 1982.

64. Neill HB, Soloway MS: Use of the tumor colony assay in the evaluation of patients with bladder cancer. *Br J Urol* 55:271, 1983.

65. Kirkel WJ, Pelgrim OE, Debruyne FMJ, Vooijs PG, Herman CJ: Soft agar culture of human transitional cell carcinoma colonies from urine. *Am J Clin Pathol* 78:690–694, 1982.

66. Fleischman J, Heston WDW, Fair WR: Renal cell carcinoma and the clonogenic assay. *J Urol* 130:1060–1062, 1983.

67. Lieber MM: In vitro chemotherapy sensitivity testing for genitourinary malignancies. In Kurth KH, Debruyne FMJ, Splinter TAW, Wagener TDJ (eds): *Progress and Controversies in Oncological Urology.* New York, Alan R Liss, 1984, pp 51–65.

68. Agrez MV, Kovach JS, Lieber MM: Cell aggregates in the soft agar "human tumor stem cell assay." *Br J Cancer* 46:880–887, 1982.

69. Allez MC, Uhl CB, Lieber MN: Improved detection of drug cytotoxicity in the soft agar colony formation assay through use of a metabolizable tetrazolium salt. *Life Sci* 31:3071, 1982.

70. Von Hoff DD: Send this patent's tumor for culture and sensitivity. *N Engl J Med* 308:154–155, 1983.

71. Selby PJ, Buik RN, Tannock I: A critical appraisal of the "human tumor stem cell assay." *N Engl J Med* 308:129–134, 1983.

72. Griffin TW, Bogden AE, Reich SD, Hunter RE, Ward A, Yu DT, Greene HL, Constaza ME: Initial clinical trials of the subrenal capsule assay as a predictor of tumor response to chemotherapy. *Cancer* 52:2185–2192, 1983.

73. Carter SK: Predictors of response and their clinical evaluation. *Cancer Chemother Pharmacol* 7:1, 1981.

74. Atassi G: Do we need new chemosensitive experimental models? *Eur J Cancer Clin Oncol* 20:1217–1220, 1984.

75. Oosterwijk E, Fleuren GJ, Zwartendijk J, de Velde J, Jonas U, Warnaar SO: The expression of renal antigens in renal cell carcinoma. *World J Urol* 2:156–158, 1984.

16

In Vitro Chemotherapy Sensitivity Testing for Renal Cell Carcinoma

Michael M. Lieber, M.D.

INTRODUCTION

Among patients who are diagnosed as having renal cell carcinoma, 20 to 30% present with macroscopic metastatic disease already clinically evident; in 1985 there are no standard successful therapies to recommend for these patients. Moreover, the majority of patients who come to nephrectomy for renal cell carcinoma now go on to die from metastatic disease (1). These unpleasant facts illustrate the current major problem with renal cell carcinoma: the majority of patients have a systemic metastatic malignant disease, either microscopic or macroscopic, when they first come to medical attention. Such a widespread systemic disease cannot be treated effectively by surgical removal of the primary tumor in the kidney. It has become widely recognized that a fundamental advance in treatment for most patients with renal cell carcinoma, a major improvement in overall prognosis, will only occur when highly active systemic treatments for this disease are identified. If such highly active systemic agents were available, patients presenting with or developing clinically evident metastatic renal cell carcinoma could be treated aggressively with appropriate chemotherapy; patients with no macroscopic evidence of metastatic disease but with locally high stage or high grade renal cell carcinoma, with a known high probability of subsequently developing metastases, could be treated systemically in a surgical adjuvant modality.

Unfortunately, metastatic renal cell carcinoma has been among the least responsive tumors to treatment with systemic chemotherapy (2), and, indeed, in 1985, there is no single agent or combination of agents which can be recommended that can promise more than a 10 or 15% objective response rate in measurable metastatic disease. Consequently, there has been intense interest in laboratory methods which might be useful for identifying new active chemotherapeutic and other systemic agents for renal cell carcinoma and, also, for laboratory methods which might provide techniques *to individualize anticancer agent selection* for the large group of patients who have renal cell carcinoma. In these regards, a number of general laboratory approaches have been used to study renal cell carcinoma, as have been applied to most other common human malignant diseases. These have included animal model systems with induced or spontaneous renal cell adenomas and carcinomas, the study of human renal cell carcinoma xenografts carried as transplants in "nude" athymic mice (3), the creation and subsequent in vitro investigation of long term continuous/permanent cell lines derived from human renal cell carcinoma (4), and the study of a number of short term assay methods in which fresh samples of human renal cell carcinoma are maintained in vitro for a period of several days to several weeks, with the response of the tumor cells to exposure to various anticancer treatments studied by a variety of end points (5). This last general approach has been an area of intensive investigation in the Urology Research Laboratory at the Mayo Clinic over the preceding 5 years. In this time period, this laboratory has studied over 500 different samples of freshly excised human renal cell carcinoma in such short term in vitro chemotherapy sensitivity assays, both for assignment of drug sensitivity among already identified and clinically used anticancer agents, and in a search among newly formulated chemicals for potentially new active therapies. These renal cell carcinoma samples have been from among over 6000 different samples of primary human carcinomas collected from the surgical practice of the Mayo Clinic over the past 5 years and studied by in vitro chemotherapy sensitivity testing in this laboratory; both urologic and nonurologic tumors have made up the panel of tumor types studied here.

SOFT AGAR COLONY FORMING ASSAYS

The major impetus for the study of short term in vitro assays for chemotherapy sensitivity testing came with the popularization of the soft agar "human tumor stem cell assay" or "clonogenic assay" by Salmon and colleagues at the University of Arizona in Tucson beginning in 1977 to 1980 (6–10). Subsequently, over 700 reports have been published in which short term in vitro assays for chemotherapy sensitivity testing have been applied to samples of fresh human tumors using methods more or less related to Salmon's (11).

In the soft agar colony formation assay of Salmon and colleagues (7, 8, 10), viable samples of cancer are obtained from the patient; these samples can be in the form of pieces of solid tumor or in the form of cells removed as malignant effusions, such as from malignant pleural or peritoneal effusions. Since the solid tumor tissue must be broken up into single cells and small cell aggregates in order to perform this in vitro assay, tumors are first disaggregated by mechanical methods (mincing, filtering) and then by exposure to enzymes in order to create dispersed tumor cell suspensions for subsequent study (12, 13). Replicate samples of tumor cells are then incubated in cell culture medium containing 0.3% agar, agarose, or methyl cellulose (14) at concentrations just sufficient to gel the medium when cooled. Significant proliferative growth of human cancer cells can occur in such "soft agar medium"; conversely, growth of normal cells contained within the tumor, such as fibroblasts, macrophages, endothelial cells, etc, does not occur in soft agar culture matrix. Indeed, so-called "anchorage independent growth" in the three-dimensional soft agar matrix has been one of the characteristics used to define the transformed or malignant phenotype in vitro (15).

Embedded in this three-dimensional soft agar, agarose, or methyl cellulose cell culture matrix, human tumor cells of various histologic types will commonly proliferate and form small colonies for 1 to 3 weeks in vitro (16–18). Inhibition of colony growth by exposure of replicate soft agar cultures to various pharmacologic concentrations of anticancer drugs and other treatments has been the most common method used to study in vitro chemotherapy sensitivity over the preceding 5 years (11, 19, 20). The use of this particular assay technique for in vitro chemotherapy sensitivity testing was markedly promoted by the favorable early reports by Salmon's group, from Von Hoff's group in San Antonio, and by others; in preliminary studies, the results of in vitro chemotherapy sensitivity testing for a number of tumor types correlated closely with patients' subsequent response to clinical treatment with the same agents (6, 10, 21–24). As one result, commercial clinical pathology laboratories offering the Salmon soft agar colony formation assay for in vitro chemotherapy sensitivity testing became common and widely promoted in the early 1980s.

The Urology Research Laboratory at the Mayo Clinic began studying the Salmon soft agar colony formation assay and applying it to human urologic malignancies in 1979. The author's group, too, were caught up in the initial burst of enthusiasm and optimism that this in vitro assay system could revolutionize the treatment of metastatic urologic malignancies, particularly renal cell carcinoma and transitional cell carcinoma, which were currently refractory to standard and experimental treatments. Moreover, in 1981, the United States National Cancer Institute (NCI) initiated a contract research program in which the Salmon soft agar colony forming assay was utilized in a screening mode to search for new active anticancer agents from among the many thousands of new chemicals submitted for consideration to the NCI each year (25, 26). It had long been a concern at NCI that the murine P-388 transplantable leukemia in vivo prescreen currently used to detect anticancer drug activity for new chemical isolates could be deficient, and that a number of useful anticancer agents for human malignancies could be simply missed by being tested only against this one murine tumor screen. Use of the Salmon in vitro assay to screen new chemical isolates was proposed, so that the compounds of interest would be tested in vitro at an arbitrary concentration (10 µg/ml) against 10 different samples of six primary human tumor types, rather than just against mice bearing transplantable murine leukemia samples in vivo (25, 26). The Urology Research Laboratory at the Mayo Clinic was selected in 1981 to be one of the four laboratories performing the soft agar colony forming assay in a drug screening mode on contract to NCI. Participation in this contract program has continued through the present time.

IN VITRO CHEMOTHERAPY SENSITIVITY TESTING   259

Exploration of the short term in vitro culture and chemotherapy sensitivity testing of samples of renal cell carcinoma using this assay method has been the highest priority. First, renal cell carcinoma is a common clinical problem at the Mayo Clinic, with approximately 130 new patients with renal cell carcinoma presenting each year for treatment. At the time of diagnosis, most renal cell carcinoma primaries are large and consequently yield a large quantity of viable malignant cells which can be studied in the laboratory. This feature contrasts sharply with the relatively few tumor cells commonly available for laboratory study from patients with prostate carcinoma or transitional cell carcinoma. Most patients with metastatic renal cell carcinoma have measurable metastases in the bones, brain, lung, or mediastinum, which make them good candidates for study in prospective phase II or phase III clinical research protocols. Finally, as noted above, there is no standard treatment now available for patients with advanced renal cell carcinoma.

Having studied over 500 different samples of human renal cell carcinoma in soft agar colony formation assays in this Laboratory through the end of 1984, the following generalizations about the assay can be stated with some confidence. Short term soft agar colony formation assays for samples of human renal cell carcinoma are a workable and promising technique to study new therapies for renal cell carcinoma in the laboratory. However, this form of in vitro chemotherapy sensitivity testing is still in a developmental phase; it is *not yet ready* for wide scale clinical application as a standard laboratory test, such as the conceptually analogous method used for bacterial culture and sensitivity testing. However, it is still a highly appropriate test for research exploitation and in vitro studies of human renal cancer.

TECHNICAL PROBLEMS WITH SOFT AGAR COLONY FORMATION ASSAYS

Limited Proliferative Potential of Renal Cell Carcinoma Samples in Short Term in Vitro Culture

The major technical limitation which handicaps the ability to perform in vitro chemotherapy sensitivity testing for the majority of samples removed from patients with renal cell carcinoma is ignorance of the cell culture medium ingredients necessary to bring about the routine successful and sustained proliferation of human renal carcinoma cells in vitro. When samples of human renal cell carcinoma are removed from surgical specimens, disaggregated by enzymatic exposure, and subsequently cultured in presently available culture media, the cells will commonly go through several cycles of cell division, resulting in an increase in colony volume of 2- to 64-fold (27). The majority of tumor samples studied show volume increases in the range of 2- to 8-fold. Subsequently, viable cell colonies can survive in vitro for a period of several weeks, but overall viability is steadily falling, usually after the first 5 to 9 days in in vitro culture.

Knowledge is lacking of which growth factors are required to maintain and, indeed, to stimulate renal cell carcinoma cells to proliferate successfully in vitro longer term. Most cell biologists believe that various peptide growth factors in the culture medium are required to stimulate cells in vitro to continue to divide. While such peptide growth factors may be available in high concentration locally within the tumor in vivo, disaggregated tumor cells in vitro encounter a totally different environment and, in general, do not proliferate at all or proliferate poorly. Single cells proliferate particularly poorly; small cell aggregates, with perhaps a more protected local environment, with perhaps enhanced local concentration of growth factors, do proliferate in vitro somewhat better (28). The radical change in the course of in vitro culture of primary tumor cells which identification of relevant peptide growth factors can make has been demonstrated in the research of Minna, Carney, and colleagues, who, by isolating the requisite peptide growth factors, have been able routinely to carry out the long term successful in vitro propagation of malignant cells from literally hundreds of samples of human lung cancer (29). The successful identification of such peptide growth factors for human renal cell carcinoma has not been carried out as yet, although some investigations of conditioned media from continuous and successfully growing renal cell carcinoma cell lines have begun. It seems likely that successful in vitro cultivation and successful short term in vitro chemotherapy sensitivity testing for samples of human renal carcinoma will proceed slowly until such peptide growth factors or other factors which will permit the reliable medium to long term cultivation of renal carcinoma cells in vitro are identified.

Difficulty in Preparing Pure Single Cell Suspensions from Fresh Human Solid Tumors Including Renal Cell Carcinoma

The basic biological premise behind Salmon's soft agar colony forming assay (the "clonogenic assay" or "human tumor stem cell assay") (9) was the basic assumption that human tumor effusions or samples of solid tumors could be processed in the laboratory by filtration, by other mechanical methods, and by exposure to enzyme cocktails to result in satisfactory preparation of "pure" single cell suspensions which would still retain their ability to proliferate in soft agar cultures. As a result, the multicell tumor cell colonies scored after 1 to 3 weeks of culture incubation would therefore derive from the clonal proliferation of single cells seeded much as in standard bacterial cultures or in soft agar cultures observed after the incubation of single cell suspensions derived from long established continuous human tumor cell lines. Unfortunately, this basic biologic premise has not turned out to be achievable in practice. If a deliberate effort is made by extensive enzymatic exposure and filtration to prepare pure suspensions of single tumor cells, their subsequent proliferative ability in soft agar cultures appears quite limited (28). Useful in vitro drug testing has not been possible with such pure single cell suspension cultures for most human solid tumors. It may work effectively with occasional samples of malignant melanoma and cells from malignant ascites from ovarian carcinoma, but, in general, cell suspensions from most human solid tumors, including renal cell carcinoma, which remain proliferative in vitro, are found to consist of a mixture of single tumor cells and *small tumor cell aggregates* (28). When cultures are studied by serial microphotography, the large cell colonies observed after 1 to 2 weeks of incubation in vitro are found to originate from the progressive enlargement of the *seeded small cell aggregates* rather than from the single cells. Thus, the fundamental basis of most short term colony forming assays in soft agar medium is not the clonal growth of single tumor cells but rather the short term enlargement of small cell aggregates initially seeded into the agar culture medium (27).

Many of the numerous early studies carried out in the initial burst of enthusiasm for Salmon's assay (in the period 1978 to 1982) (30) were performed by investigators totally unaware of the problem of "contamination" of their cultures by tumor cell aggregates, and, therefore, such early studies did not control for the presence of such cell aggregates. Thus, so-called "clonal growth" of tumor cells reported in soft agar or agarose cultures for a large number of human tumors (19) (as well as benign neoplasms and normal tissues) must be regarded with a large degree of skepticism (28, 31) since the observed colony formation could simply have resulted from the modest enlargement of cell aggregates initially seeded rather than from the clonal growth of single tumor cells that was assumed. A further complicating factor is the fact that small tumor cell aggregates have virtually the same optical density as the agar or agarose culture medium when they are first seeded. Consequently, scanning the culture dishes at low power magnification immediately after culture initiation generally fails to reveal the presence of the small tumor cell aggregates because of the lack of contrast between the cell aggregates and the culture medium. However, as the cell aggregates age, and, indeed, die, their optical density increases and they therefore become visible when the plates are scanned and counted. To the uninitiated, it appears that cell colonies have formed that were not present previously; in fact, it is only "optical aging" of the cultures. Again, this particular technical artifact was not appreciated by the early proponents of this assay method and was not controlled for in earlier studies.

Artifacts Induced and Generated by the Presence of the Cell Aggregates

Because the end point for soft agar colony forming assays has been the counting of cell aggregates present at the end of incubation, and comparing the number of arbitrary size colonies between control and drug-exposed culture dishes, the invariable presence of cell aggregates in cell cultures of human renal cell carcinoma and other fresh solid tumor samples causes a major problem. As a result, much technical effort has gone into developing methods to assess the presence of cell aggregates objectively and to control for their presence in performing in vitro chemotherapy sensitivity testing using Salmon's method. A major advance has been the recognition that nonviable cell aggregates persist in these agar cultures, basically held in place by the three-dimensional gel matrix. Such dead tumor cell aggregates or colonies cannot be distinguished from viable colonies by standard optical observations. The application of vital staining to assessment of such cultures and to in vitro chemotherapy sensitivity assays of this type, therefore, represented one important advance. The most widely used vital dye has been the tetrazolium compound, INT, a colorless chemical which, when reduced by living cells, turns into a brick red-colored stain which makes previously transparent, viable cell colonies markedly visible and contrasts them with the transparent cell culture medium (32). The use of the vital stain INT allows the selective staining of viable cell aggregates or colonies and their differentiation from nonviable cell aggregates present in the same culture plates. Moreover, contrasting colonies stained by INT can be counted by a computerized image analyzer. The use of a vital stain for identifying and quantitating viable cell aggregates has markedly increased the sensitivity of standard soft agar or agarose cultures for chemotherapy testing (25, 26, 32, 33).

Most important, viable colony staining has eliminated "false negative" drug sensitivity testing which commonly resulted when cell aggregates were killed by exposure to anticancer drug but persisted in the agar culture and were scored as viable surviving colonies. Since investigators in the vast bulk of the early studies performed in the 1978 to 1982 era were not aware of this technical problem and did not use vital staining, in vitro sensitivity data reported in early studies must necessarily be regarded with some skepticism and, in particular, are biased toward showing drug resistance in vitro because of the nature of this artifact. Most laboratories performing in vitro chemotherapy sensitivity testing now use a "positive cytotoxic" control compound, a highly lethal agent such as abrin or mercuric chloride, to control for this particular artifact.

Current Need for Large Tumor Sample Volumes

An ideal test for clinical in vitro chemotherapy sensitivity testing should use a small sample of tumor cells. A test which could use a small needle biopsy core or aspiration sample would be desirable since tumor tissue from deep seated primaries or metastases could be studied with a minimum of invasive surgical intervention. Unfortunately, this circumstance is not the case with present in vitro chemotherapy sensitivity tests. For example, for standard soft agar colony formation assays, a piece of viable non-necrotic tumor tissue 2 to 3 cm^3 in size is required for preparation of cell suspensions, in order to provide enough cells to test a significant number of drugs with the appropriate controls and replicate plates. Thus, for example, for human renal cell carcinoma, surgically excised large pulmonary metastases, or large lymph node metastases, or the primary tumor with at least 2 to 3 cm^3 of non-necrotic tissue must be obtained for in vitro chemotherapy sensitivity studies to be performed in 1985. Such large volumes of tumor tissue are required because approximately 5×10^5 viable tumor cells are required for each culture dish of the assay; approximately 100 dishes are needed to perform a standard assay involving multiple control dishes, positive cytotoxic control compounds, and replicate drug exposure dishes. The requirement for this quantity of renal cell carcinoma makes formal open surgical intervention necessary in order to carry out studies of this tumor type. Therefore, most studies have in fact been performed with pieces of primary tumors removed at the time of nephrectomy (34, 35), since in the developmental stages of this assay methodology, it has not seemed ethically justifiable to recommend that patients undergo thoracotomy, exploratory laparotomy, or, indeed, craniotomy to obtain tumor tissue simply to perform these experimental studies. In this regard, in vitro chemotherapy sensitivity testing for patients who have malignant effusions, either pleural or peritoneal, in which a large number of viable tumor cells can be simply recovered by thoracentesis or paracentesis, represents a more ideal circumstance for study by this experimental assay method. Unfortunately, such effusions are not commonly present for patients with metastatic renal cell carcinoma.

Problems with Pharmacologic Modeling

Exposure of fresh human tumor cell suspensions in vitro to anticancer drugs also requires major assumptions and simplifications. At the most fundamental level, the concentration of an activated anticancer drug which is actually "seen" by tumor cells in vivo is basically unknown. Although there is much pharmacokinetic information available on the concentration of various species of anticancer drugs circulating in the plasma after different modes of drug delivery, the actual concentration of active drug which is presented to the tumor cells in vivo, within the actual circulatory confines of the tumor, is simply not known. Moreover, other fundamental aspects of the environment in which tumor cells contact anticancer drugs, such as the pH or oxygen concentration, are also not known for the vast majority of tumor types or locations. Consequently, markedly arbitrary and simplifying assumptions must be made in exposing tumor cells in vitro to anticancer drugs. First, some arbitrary assessment must be made about how long the tumor cells should be exposed to the anticancer drug. A large number of different methods have been used. When the Salmon assay began, exposure of tumor cells in suspension to a drug for 1 hour in vitro was used, with the cells subsequently being washed and seeded into virgin cell culture medium (9, 10). More recently, most laboratories have switched to exposing the cells "continuously" to anticancer drug by mixing it permanently into the cell culture medium or applying it onto the surface of the culture plates (33, 36). Obviously, such methods of exposing cells to drug are a simplification of the varying concentration and time of exposure that tumor cells "see" drugs in vivo. To account somewhat for such variations, tumor cells are usually exposed in vitro to several orders of magnitude of drug concentration, bracketed around achievable serum concentration resulting from standard clinically used drug delivery protocols. Thus, for example, if a peak safely achievable serum concentration of cis-platinum is about 4 μg/ml, the response of tumor cells is studied in vitro at 40, 4, and 0.4 μg/ml so that a small dose-response curve is generated for the individual tumor cell samples. The generation of such dose-response curves is quite important but further increases the number of samples, the quantity of tumor cells, and the number of plates to be studied for a successful assay in vitro to be performed. Moreover, picking the significant level of colony inhibition to use to assign "in vitro sensitivity" remains arbitrary.

As just described, the testing of single agents in this assay is artificial and markedly simplified. Furthermore, no one has yet worked out a satisfactory comprehensive rationale for testing the possible synergistic effects of *drug combinations* in soft agar colony forming assays for primary human tumor cells. Clinically, administration of two or more drugs in synergistic combination often has been the most effective chemotherapy strategy. No one has a proven model of how to mirror the effects of multiple drug scheduling and combination in vitro. In addition, for a large number of anticancer drugs, particularly new agents, the exact active cytocidal molecular species which the tumor cell "sees" in vivo may be different from the chemical species present in the drug vial used to create the in vitro formulations. There has been some research in modifying the soft agar colony formation assay through the use of activating systems, either microsomal preparations or hepatocytes, in order to activate or inactivate drugs such as might be done in vivo by the liver, etc (37–39). However, again, this is at best a rough first approximation of in vivo effects. Much more laboratory work is needed in order to create an in vitro drug testing environment more representative of the tumor cell environment in vivo.

Finally, quite a major problem, particularly regarding in vitro chemotherapy sensitivity testing for renal cell carcinoma, is the primary dearth of known clinically active drugs for this particular tumor type. It makes little sense to perform elaborate and quite expensive in vitro chemotherapy sensitivity testing as a "standard laboratory test" when clinically active drugs are so uncommon.

RESULTS

Despite all of these caveats, a large volume of experimental work has been performed in the in vitro chemotherapy sensitivity testing of renal cell carcinoma using assay systems similar to that discussed above (3, 5, 34, 35, 40). As noted before, the author's laboratory has studied more than 500 different samples of human renal cell carcinoma in assays of this type over the preceding 5 years. From this experience, the following generalizations can be made.

1. Renal cell carcinoma is an excellent tumor type to study in soft agar colony formation assays. A large sample of healthy non-necrotic tumor tissue free of microbial contamination *is* commonly available from renal cell carcinoma primaries. Using standard enzymatic digestion techniques, a large number of viable and proliferative single cells and small cell aggregates can be prepared from renal cell carcinomas. Most important, depending on the end point selected to quantitate the extent of proliferation, using the culture media formulations currently available, short term in vitro proliferation of cells from renal cell carcinoma samples can be seen in from 50 to 80% of tumor samples studied (34).

Such a high percentage of successful short term culturability is quite promising for the future use of this assay, both for individualized in vitro chemotherapy testing among known anticancer drugs and for use of this assay method in the screening for new anticancer agents for renal cell carcinoma.

2. In vitro chemotherapy sensitivity testing using the soft agar colony formation assay can, in fact, be performed using the standard culture methods discussed above. The most recent relevant report on renal cell carcinoma from this laboratory was presented in *The Journal of Urology* in February, 1984 (34). This report described 206 samples of human renal cell carcinoma studied here from February, 1981, until March, 1983. Fifty percent of available tumor tests showed colony formation and gave clinical drug sensitivity information. Two-thirds of tumors were resistant to all drugs tested, despite a median number of different drugs tested per tumor of about 15. Six percent of tumors were remarkably sensitive to numerous anticancer drugs in vitro. Testing at clinically achievable fixed concentrations, the most active drugs in vitro were teniposide, actinomycin D, bleomycin, hydroxyurea, mitoguanisone dihydrochloride (methyl-GAG), mitomycin C, and L-alanosine. Fourteen other drugs showed low in vitro cytotoxicity (Table 16.1). Since February, 1983, somewhat more successful testing of human renal cell carcinoma samples has been achieved in this laboratory on a "percentage success" basis.

3. Renal cell carcinoma is a quite useful human tumor type to use in a screening panel to detect new anticancer drugs. From 1981 through 1984, renal cell carcinoma has been one of six tumor types successfully used in the National Cancer Institute Drug Screening contract program using this assay method (along with melanoma, breast, lung, ovarian, and colorectal carcinomas) (25, 26). Since short term cultures of human renal cell carcinoma do proliferate reliably in this assay, the use of this in vitro modeling system for screening for new anticancer agents which might be active against human renal cell carcinoma in vivo is a very attractive possibility.

New Technical Improvements and Modifications in Soft Agar Colony Forming Assays

The discovery of the numerous technical problems in performing soft agar colony formation assays described above recently has led to a large number of studies in which technical modifications of the basic "human tumor stem cell assay" have been made in order to control for or eliminate some of the problems. Multiple changes have been made in the method of tumor cell disaggregation in order to attempt to eliminate or control for the small cell aggregates present (12, 13, 33). The use of vital staining with drugs such as INT has been popularized and is widely used (25–27, 32, 33). Additional methods for assessing cytotoxic drug end points in vitro using other vital stains have been popularized by Weisenthal and colleagues (41, 42). Use of micropipettes rather than Petri dishes to grow tumor cells in vitro has been described recently by Von Hoff (43).

Table 16.1
Renal Cell Carcinoma: Soft Agar Colony Formation Assay, Mayo Clinic
February 1, 1981 to March 1, 1983[a]

Drug[b]	Drug Concentration (μg/ml)	Overall Drug Activity	
		Activity (%) (>70% Inhibition of Colony Formation)	Tumors Sensitive/Total No. of Successful Drugs Tested
VM-26	10.0	28	(11/40)
Actinomycin D	0.01	20	(8/40)
Bleomycin	2.0	18	(8/45)
Hydroxyurea	60.0	18	(7/38)
MGBG (Methyl-GAG)	5.0	17	(11/63)
Mitomycin C	0.4	12	(8/68)
L-Alanosine	50.0	12	(9/77)
Methyl-CCNU	1.5	9	(3/34)
Adriamycin	0.6	7	(4/58)
AZQ	1.0	6	(4/68)
DAG	2.0	6	(4/62)
ICRF-159	0.38	6	(3/53)
Dacarbazine (DTIC)	5.0	6	(3/52)
Vinblastine	0.05	5	(3/63)
BCNU	2.0	5	(2/42)
VP-16-213	10.0	2	(1/49)
Bisantrene	0.5	2	(1/51)
PALA	200.0	0	(1/45)
Cis Platinum	1.5	0	(0/51)
Triazinate	40.0	0	(0/36)
Procarbazine	5.0	0	(0/42)

[a] From Lieber MM: Soft agar colony formation assay for in vitro chemotherapy sensitivity testing of human renal cell carcinoma: Mayo Clinic experience. *J Urol* 131:391, 1984.

[b] Drug abbreviations used: VM-26, tenoposide (NSC-122819); MGBG, mitoguanazone dihydrochloride (NSC-32946); methyl-CCNU, semustine (NSC-95441); AZQ, diaziquone (NCS-182986); DAG, 1,2:5,6-dianhydrogalactitol (NSC-132313); ICRF-159, (NSC-129943); BCNU, carmustine (NSC-409962); VP-16-213, etoposide (NSC-141540); PALA, (NSC-224131); Triazinate, soluble Baker's antifol (NSC-139105).

In the traditional assay methodology (9), the drug effect end point is ascertained by simply counting the number of colonies of a certain size, usually 60 μm in diameter, present after the time of incubation. Counting these small colonies in hundreds of Petri dishes is quite demanding technically and can only be reliably performed by a computerized image analysis system (44), which is quite expensive. Because of these colony enumeration problems and additional problems with cell aggregates, there has been interest of late in using a radically different end point from optically counting colonies of a certain size to assess tumor cell growth and in vitro chemotherapy sensitivity. Most popular have been experimental methods in which radioactive thymidine is placed into the culture dishes with the extent of incorporation of the label into DNA is taken as an index of cell proliferation; inhibition of thymidine uptake by exposure to anticancer drugs is taken as a valid index of anticancer drug effect similar to comparing the number of cell colonies of a certain size in the control and drug-treated plates (45–49). This methodology is particularly popular now since it appears to obviate the problems in preparing uniform single cell tumor suspensions and cultures. The author's laboratory has intensively investigated the thymidine incorporation methodology described originally by Kern and colleagues at the University of California, Los Angeles (49). In a series of several hundred primary human tumors studied by this method, the author's group found the results of colony formation and drug sensitivity testing to correlate well when either the optical colony counting assay performed by the computerized image analyzer or the thymidine assay are compared on replicate samples of the same tumor (47). Since Kern's thymidine incorporation assay is completed 4 days after tumor removal from the patient and does not require an expensive computerized image analyzer, this particular methodology shows substantial promise for expanding the scope of the assay method. Another important feature is that the thymidine incorporation end point can commonly be performed successfully with 2- to 5-fold fewer tumor cells per dish and still yield enough thymidine uptake per dish for measuring drug effects.

Another technical modification in assessing the assay end point which also appears promising for increasing the evaluability and clarity of in vitro chemotherapy sensitivity testing utilizes the Omnicon FAS-II computerized image analyzer, which has been used previously to count the colonies in the plates (44), to measure three-dimensional volumes of the cell colonies after they have been vitally stained with INT (27, 50). The software furnished with this image analyzer computer can automatically size each stained individual tumor cell colony, compute a three-dimensional volume for the colony, and subsequently tabulate the integrated volumes for different colony sizes for the entire culture dish. In the Mayo Clinic experience with over 400 human tumor samples cultured by standard methods and analyzed by this method, computerized volume analysis gave an improved quantitation and understanding of the extent of tumor colony enlargement and proliferation in soft agar cultures compared to simply counting the number of colonies of a certain size (27). The use of computerized volume analysis also allows a quantitative index of the number and size of tumor cell aggregates initially seeded into the agar.

As of autumn 1984, the author believes these new technical methods for assessing assay end point—that is, some form of thymidine incorporation end point, or some form of computerized colony counting and volume analysis—will provide for a higher degree of evaluability and for harvesting more quantitatively significant biologic information about what is happening in the culture plates than has been available heretofore.

CONCLUSION

Major changes in the treatment and prognosis for patients with renal cell carcinoma depend on the identification of highly active chemotherapeutic agents for treating this disease in its metastatic forms. It seems possible that soft agar colony formation assays of human renal cell carcinoma will help us along the road to this important goal. First, this laboratory method does allow for the direct individualized study of tumor cells freshly removed from primary or metastatic human renal carcinoma cell samples. Use of such cell substrates seems more desirable in the search for new anticancer agents than, for example, using animal-derived renal cell carcinoma models such as from the mouse, rat, or hamster, or from studying human renal carcinoma cell lines maintained in continuous culture for a long time. Such continuous cell lines have been intensely selected for rapid growth in vitro and, in the author's experience as well as that of many others, are generally sensitive to a large number of anticancer agents in vitro at low concentration. Indeed, continuous human cancer cell lines from many tissue sources, as yet and in general, have not been particularly helpful in the search for new anticancer agents. The maintenance of human renal carcinoma samples by serial growth as xenografts in nude athymic mice or other immuno-suppressed animals is also a promising method for maintaining samples of human renal carcinoma in the laboratory for study against various proposed anticancer modalities (23). It is important to note that human renal cell carcinoma xenograft cells grow particularly well in soft agar cultures. The same property that allows tumor cells to proliferate rapidly in "nude" mice appears to be the same property which allows tumor cells to proliferate well in soft agar cultures. Consequently, soft agar colony formation assays in vitro are a useful method for studying the response of xenograft renal cell carcinoma cells to anticancer drug treatments, particularly so since nude mice are so expensive and drug treating large cohorts of nude mice bearing xenografts in vivo rapidly becomes prohibitively expensive.

Many human tumor types, such as brain tumors, sarcomas, and prostate adenocarcinomas, proliferate exceptionally poorly in soft agar colony formation assays with current techniques and at the present time cannot be studied successfully in vitro by this methodology. Transitional cell carcinomas of the urinary tract proliferate moderately well in vitro in the soft agar colony formation assay (51), but studies of this tumor type in this assay are usually limited by the small quantity of viable tumor cells available in biopsies or by bladder barbotage. In contrast, fresh surgical samples of human renal cell carcinoma generally do grow quite well in soft agar cultures, nearly as well as malignant melanoma cells and cells from ovarian carcinoma effusions, which are the most proliferate tumor cell types studied in this assay at present. Finally, as described above, it already has been demonstrated that samples of renal cell carcinoma studied in vitro by this culture technique can be effectively tested for anticancer drug sensitivity against standard agents (34) and have been successfully used in a screening mode as part of the United States National Cancer Institute Drug Screening contract program over the preceding 4 years (25, 26).

Thus, soft agar colony formation assays for studying renal cell carcinoma in vitro already are a useful laboratory research method for investigating various aspects of this disease, particularly sensitivity to anticancer treatments. Much experimental effort has gone into the study of this system already, so that firm technical guidelines exist for new investigators who wish to study these methods. With the increasing use of a thymidine incorporation assay end point, practical performance of the assay requires much less capital investment than when using the older colony counting end point that requires a computerized image analyzer.

Nevertheless, in vitro chemotherapy sensitivity testing for human renal cell carcinoma using this methodology (or others) is still a laboratory research tool. There is no intellectual justification now for urologic clinicians or medical oncologists to regard in vitro chemotherapeutic sensitivity testing for renal cell carcinoma (or other urologic malignancies) as a standard or proven clinical tool which should be used in the routine evaluation of patients with advanced renal cell carcinoma. This "hoped for" eventuality simply is not demonstrated at the present time. There is no justification to perform open surgery to obtain tumor samples to carry out this investigational assay based on the current state of the art unless this surgery is part of a *formalized clinical research protocol* in which patients render formal informed consent and realize the experimental nature of the procedure they are undergoing. Before urologic clinicians rush to adopt this type of in vitro chemotherapy sensitivity testing, they should await the publication of controlled clinical studies in which patients are successfully assigned chemotherapy treatment based on such in vitro assays. Such studies would need to demonstrate that an in vitro assay of this type is more successful than a medical oncologist picking agents empirically before the assay should be considered to be clinically useful (52–54).

In vitro chemotherapy sensitivity testing with freshly isolated tumor cells as an intellectual discipline and experimental tool has been marked by frequent pendulum swings in enthusiasm. Initially, in the 1977 to 1982 era, this technique promised to be a laboratory test of standard applicability which would revolutionize and rationalize advanced cancer treatment (9, 30). More recently, the pendulum has swung the other way, and critiques of the methodology have been published (31, 55–60). It is certainly clear now that the high praise for this assay methodology and, certainly, its commercial marketing were highly premature and should have awaited more definitive clinical trials of the assay. Nevertheless, the initial enthusiasm rapidly led to intensive investigation of the methodology and the recognition of the technical problems in performing the assay which would have taken years otherwise, without the burst of initial excitement generated by the assay's proponents. As the dust settles now 5 years later, it seems certain that a reliable laboratory method for evaluating individual samples of freshly excised renal cell carcinoma (e.g., reference 61), both for proliferative potential and for chemotherapy selection and screening, has been one of surviving achievements of this general approach to the in vitro study of human cancer.

BIBLIOGRAPHIC NOTE

Since in vitro chemotherapy sensitivity testing using the soft agar colony formation assay is such an active area of current laboratory research, most of the relevant published material is scattered in various primary cancer research journals. At the same time many of the published primary articles from 2 to 3 years ago have been made outdated by the rapid technical evolution of this field. Therefore, the new monograph, *Human Tumor Cloning*, by Salmon and Trent published in October, 1984, is the best available single volume current introduction to this field (20). The rapid rate of evolution of in vitro assays can be demonstrated by comparing this volume with Salmon's *Cloning of Human Tumor Stem Cells* published 4 years previously (9). Studies of this assay method applied to human transitional cell carcinoma are reviewed in reference 51. A good concise review article particularly focusing on urologic aspects of in vitro chemotherapy testing has recently been published by Fleischmann (5). A good general review article is that by Johnson and Rosoff (19). The recent all-inclusive bibliography compiled by Von Hoff provides a comprehensive survey of this field (11).

REFERENCES

1. McNichols DW, Segura JW, DeWeerd JH: Renal cell carcinoma: long-term survival and late recurrence. *J Urol* 126:17, 1981.
2. Harris DT: Hormonal therapy and chemotherapy of renal-cell carcinoma. *Semin Oncol* 10:422, 1983.
3. Kurth KH, van Dongen JW, Romijn JC, Lieber MM, Schroeder FH: Assay evaluability of drug testing systems determined with human renal carcinoma cell lines. *World J Urol* 2:146–155, 1984.
4. Williams RD: Human urologic cancer cell lines. *Invest Urol* 17:359, 1980.
5. Fleischmann J, Heston WDW, Fair WR: In vitro assays for directing therapy of genitourinary cancers. In Ratliff TL, Catalona WJ (eds): *Urologic Oncology.* Boston: Martinus Nijhoff, 1984, p 89.
6. Alberts DS, Salmon SE, Chen HSG, Surwit EA, Soehnlen B, Young L, Moon TE: In vitro clonogenic assay for predicting response of ovarian cancer to chemotherapy. *Lancet* 2:340, 1980.
7. Hamburger AW, Salmon SE: Primary bioassay of human tumor stem cells. *Science* 197:461, 1977.
8. Hamburger AW, Salmon SE, Kim MB, Trent J, Soehnlen BJ, Alberts DS, Schmidt JH: Direct cloning of human ovarian carcinoma cells in agar. *Cancer Res.* 38:3438, 1978.
9. Salmon SE (ed): Cloning of human tumor stem cells. *Prog Clin Biol Res* 48:12, 1980.
10. Salmon SE, Hamburger AW, Soehnlen B, Durie BGM, Alberts DS, Moon TE: Quantitation of differential sensitivity of human-tumor stem cells to anticancer drugs. *N Engl J Med* 298:1321, 1978.
11. Von Hoff DD: *Human Tumor Cell Cloning, Bibliography.* Houston, Triton Biosciences, 1983.
12. Slocum HK, Pavelic ZP, Rustum YM: An enzymatic method for the disaggregation of human solid tumors for studies of clonogenicity and biochemical determinants of drug action. Salmon SE (ed): *Cloning of Human Tumor Stem Cells.* New York, Alan R Liss, p 339.
13. Slocum HK, Pavelic ZP, Rustum YM, Creaven PJ, Karakousis C, Takita H, Greco WR: Characterization of cells obtained by mechanical and enzymatic means from human melanoma, sarcoma and lung tumors. *Cancer Res.* 41:1428, 1981.
14. Buick RN, Stanisic TH, Salmon SE, Trent JM, Krasovich P: Development of an agar-methyl cellulose clonogenic assay for cells in transitional cell carcinoma of the human bladder. *Cancer Res.* 39:5051, 1979.
15. MacPherson I, Montagnier L: Agar suspension culture for the selective assay of cells transformed by polyoma virus. *Virology* 23:291, 1964.
16. Courtenay VD, Mills J: An in vitro colony assay for human tumours grown in immune-suppressed mice and treated in vivo with cytotoxic agents. *Br J Cancer* 37:261, 1978.
17. Tveit KM, Endresen L, Rugstad HE, Fodstad O, Pihl A: Comparison of two soft-agar

methods for assaying chemosensitivity of human tumors in vitro: malignant mela-nomas. *Br J Cancer* 44:539, 1981.

18. Tveit KM, Fodstad O, Pihl A: Cultivation of human melanomas in soft agar. Factors influencing plating efficiency and chemosensitivity. *Int J Cancer* 28:329, 1981.

19. Johnson PA, Rossof AH: The role of the human tumor stem cell assay in medical oncology. *Arch Intern Med* 143:111, 1983.

20. Salmon SE, Trent JM (eds): *Human Tumor Cloning.* Orlando, Grune and Stratton, 1984.

21. Alberts DS, Leigh S, Surwit EA, Serokman R, Moon TE, Salmon SE: Improved survival of patients with relapsing ovarian cancer treated on the basis of drug selection following human tumor clonogenic assay. In Salmon SE, Trent JM (eds): *Human Tumor Cloning.* Orlando, Grune and Stratton, 1984, p 509.

22. Moon TE, Salmon SE, White CS, Chen HS, Meyskens FL, Durie BG, Alberts DS: Quantitative association between the in vitro human tumor stem cell assay and clinical response to cancer chemotherapy. *Cancer Chemother. Pharmacol.* 6:211, 1981.

23. Von Hoff DD, Casper J, Bradley E, Sandbach J, Jones D, Makuch R: Association between human tumor colony-forming assay results and response of an individual patient's tumor to chemotherapy. *Am J Med* 70:1027, 1981.

24. Von Hoff DD, Clark GM, Stogdill BJ, Sarosdy MF, O'Brien MT, Casper JT, Mattox DE, Page CP, Cruz AB, Sandbach JF: Prospective clinical trial of a human tumor cloning system. *Cancer Res.* 43:1926, 1983.

25. Shoemaker RH, Wolpert-DeFilippes MK, Kern DH, Lieber MM, Makuch RW, Melnick NR, Miller WT, Salmon SE, Simon RM, Venditti JM, Von Hoff DD: Application of a human tumor colony forming assay to new drug screening. *Cancer Res.* 45:2145–2153, 1985.

26. Shoemaker RH, Wolpert-DeFilippes MK, Melnick NR, Venditti JM, Simon RM, Kern DH, Lieber MM, Miller WT, Salmon SE, Von Hoff DD: Recent results of new drug screening trials with a human tumor colony forming assay. In Salmon SE, Trent JM (eds): *Human Tumor Cloning.* Orlando, Grune and Stratton, 1984, p 345.

27. Alley MC, Lieber MM: Measurement of human tumor cell colonies in soft agarose cultures using computerized volume analysis. *Br J Cancer* 52:205–214, 1985.

28. Agrez MV, Kovach JS, Lieber MM: Cell aggregates in the soft agar "human tumor stem cell assay." *Br J Cancer* 46:880, 1982.

29. Carney DN, Nau MM, Minna JD: Variability of cell lines from patients with small cell lung cancer. In Salmon SE, Trent JR (eds): *Human Tumor Cloning.* Orlando, Grune and Stratton, 1984, p 67.

30. Editorial. *JAMA* 242:501, 1979.

31. Editorial: clonogenic assays for the chemotherapeutic sensitivity of human tumours. *Lancet* 1:780, 1982.

32. Alley MC, Uhl CB, Lieber MM: Improved detection of drug cytotoxicity in the soft agar colony formation assay through use of a metabolizable tetrazolium salt. *Life Sci.* 31:3071, 1982.

33. Alley MC, Lieber MM: Improved optical detection of colony enlargement and drug cytotoxicity in primary soft-agar cultures of human solid tumor cells. *Br J Cancer* 49:225, 1984.

34. Lieber MM: Soft agar colony formation assay for in vitro chemotherapy sensitivity testing of human renal cell carcinomas: Mayo Clinic experience. *J Urol* 131:391, 1984.

35. Lieber MM, Kovach JS: Soft agar clonogenic assay for primary human renal carci-noma: in vitro chemotherapeutic drug sensitivity testing. *Invest Urol* 19:111, 1981.

36. Alley MC, Lieber MM: Drug application to the surface of soft-agarose cell cultures. In Salmon SE, Trent JM (eds): *Human Tumor Cloning.* Orlando, Grune and Stratton, 1984, p 205.

37. Alley MC, Powis G, Appel PL, Kooistra KL, Lieber MM: Activation and inactivation of cancer chemotherapeutic agents by rat hepatocytes cocultured with human tumor cell lines. *Cancer Res.* 44:549, 1984.

38. Lieber MM, Ames MM, Powis G, Kovach JS: Anticancer drug testing in vitro: use of an activating system with the human tumor stem cell colony assay. *Life Sci* 28:287, 1981.

39. Lieber MM, Ames MM, Powis G, Kovach JS: Drug sensitivity testing in vitro with a

liver microsome "activated" soft agar human stem cell colony assay. In Fidler IJ, White RJ (eds): *Design of Models for Testing Cancer Therapeutic Agents*. New York, Van Nostrand Reinhold, 1982, p 12.

40. Sarosdy MF, Lamm DL, Radwin HM, Von Hoff DD: Clonogenic assay and in vitro chemosensitivity testing of human urologic malignancies. *Cancer* 50:1332, 1982.

41. Weisenthal LM, Dill PL, Kurmich NB, Lippman ME: Comparison of dye exclusion assays with a clonogenic assay in the determination of drug-induced cytotoxicity. *Cancer Res* 43:258, 1983.

42. Weisenthal LM, Marsden JA, Dill PL, Macaluso CK: A novel dye exclusion method for testing in vitro chemosensitivities of human tumors. *Cancer Res* 43:749, 1983.

43. Von Hoff DD: Plating efficiencies of human tumors in capillaries versus Petri dishes. In Salmon SE, Trent JM (eds): *Human Tumor Cloning*. Orlando, Grune and Stratton, 1984, p 153.

44. Kressner BE, Morton RRA, Martens AE, Salmon SE, Von Hoff DD, Soehnlen B: Use of an image analysis system to count colonies in stem cell assays of human tumors. In Salmon SE (ed): *Cloning of Human Tumor Stem Cells*. New York, Alan R Liss, 1980, p 179.

45. Friedman HM, Glaubiger DL: Assessment of in vitro drug sensitivity of human tumor cells using (^{3}H)thymidine incorporation in a modified human tumor stem cell assay. *Cancer Res.* 42:4683, 1982.

46. Group for Sensitivity Testing of Tumors (KSST): In vitro short-term test to determine the resistance of human tumors to chemotherapy. *Cancer* 48:2127, 1981.

47. Jones CA, Tsukamoto T, Uhl CB, Alley MC, Lieber MM: Soft agarose culture human tumor colony forming assay for drug sensitivity testing: [^{3}H]-thymidine incorporation vs colony counting. *Br J Cancer* 52:303–310, 1985.

48. Shrivastav S, Bonar RA, Stone KR, Paulson DF: An in vitro assay procedure to test chemotherapeutic drugs on cells from human solid tumors. *Cancer Res.* 40:4438, 1980.

49. Tanigawa N, Kern DH, Hikasa Y, Morton DL: Rapid assay for evaluating the chemosensitivity of human tumors in soft agar culture. *Cancer Res* 42:2159, 1982.

50. Thomson SP, Buckmeier JA, Sipes NJ, Meyskens FL Jr, Hickie RA: Colony size, linearity of formation, and drug survival curves can depend on the number of cells plated in the clonogenic assay. In Salmon SE, Trent JM (eds): *Human Tumor Cloning*. Orlando, Grune and Stratton, 1984, p 37.

51. Lieber MM: In vitro culture and chemotherapy sensitivity testing of human transitional cell carcinoma. *Urol Clin North Am* 11:725–733, 1984.

52. Carter SD: Predictors of response and their clinical evaluation. *Cancer Chemother. Pharmacol.* 7:1, 1981.

53. Salmon SE: Preclinical and clinical applications of chemosensitivity testing with a human tumor colony assay. In Salmon SE, Trent JM (eds): *Human Tumor Cloning*. Orlando, Grune and Stratton, 1984, p 499.

54. Salmon SE, Alberts DS, Meyskens FL Jr, Moon TE: Human tumor stem-cell assay (letter to the editor). *N Engl J Med* 308:1478, 1983.

55. Bertoncello I, Bradley TR, Campbell JJ, Day AJ, McDonald IA, McLeish GR, Quinn MA, Rome R, Hodgson GS: Limitations of the clonal agar assay for the assessment of primary human ovarian tumor biopsies. *Br J Cancer* 45:803, 1982.

56. Lieber MM: Soft agar colony formation assays for in vitro chemotherapy sensitivity testing of human solid tumors cells: practical problems. *Am Assoc Clin Chem* 5:1, 1983.

57. Lieber MM, Kovach JS: Soft agar colony formation assay for chemotherapy sensitivity testing of human solid tumors. *Mayo Clin Proc* 57:527, 1982.

58. Rupniak HT, Hill BT: The poor cloning ability in agar of human tumor cells from biopsies of primary tumors. *Cell Biol Int Reps* 4:479, 1980.

59. Selby P, Buick RN, Tannock I: A critical appraisal of the "human tumor stem-cell assay." *N Engl J Med* 308:129, 1983.

60. Von Hoff DD: "Send this patient's tumor for culture and sensitivity." *N Engl J Med* 308:154, 1983.

61. Strayer DR, Weisband J, Carter WA, Brodsky I: Sensitivity of renal cell carcinoma to leukocyte interferon in the human tumor clonogenic assay and clinical correlations. In Salmon SE, Trent JM (eds): *Human Tumor Cloning*. Orlando, Grune and Stratton, 1984, p 585.

17

Immunotherapy in the Treatment of Metastatic Renal Adenocarcinoma

J. Edson Pontes, M.D.

INTRODUCTION

Metastatic renal cell carcinoma is present in approximately 30% of patients when initially seen with this disease (1). Additionally, another 50% of patients without evidence of metastases initially will develop metastatic disease later (1). Treatment of metastatic disease has been largely unsuccessful due to the fact that these tumors are resistant to all types of chemotherapeutic agents tested thus far (1). Hormonal therapy, thought to be effective initially, has also been shown to be of little value in the treatment of metastatic renal cell carcinoma, with a response rate of approximately 11% (2).

INFLUENCE OF IMMUNOLOGIC FACTORS IN RENAL CELL CARCINOMA SPONTANEOUS REGRESSION

The initial reports of spontaneous regression of renal cell carcinoma dealt with the primary lesion as authors observed either fibrotic, calcified, or cystic areas in the primary tumor. In 1973, Nauts reviewed the literature on the influence of host factors in renal cell carcinoma and cited 7 cases of spontaneous regression of the primary tumor and 41 cases of spontaneous regression of pulmonary lesions (3). It appears by the description that most cases of "spontaneous" regression of the primary tumor were due to other factors, such as blood supply and healing of necrotic areas, rather than to immunologic factors. Perhaps the first description of spontaneous disappearance of pulmonary metastasis following nephrectomy was reported by Bumpus in 1928 (4). Since then, 69 cases of spontaneous regression of metastasis following nephrectomy have been described, although only 22 have had histologic confirmation (5). The precise mechanism of spontaneous regression is unknown; however, changes in the immunologic system following excision of tumor bulk, surgical trauma, hormonal alteration, and infection with fever have been proposed as potential mechanisms (5). Spontaneous regression has been reported mainly following surgical excision of the primary. However, occasionally it has been observed without surgical manipulation, and recently it has been described after radiation therapy of a dominant metastasis (6). Regression of metastasis has also been reported following infection with fever associated with either abscess formation after surgical resection or infection located elsewhere. Nauts reported 29 such cases collected from the world literature (3).

IMMUNOTHERAPY FOR RENAL CELL CARCINOMA

Historical Background

Coley was perhaps the first person to use immunotherapy in the treatment of malignant disease (7). After initial trials of producing erysipelas in cancer patients proved to be both troublesome and dangerous, he started to use a mixture of toxins obtained from bacterial products. Eight cases of adenocarcinoma of the kidney and three Wilms' tumors were treated with Coley's toxin (8, 9). Four complete responses were observed among the patients with renal cell carcinoma and one among the patients with Wilms' tumor (8, 9) Three other cases have been reported as being treated with bacterial or parasite products with complete disappearance of the disease (10–12). The precise mechanism of tumor disappearance following injection of toxins is not clear, although a combination of systemic reaction caused by the products plus the possibility of shared antigens which are present in the toxins with those of the tumor has been proposed. Since these initial trials, several methods have been proposed for the treatment of metastatic renal cell carcinoma.

Arterial Embolization of Renal Cell Carcinoma

Preoperative embolization of primary renal cell carcinoma has been thought to stimulate an immune response in patients, but has been associated with controversial results. Based on the experience of Almgard and associates (11), in which many patients' metastatic disease stabilized after embolization of renal tumors, Swanson and associates (12) used this method in conjunction with hormonal therapy to treat a group of patients with metastatic renal cell carcinoma. Nephrectomy was performed approximately 1 week following infarct, followed by progestational agents (Depo-Provera, 400 mg intramuscularly twice a week) (12). Seven complete and eight partial responders were reported. Equally, McDonald (13) reported seven complete responses and five partial responses among 50 patients treated by this method. In the recent report of nine patients treated by embolization, deKernion observed two responses (1). Recently, however, Mebust and associates found no evidence of benefit from renal infarct in patients with metastatic renal cell carcinoma (14). Although augmentation of natural killer activity has been demonstrated following renal infarct (15), in an experimental model, Pontes et al were unable to demonstrate any improvement in cellular immunity following renal tumor infarct (16). Although the data on this type of approach are inconclusive as related by the results, it is clear that a small number of patients have benefitted from this approach. Recently, Varma et al have embolized a group of patients with lytic lesions in their pelvic bones from metastatic renal cell carcinoma with good objective results (17).

Biologic Response Modifiers and Nonspecific Immunotherapy

Several attempts to use nonspecific immunotherapy or biologic modifiers have been met with varying degrees of success in metastatic renal cell carcinoma. Bacillus Calmette-Guérin (BCG) has probably been the most commonly used agent in nonspecific immunotherapy. The activity of this agent in metastatic renal cell carcinoma is controversial. While Morales and associates (18, 19) have found BCG effective as an adjunctive therapeutic agent following nephrectomy and useful in a small group of patients with metastatic disease, Brossman (20) found no difference among two groups of patients with metastatic disease treated with this agent. The administration of lymphokines, such as transfer factor, has been of little value in metastatic renal cell carcinoma. Montie and associates (21, 22), however, have reported about 14% response rate when combining transfer factor with BCG and 19% response when transfer factor is combined with BCG, hormonal therapy, and chemotherapy. Recently, α-interferon has been used in the treatment of metastatic renal cell carcinoma with initial success. In two different trials, the response rate has been reported to be between 14 and 26% (23, 24). The efficacy of α-interferon was not increased by combination with vinblastine, although toxicity was significantly greater (25). Recent experimental work in a metastatic sarcoma model has shown that the combination of sensitized syngeneic lymphocytes plus interleukin-2 can significantly prevent metastasis in this model (26). Similar work using the renal cell carcinoma model is presently under way in the research laboratories at the Cleveland Clinic.

Specific Immunotherapy

PASSIVE IMMUNOTHERAPY

Horn and Horn (27) reported the treatment of metastatic renal cell carcinoma by means of serotherapy. They transferred serum from a relative of a previously cured renal cell carcinoma patient to another with metastatic disease with excellent objective response (27). Similar attempts of serotherapy have been reported elsewhere (28). Because of the difficulties involved with such an approach, it cannot be widely used. Most other attempts at passive immunotherapy have included the use of syngeneic immune ribonucleic acid (immune RNA). Immune RNA has usually been obtained from lymphocytes of sheep immunized with the patients tumor. In a phase II study, Ramming and deKernion

(29) demonstrated a few minimal responses to this modality of treatment. A subsequent follow-up study failed to confirm the efficacy on survival, and the authors concluded that immune RNA, administered intracutaneously, has no proven value (30). The main problem with the administration of immune RNA has been the enzymatic degradation caused by human ribonucleases (1).

Another approach for the use of immune RNA has recently been proposed by Richie and associates (31, 32). These authors primed patients' lymphocytes in vitro with immune RNA and used these lymphocytes as effector cells. In a group of 27 patients with metastatic renal cell carcinoma, one complete response and five partial responses were observed.

ACTIVE IMMUNOTHERAPY

Attempts to stimulate a specific antitumor response by means of actively immunizing the host with his own tumor has been proposed by several authors. The concept of exposing the host to a tumor-associated antigen is the goal with most of the preparations. The difficulty, however, lies in the fact that tumor-associated antigens are usually weak antigens and the tumor is heterogeneous.

Perhaps the best known attempt to produce an immunologic response is the work reported by Tykka and associates (33) using polymerization of the tumor into small particles by the addition of ethylchoroformiate plus purified derivative (PPD) or *Candida* as the adjuvant. Thirty-one patients with metastatic renal cell carcinoma were treated, and seven were alive after 5 years. Among 16 patients with lung metastasis, only 6 showed complete disappearance of lesions. In a comparison with a similar group of patients treated by standard means, there was a statistical survival advantage among the immunotherapy group. Although the results are significant, it is important to point out that the study was not prospectively randomized, and therefore, factors such as patient selection and repeated surgical excision of metastatic tumors may have influenced the results (34). However, the responses in the immunotherapy group were well documented and, without question, the results of stimulation of immunologic factors.

Using a similar approach, Neidhart and associates (35) observed 2 complete responses and 2 partial responses among 30 patients treated. In comparison with the historical control group, there was improvement in survival rate in the treated patients.

Another approach to the development of active immunotherapy has been used by Brown and associates (36), who coupled autologous radiated cells to dimethyldioctadecyl ammonium bromide (DDA) to treat 27 patients with metastatic renal cell carcinoma and observed 3 complete responses.

McCune and associates (37) have used autologous radiated cells mixed with *Corynebacterium parvum* as an adjuvant to treat four patients in a phase I study and noted only minimal toxicity with one long term response. Subsequently, in a phase II study, they treated 14 patients and observed 4 objective responses (38). Among the latter group, they observed that in some patients, while some metastases were regressing, others were progressing, suggesting the possibility of antigenic heterogeneity of the metastasis due to clonal selection.

Recently, a collaborative study between the University of Rochester, New York (C McCune), the University of California at Los Angeles (J deKernion), and Roswell Park Memorial Institute in Buffalo, New York (JE Pontes) has been completed in which the effectiveness of a specific immunotherapy protocol versus traditional hormonal therapy was studied. A total of 60 patients was evaluable for analysis. Although approximately 15 to 20% of patients in the immunotherapy arm have shown objective responses including some long term complete responses, there was no statistical difference between the two groups.

As a continuation of the studies conducted by the same group, a phase II study was completed using small doses of cyclophosphamide prior to immunotherapy in an attempt to suppress suppressor cells. Among 22 patients entered in this phase II study, 16 were evaluable, and 4 (25%) have shown objective partial response. Interestingly, 3 of the 4 patients who were responders were those whose skin tests against their own tumors became positive.

There appears to be a response rate to the immunotherapy program which is reflected in a better survival among these patients when compared to patients treated by conventional means.

FUTURE PROSPECTS

It is evident that a small but significant number of patients receiving specific immunotherapy will exhibit a positive clinical response. In laboratory tests, using an in vitro cytotoxicity assay in an autochthonous system, investigators are able to demonstrate an increase of specific lymphocyte cytotoxicity against tumor cells while natural killer activity remains unaffected. The preliminary evidence from the skin test reaction against their own tumors may give a clue as to which patients most likely will respond to specific immunotherapy. It is possible, also, that by using biologic response modifiers, such as interferon, which affects natural killer activity, further improvement in response will take place. Finally, the recent evidence that lymphocytes sensitized in vitro to interleukin-2 and reinjection of these lymphocytes in the host will lead to disappearance of metastatic disease deserves further clinical trials.

REFERENCES

1. deKernion JB: Treatment of advanced renal cell carcinoma. Traditional methods and innovative approaches. *J Urol* 130:2, 1983.
2. Raghavaiah NV: Hormone treatment of advanced renal cell carcinoma. *Urol* 19:123, 1982.
3. Nauts HC: *Enhancement of Natural Resistance to Renal Cancer: Beneficial Effects of Concurrent Infections and Immunotherapy with Bacterial Vaccines.* Mongraphy 12. New York, New York Cancer Research Institute, 1973.
4. Bumpus HC Jr: The apparent disappearance of pulmonary metastases in a case of hypernephroma following nephrectomy. *J Urol* 20:185, 1928.
5. Katz SE, Shapira L: Spontaneous regression of genitourinary cancer—an update. *J Urol* 128:1, 1982.

6. Fairlamb DJ: Spontaneous regression of metastases of renal cancer: a report of two cases including the first recorded regression following irradiation of a dominant metastasis and review of the world literature. *Cancer* 47:2101, 1981.

7. Coley WB: The treatment of inoperable sarcoma by bacterial toxins (the mixed toxins of the *Streptococcus erysipelas* and the *Bacillus prodigiosus*). *Proc R Soc Med Surg* 3 (no. 3):1, 1909–1910.

8. Coley WB: The treatment of malignant inoperable tumors with the mixed toxins of the *erysipelas* and *Bacillus prodigiosus*. Weissersbruchm (ed): Brussels, 1914, p 119.

9. Coley WB: Wilms' tumor. *Am J Surg* 29:463, 1935.

10. Lageze P, Durand L, Chassagnon C: Nouvelle observation d'une image pulmonaire dite "en lacher di ballons" ayant disparu apres exercice d'un cancer primitif du rein. *Lyon Med* 203:447, 1960.

11. Almgard LE, Fernstrom J, Haverling M, Ljungquist A: Treatment of renal cell carcinoma by embolic occlusion of the renal circulation. *Br J Urol* 65:474, 1973.

12. Swanson DA, Wallace S, Johnson DE: The role of embolization and nephrectomy in the treatment of metastatic renal carcinoma. *Urol Clin North Am* 7:719, 1981.

13. McDonald MW: Current therapy for renal cell carcinoma. *J Urol* 127:211, 1982.

14. Mebust WK, Weigel JW, Lee KR, Cox GG, Jewell WR, Krishnan EC: Renal cell carcinoma—angioinfarction. *J Urol* 131:231, 1984.

15. Bakke A, Gothlin JH, Haukaas SA, Kalland T: Augmentation of natural killer cell activity after arterial embolization of renal carcinoma. *Cancer Res* 42:3880, 1982.

16. Pontes JW, Goldrosen M, Murphy GP: Immunological response to tumor ischemia in a murine renal cell carcinoma model. *Oncology* 40:63, 1983.

17. Varma J., Huben RP, Wajsman Z, Pontes JE: Therapeutic embolization of pelvic metastasis of renal cell carcinoma. *J Urol* 131:647, 1984.

18. Morales A, Wilson JL, Pater JL, Loeb M: Cytoreductive surgery and systemic Bacillus Calmette-Guérin therapy in metastatic renal cancer: a phase II trial. *J Urol* 127:230, 1982.

19. Morales A, Eidinger D: Bacillus Calmette-Guérin in the treatment of adenocarcinoma of the kidney. *J Urol* 155:377, 1976.

20. Brossman S: Non-specific immunotherapy in GU cancer. In *Proceedings of Chicago Symposium*. Chicago, Franklin Institution Press, 1977, p 97.

21. Montie JE, Bukowski RM, Deodhar SD, Hewlett JS, Stewart BH, Straffon RA: Immunotherapy of disseminated renal cell carcinoma with transfer factor. *J Urol* 117:553, 1977.

22. Montie JE, Buowski RM, James RE, Straffon RA, Stewart BH: A critical review of immunotherapy of disseminated renal carcinoma. American Urological Association, Boston, 1981, abstract 338, p 176.

23. Quesada JR, Swanson DA, Trindade A, Gutterman JV: Renal cell carcinoma: anti-tumor effects of leukocyte interferon. *Cancer Res* 43:940, 1983.

24. deKernion JB, Sarna G, Figlin R, Lindner A, Smith RB: The treatment of renal cell carcinoma with human leukocyte alpha-interferon. *J Urol* 130:1063, 1983.

25. Figlin R, deKernion J, Maldazys J, Sarna G: Treatment of renal cell carcinoma with interferon and vinblastine in combination: a phase I–II trial. *Cancer Treat Rep* 69:263, 1985.

26. Mule JJ, Shu S, Schwarz SL, Rosenberg SH: Adoptive immunotherapy of established pulmonary metastasis with LAK cells and recombinant interleukin-2. *Science* 225:1487, 1984.

27. Horn L, Horn HL: An immunological approach to the therapy of cancer. *Lancet* 2:466, 1971.

28. Hellstrom I, Hellstrom KE: Some aspects of human tumor immunity and their possible implication for tumor prevention and therapy. *Front Radiat Ther Oncol* 7:3, 1972.

29. Ramming KP, deKernion JB: Immune RNA therapy for renal cell carcinoma: survival and immunological monitoring. *Ann Surg* 186:459, 1977.

30. deKernion JB, Ramming K: Therapy of renal adenocarcinoma with immune RNA. *Invest Urol* 17:378, 1980.

31. Richie JP, Wang BS, Steele GD Jr, Wilson RE, Mannick JA: In vivo and in vitro effects of xenogeneic immune ribonucleic acid in patients with advanced renal cell carcinoma: a phase I study. *J Urol* 126:24, 1981.

32. Richie JP, Steele GD Jr, Wilson RE, Ervin T, Wang BS, Mannick JA: Current treatment of metastatic renal cell carcinoma with xenogeneic immune ribonucleic acid. *J Urol* 131:236, 1984.

33. Tykka H, Oravisto KJ, Lehtonew T, Sarna S, Tallberg T: Active specific immunotherapy of advanced renal cell carcinoma. *Eur Urol* 4:250, 1978.

34. Tykka H: Active specific immunotherapy with supportive measures in the treatment of advanced palliatively nephrectomised renal adenocarcinoma. A controlled clinical study. *Scand J Urol Nephrol (Suppl)* 63:1, 1981.

35. Neidhart JA, Murphy SG, Hennick LA, Wise HA: Active specific immunotherapy of metastatic human cell carcinoma with aggregated tumor antigen adjuvant. *Cancer* 46:1128, 1980.

36. Brown GL, Peters PC, Prager MS, Baechter S: Specific immunotherapy of metastatic human cell carcinoma. In American Urological Association Abstracts, Boston, 1981, Abstract 337, p 176.

37. McCune CS, Patterson WB, Henshaw EC: Active specific immunotherapy with tumor cells and *Corynebacterium parvum*. A phase I study. *Cancer* 43:1619, 1979.

38. McCune CS, Shapira DV, Henshaw EC: Specific immunotherapy of advanced renal carcinoma: evidence for polyclonality of metastasis. *Cancer* 47:1984, 1981.

18

Immunotherapy in Metastasizing Hypernephroma with Autologous Tumor Cells

Karl F. Klippel, M.D.

Hypernephroma metastases are the most common radioresistant tumors; 90% are not affected by cytostatic drugs. The mortality among patients suffering from renal adenocarcinoma varies appreciably in different series due to different criteria for selection as well as various modes of treatment. Five-year survival rates ranging from 5 to 10% (1) to 90% (2) have been reported though in large patient series rates are 20–50% (3, 4). The overall prognosis of the clinical series is primarily dependent on how many patients with metastasizing carcinoma are included. In different studies distant metastases have been detected in 25 to 68% of the patients before treatment (5). Irrespective of the form of treatment, results are poor in cases of metastatic disease. It was impossible to gain a prolonged lifetime in patients tested with gestagen preparations. Once metastasis has begun, people are generally expected to live for another 1 to 2 years (6). None of the patients treated by cytostatic drugs, radiotherapy, and surgery lived for 5 years.

Tykkä (7) was the first to report on the total remission of metastasizing hypernephroma using autologous vaccine immunotherapy. In 1978, the same group reported on a randomized study of metastatic hypernephroma. After excision of the tumor, patients were injected with autologous tumor cells, together with Bacille bilie de Calmette-Guérin (BCG) or *Candida* antigens, which are unspecific immunostimulators. Of these patients 23.6% lived for more than 5 years, whereas only 4.3% of the conventionally treated patients were alive at 5 years.

Most of the "long term" survivors in nonimmunotherapy-treated series with metastasized tumors have received active surgical treatment of solitary metastases as well as extirpation of the primary tumor (8, 9).

Patients with solitary metastases are the only group among those with metastatic disease who do not have the usual poor prognosis.

Of all patients with renal cell carcinoma, approximately 2 to 4% exhibit only solitary metastases. When treated by active surgery the 5-year survival rate is considerably better than that of other patients suffering from metastasized disease (10). In the series of 59 cases compiled from the literature by Middleton (5), the 5-year survival rate was 34%, and in the material compiled by Skinner (3) 34 patients (14.7%) with solitary metastases survived for 5 years. In Tolia and Whitmore's series (11) of 19 patients, the 5-year survival rate was 35%. All of the authors stress that, in spite of a primary remission of metastases, the tumor will usually reappear and the patient will die of cancer.

In many of the previously described cases, a solitary metastasis has appeared only after nephrectomy, even though the nephrectomy was regarded as radical at the time.

Due to the poor prognosis of patients suffering from metastasized renal cell carcinoma, no standard modality of treatment has been established. Radical nephrectomy has not been shown to improve the final prognosis, although it may provide some palliative effect in decreasing the clinical symptoms. In many clinics it is not considered indicated to remove the primary tumor in patients with verified distant metastases (5) and these patients are all intended to have other forms of treatment.

Irradiation, hormonal treatment, chemotherapy, and, lately, various immunologic therapy regimens are most frequently employed (12). Some patients are also left without any active treatment (13). In this respect there has developed a move toward more active surgical treatment since adjunctive nephrectomy is regarded as supporting the effect of adjuvant therapies by decreasing the tumor mass and by improving the immunologic defense mechanism of the patient (14).

The prognosis is as poor when carcinomatous cell tissue is left locally in the field of operation as in patients with distant metastases (15). Overall, the prognosis of advanced renal cell carcinoma is so poor that these patients have been regarded as practically incurable by current treatments. In the few cases of cure it is possible that a special character of the tumor or the individual constitution of the patient was more decisive than the actual treatment applied (6).

CLINICAL CONCLUSIONS: THE NEED FOR AN EFFECTIVE IMMUNOTHERAPY

Patients with stage IV renal cancer have a very poor prognosis irrespective of histologic tumor grade. Nephrectomy alone does not increase survival. In their series Robson et al (16) saw no survivors 3 years or more postoperatively. At the time of surgery approximately half of the patients have already developed distant metastases. Unfortunately renal cell cancer is characterized by a distinct resistance to conventional modes of therapy. Studies concerning chemotherapeutic treatments have been very discouraging. It is difficult to obtain curative effects with irradiation and it does not prolong survival. The author has found radiation therapy to be a potent measure in the palliation of metastases-induced bone pain. Promising results with immunotherapy reported by Skinner et al (9), Neidhart et al (17), Tykkä et al (18), and Shapira et al (19) led to a phase II clinical trial at the Mainz University Department of Urology in 1976, after a pilot study had been initiated, and follow-up continues to the present (20).

MAINZ UNIVERSITY CLINICAL TRIAL

Patients and Methodology

A total of 53 patients with stage IV renal cancer have been treated by immunotherapy after palliative nephrectomy since 1976. Of these, 32 patients had distant lesions to one organ system only, including lung, liver, bone, and brain. Twenty-one patients had metastases involving more than one organ system (Table 18.1). There was no predominance of any one histologic grade (Table 18.1).

Preparation of Vaccine

Viable tumor material was obtained at surgery and processed immediately under sterile conditions. Single cell suspension was prepared by teasing the tumor tissue through a 60-mesh steel grid. Tumor cells were washed twice in Dulbecco's minimum essential tissue culture medium (DMEM), pelleted at $400 \times g$ for 10 minutes, and resuspended in a dilute *Candida* antigen mixture. Gamma irradiation with 100 Gy yielded the ready-for-use vaccine which was aliquoted and stored in liquid nitrogen until further use. Cells were frozen at a controlled rate of 1°C/minute to avoid excessive damage (Fig. 18.1).

Treatment Protocol

Patients received two cycles of vaccinations with four injections each, the first one beginning 2 weeks after operation. The second set of

Table 18.1
Immunotherapy of Renal Cell Cancer (Stage IV, $n = 53$)[a]

$T_{34} = 53$	I = 16	Single organ = 32
$M_+ = 53$	II = 17	Lung 26
$N_+ = 20$	III = 20	Bone 2
		Lymph node 2
		Skin 1
		Thyroid 1
		Multiple organs = 21
		Liver 3
		CNS 3

[a] From Schärfe T, Becht E, Klippel KF, Jacobi GH, Hohenfellner R: Active immunotherapy of stage IV renal cell cancer using autologous tumor cell. In Klippel KF, Gardilcic S (eds): *Immunotherapy in Urology.* Munich, Zuckschwerdt-Verlag, 1984, vol 9, p 59.

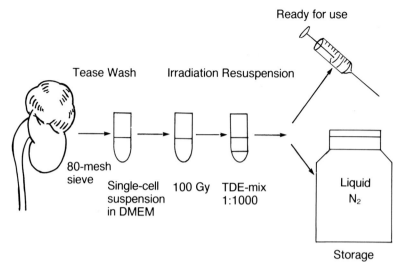

Figure 18.1. Preparation of vaccine. (From Schärfe T, Becht E, Klippel KF, Jacobi GH, Hohenfellner R: Active immunotherapy of stage IV renal cell cancer using autologous tumor cell. In Klippel KF, Gardilcic S (eds): *Immunotherapy in Urology.* Munich, Zuckschwerdt-Verlag, 1984, vol 9, p 59.)

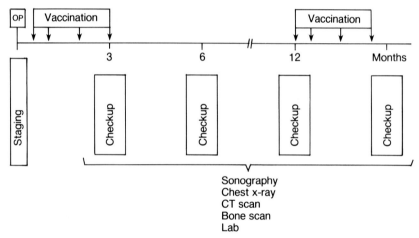

Figure 18.2. Vaccination schedule. (From Schärfe T, Becht E, Klippel KF, Jacobi GH, Hohenfellner R: Active immunotherapy of stage IV renal cell cancer using autologous tumor cell. In Klippel KF, Gardilcic S (eds): *Immunotherapy in Urology.* Munich, Zuckschwerdt-Verlag, 1984, vol 9, p 59.)

injections is continued 1 year after surgery (Fig. 18.2). The vaccine is injected intracutaneously into the volar forearm using 0.5 ml of vaccine at a cell concentration of 5×10^6 cells/ml in dilute Trichophyton Caudida Epidermis (TCE) mix (TCE mix = 1:1000 in saline).

Patients were vaccinated on days 0, 14, 30, and 60. They were seen at 3-month intervals and examined for tumor progress or regression by abdominal sonography, chest x-rays, bone scans, overall performance, and routine laboratory work (serum creatinine, blood urea nitrogen, electrolytes, protein, glucose, alkaline phosphatase).

Results

In this trial, 9 of 53 patients had objective regression of tumor burden. Of these, 3 had complete remission with a follow-up period of 48 months, and 6 had a partial remission with a follow-up of 60 months. Eighteen patients are stable with their disease, showing no increase in tumor mass (Tables 18.2 and 18.3). Twenty-six patients had progressing disease; 17 of them died within 12 months after diagnosis of their tumor. Patients with multiple metastases confined to one organ system have done better with immunotherapy than those with disseminated tumor spread. Among therapy responders, dedifferentiated tumors prevailed. The longitudinal evaluation of therapy responders showed an increase in tumor volume after the first vaccination cycle, converting to a definite complete remission with the second set of injections (Fig. 18.3). These patients have remained tumor free for more than 49 months so far.

In patients with partial remission, no distinct increase in tumor burden was observed. Rather, metastases decreased in size and number gradually over several months. Relapse then usually occurred at a different organ site. Two patients developed CNS lesions to which they succumbed (Fig. 18.4).

Those lesions that were seen to regress readily upon immunotherapy were, in most cases, confined to the lung. In one case the patient had tumor spread to both liver and lung. In the latter patient all lesions vanished completely and she has been free of disease for more than 72 months so far.

Table 18.2
Responsiveness to Therapy and Tumor Spread[a]

	Complete Remission	Partial Remission	Stable	Progress
Single organ metastases	1	5	13	13
Multiple organ metastases	2	1	4	14

[a] From Schärfe T, Becht E, Klippel KF, Jacobi GH, Hohenfellner R: Active immunotherapy of stage IV renal cell cancer using autologous tumor cell. In Klippel KF, Gardilcic S (eds): *Immunotherapy in Urology.* Munich, Zuckschwerdt-Verlag, 1984, vol 9, p 59.

Table 18.3
Distribution of Histologic Tumor Grade[a]

Response (n = 9)	Stable (n = 18)	Progress (n = 26)
Complete		
G I: 0		
G II: 1	G I: 8	G I: 6
G III: 2	G II: 4	G II: 9
Partial	G III: 6	G III: 11
G I: 1		
G II: 2		
G III: 3		

[a] From Schärfe T, Becht E, Klippel KF, Jacobi GH, Hohenfellner R: Active immunotherapy of stage IV renal cell cancer using autologous tumor cell. In Klippel KF, Gardilcic S (eds): *Immunotherapy in Urology.* Munich, Zuckschwerdt-Verlag, 1984, vol 9, p 59.

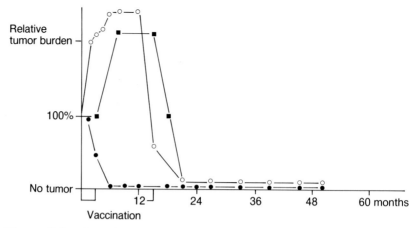

Figure 18.3. Complete responders—follow-up. (From Schärfe T, Becht E, Klippel KF, Jacobi GH, Hohenfellner R: Active immunotherapy of stage IV renal cell cancer using autologous tumor cell. In Klippel KF, Gardilcic S (eds): *Immunotherapy in Urology.* Munich, Zuckschwerdt-Verlag, 1984, vol 9, p 59.)

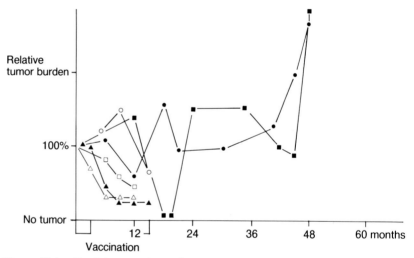

Figure 18.4. Partial responders—follow-up. (From Schärfe T, Becht E, Klippel KF, Jacobi GH, Hohenfellner R: Active immunotherapy of stage IV renal cell cancer using autologous tumor cell. In Klippel KF, Gardilcic S (eds): *Immunotherapy in Urology.* Munich, Zuckschwerdt-Verlag, 1984, vol 9, p 59.)

Severe side effects have not been seen with immunization. Local erythema at the injection sites is common and appears 48 hours after vaccination. The cutaneous reaction in no instance required treatment or suspension of immunotherapy. Usually swelling and itching vanish spontaneously within 2 or 3 days. In addition, a slight temperature (less than 38°C) or malaise was observed occasionally and passed within a week.

The author's group was not able to discover any correlation between cutaneous allergic reactions to the vaccine and tumor response.

RESULTS OF A PILOT STUDY STARTED IN 1976

Immunization

Autologous or allogenic tumor cells (5×10^6 to 10×10^6) were injected together with the immunostimulator, Keyhole Limpet Hemocyanin (KLH) (Calbiochem 374805, A grade), or with *Candida* antigens (Candidin 1:100). Patients who were treated with immunostimulator KLH (0.5 mg) were treated or presensitized with KLH 4 weeks previously.

Skin Reactions

Six to 12 hours after treatment a localized erythema was noted at the injection site (lower left arm), together with slight itching and a subfebrile temperature. After the injections, the axillary lymph nodes in nearly all patients were palpable as big stringy objects. All of these acute reactions disappeared within 5 to 6 days after the injections. The local induration, partly with hyperpigmentation, subsided after 4 to 6 weeks.

Choice of Patients

Patients were picked at random. Written consent for therapy was given by all patients. The following parameters were tested immunologically:

1. Electrophoresis
2. Immunoglobulins
3. T cells (rosette test)
4. B cells (immunofluorescent test with anti-light chain immunoglobulin;
5. Dinitrochlorobenzene test
6. Lymphocyte stimulations: phytohemagglutinin (PHA), pokeweed mitogen (PWM), concanavalin A (Con A)
7. *Candida* antibody titer: immunofluorescence, hemagglutination titer (Hoffman-La Roche).

All patients were seen on a regular basis in the tumor clinic. During those visits routine tests, such as full blood count (Fbc), electrolytes, phosphatases, creatinine and protein, carcinoembryonic antigen, and urinalysis, were performed.

Chest x-rays were made monthly or every 3 months, urograms were made twice a year, and a whole body bone scan was performed yearly. If necessary, additional studies, such as computed tomograms or ultrasonograms, were done.

Case Histories

ES, FEMALE, 39 YEARS OLD

After preoperative radiation with 4000 rad, stage of tumor $P_3 N_0 M_2$, a total tumor nephrectomy was carried out in March 1977 (left kidney). The patient was given daily injections into the right thigh, of 5×10^6 tumor cells plus 5 mg of KLH for 14 days following the operation.

Monthly routine chest x-rays showed stabilization of metastases for 4 months. Because the patient had a very severe local reaction (erythema 4 × 8 cm) and painful induration, she refused further injections. Polychemotherapy was started in July 1977. Following this, metastases in the lung spread rapidly and the patient died in December 1977.

KR, FEMALE, 50 YEARS OLD

After preoperative radiation with 4000 rad, stage of tumor P_3 N_0 M_2, a total tumor nephrectomy was carried out in December 1976. Two lung metastases were first seen on an x-ray taken in October 1977. First injections of 5 mg of KLH (intradermal) were given in December 1977. This was followed by injections of 4×10^6 allogenic tumor cells plus 5 mg of KLH in January 1978. An x-ray taken in February 1978 showed shrinking of metastases, and in March 1978 and again in April 1978 metastases were not visible.

Tomography of the lungs done in December 1978 showed no sign of metastases. A booster of 1 mg of KLH was given dermally, followed by a strong skin reaction. The patient had an apoplectic attack in the late part of October which left her with hemiparesis of the left side. The computed tomogram showed a single brain metastasis with no localization on electroencephalography. Furthermore, it showed enlargement of the right single kidney. The whole body bone scan was negative, and the mediastinal tomogram showed enlarged lymph nodes, which could possibly be metastases. There is now no known localization of metastases, and 9 years after immunization, the patient is still alive with a known brain metastasis, an enlarged kidney, and possible lymph node metastases.

EJ, MALE, 37 YEARS OLD

After preoperative radiation with 3600 rad, stage of tumor P_1 N_2 M_2 (lung metastases), a total tumor right nephrectomy was carried out in November 1978. After immunization with 5 mg (intradermal) of KLH, an injection of 2×10^6 syngeneic cells followed in December 1978. In January 1979, no further metastases showed on chest x-rays. In February 1979, however, after a second injection of 3.5×10^6 plus 1 mg of KLH, lung metastases were showing in their original location and in greater numbers. In April 1979, the patient had multiple pulmonary metastases.

Regression of all metastases was noted in December 1980, 2 years after starting the immunotherapy. The patient now is in very good general condition and able to work full time. In June 1983, a solitary lesion in the lung appeared, which was operated and used for new vaccination. To the time of writing (September 1985), the patient is still alive.

OW, MALE, 62 YEARS OLD

After orthopaedically treating a spontaneous fracture of the left humerus with known osteolysis of the scapula, an operation was carried out only to find a right hypernephroma. After preoperative radiation with 4000 rad a total tumor right nephrectomy was carried out in November 1976 (stage of tumor $P_1 V_1 N_0 M_{1D}$).

Because of osteolysis in the left shoulder joint, a disarticulation had to be performed, as there were still more osteolyses in the scapula and several ribs. Following this, the patient was presensitized with 5 mg of KLH intradermally. He was injected with 5×10^6 allogenic hypernephroma cells plus KLH in February 1979. Despite this, metastases kept progressing, and the patient died 6 months after starting immunotherapy and 3 years after palliative tumor nephrectomy.

WJ, MALE, 44 YEARS OLD

After extirpation of a single metastasis located at the front of the skull cap, the following electroencephalogram and computed tomogram of the skull showed no irregularity.

Because right hypernephroma was seen after angiography and multiple metastases were known to be in lung and bones, embolization of the right kidney artery with histoacryl was carried out. The number of metastases in the lung doubled between April 1978 and August 1978. The number of metastases stayed stable after immunization with 5 mg of KLH given in December 1978. January 1979 saw rapid growth of lung metastases and relapse in the front skull cap. A computed tomogram showed atrophy of the brain with no sign of metastases. The patient became tachycardiac and dispneic as a result of enormous growth of the metastases. Injection of 10×10^6 allogenic-radiated hypernephroma cells plus KLH was given intradermally on February 1, 1979. After added treatment with testosterone and digitalis, metastases stabilized in December 1979. The patient died in February 1980 following cancerous cachexia.

GS, FEMALE, 44 YEARS OLD

A total tumor nephrectomy was carried out March 20, 1979 (Fig. 18.1, left kidney). During the operation, a single metastasis was seen in the liver and multiple metastases were known to be in the lungs. Histopathology showed cancer stage $P_3 G_3 V_1 M_{1d}$. Metastases in the lungs increased significantly in size and number, 4 weeks after the operation. Injection of 5×10^6 autologous tumor cells plus 0.2 ml of Candidin was given 5 weeks after the operation. The patient experienced a slight skin reaction; immunoglobulin (Ig) titer against *Candida albicans* 1:80, and IgM 1:640. Restimulation with *Candida* antigen 1:10 was performed in May 1979; *Candida* titer IgG 1:640 and IgM 1:1.280 were found following restimulation.

A computed tomogram of the liver in July 1979 showed liver metastasis still existing. In August 1979 restimulation was done with 5×10^6 autologous cells plus Candidin 1:100 given intradermally. The patient underwent restimulation with autologous cells every 3 months until December 1980. The running computed tomograms of the liver and 6-weekly chest x-rays showed stabilization of lung metastases until August 1980. At that time there was a cystic change of known liver metastasis. There was continuous regression of lung metastases after this. After numerous chest x-rays in December 1980, no metastases were seen in the lungs. The patient gained 10 kg in weight, felt physically fit, and was doing a full time job. In February 1982 the liver lesion was punctured by the radiologist, and there were no signs of tumor cells. The patient is still doing well.

MF, FEMALE, 48 YEARS OLD

In 1975 a tumor nephrectomy was carried out for hypernephroma of the left kidney. In July 1979 liver metastases were found by liver scan, computed tomogram, angiography, and ultrasound. Nonspecific immunotherapy was started in March 1980 with 5 mg of KLH given intradermally, followed by 4×10^6 allogenic radiated tumor cells. Bone destruction was found in the right humerus head in the form of a bone metastasis. After removal of the metastasis, the humerus head was replaced with a prosthesis. A computed tomogram in August 1980 showed no visible liver metastasis. The single right kidney showed tumor-like changes in some areas. A subsequent angiogram showed none of the earlier liver metastases, but definite pathologic findings were seen in the right kidney. Metastases in this patient were stable for 10 months. She died of progressive bone metastasis (Table 18.4).

The outcome of these seven patients in the pilot study clearly indicates the need for more investigations of the future possibilities of immunotherapy in hypernephroma patients.

Tunn and co-workers (21) tried to optimize immunotherapy by cell classification using a cell sorter computer (Histomat). They selected for the autologs vaccine primarily grades 2 and 3 tumor cells from the original tumor with favorable results concerning the antibody titers in the patients.

Nakano and co-workers (22) were able to show a high tumor cell lysis rate by blood lymphocytes when cultured in interleukin-2. They suggest that interleukin-2 might become a useful agent for patients with renal cell carcinoma.

DISCUSSION

In stage IV renal cell cancer, poor prognosis with a mean survival of less than 12 months postoperatively is combined with an inherent resistance to conventional modes of tumor therapy (2, 5, 8, 12–14, 17, 22–25). Observations correlating tumor-specific cytotoxicity and other immune parameters with tumor burden and prognosis (3, 7, 9, 11, 18, 21, 26) suggested that functions of the immune system are involved in tumor control. Observations linking impaired immune function to tumor stage and poor prognosis indicated that stimulation of the immune system, whether adoptive or active tumor-specific, might be beneficial in tumor therapy. Concepts using adoptive immunotherapy were reported by Morales and Eidniger (25), who saw 4 temporary remissions in 10 patients treated with BCG. On the other hand, Skinner et al (9), describing the use of immune RNA as adoptive tumor-specific treatment, showed an improved survival and a stabilization of metastatic

Table 18.4
Results of Pilot Study

Patient	Age	Sex	Operation	Metastases	Start Immunotherapy Postoperatively	Cells	Complete Remission	Partial Remission	Progress	Follow-up (months)	Status
ES	39	F	3/77	Lung	2 weeks	Autologous	No	No	Yes	9	Dead
OW	62	M	11/76	Bone	27 months	Allogenic	No	No	Yes	34	Dead
WJ	44	M	Embolization 4/78	Bone Lung	13 months	Allogenic	No	No	Yes	22	Dead
KR	50	F	12/76	Lung, CNS, bone	12 months	Allogenic	No	Yes	No	124	At risk (60%)[a]
EJ	37	M	11/78	Lung	2 weeks	Autologous	Yes	No	No	100	At risk (100%)
GS	44	F	3/79	Lung, liver	5 weeks	Autologous	Yes	No	No	97	At risk (100%)
MF	48	F	6/75	Lung, bone, Kidney	5 years	Allogenic	No	Yes	Yes	111	Dead (80%)

[a] Percent: Karnofsky index.

growth. Transfer-induced restoration of immune defects in patients with renal cell cancer brought about stabilization of disease in approximately 20% of the patients. Active tumor-specific immunotherapy with autologous tumor material promised to be very effective.

Investigations by Tykkä (7, 18) as well as Neidhart et al (17) showed excellent results in respect to 5-year survival (23.6% versus 4.3% in the control group). Approximately 20% of the patients had objective tumor regression, which is beyond the spontaneous course of disease (20). Interestingly, all authors described lung metastases as being the ones most responsive to immunotherapy. Whether this is due to some specific mechanism facilitated by the pulmonary tissue or lying within the specific nature of pulmonary lesions is not known. In the author's patients pulmonary metastases have been the ones to respond best, although he has definitely seen that in three cases liver metastases decreased and vanished after cystic degeneration. These lesions had been confirmed to be metastatic tissue by intraoperative or percutaneous biopsy.

In their latest report Tallberg et al (26) described in a 13-year followup a highly significant difference between the calculated life expectancy of the immunotherapy group (44.5 months) versus the control group (19.0 months).

Studies are under way to investigate immune mechanisms possibly related to or responsible for tumor surveillance, including tumor-specific cytotoxicity, NK cell activity, and humoral blocking factors in patients undergoing immunotherapy. It is hoped that these parameters will make therapy monitoring possible, resulting in more effective vaccines and vaccination protocols.

Although parameters monitoring the effectiveness of mechanisms of therapy have not been identified, the author concludes that immunotherapy for stage IV renal cell cancer is justified considering that no other treatment mode is presently available. An objective response rate of approximately 20% and significantly prolonged survival are achieved without compromising life quality. The authors group have not seen adverse side effects or tumor enhancement with their treatment protocol. Whether new perspectives of adoptive immunotherapy with tumor-specific monoclonal antibodies or combination of immuno- and chemotherapy will be able to yield higher scores remains to be seen. Careful investigations of tumor biology and tumor kinetics will be necessary for the development of therapeutic protocols that take into consideration specific characteristics of the individual tumor.

Notwithstanding problems in the design of previous trials, the treatment failures that have been seen, and the theoretical reservations concerning the ultimate role that immune response manipulation may have in successful cancer therapy, the absence of any other effective therapy in the management of metastatic disease in kidney cancer underscores the need to develop new and effective treatment approaches (23).

REFERENCES

1. Cahill G: Cancer of the kidneys, adrenals and testes. *JAMA* 138:357, 1948.
2. Foot N, Humphreys G, Whitemore W: Renal tumors, pathology and prognosis in

295 cases. *J Urol* 66:190, 1951.

3. Skinner D, Colvin R, Vermillon C, Pfister R, Leadbetter W: Diagnosis and management for renal cancer. *Cancer* 28:1165, 1971.

4. Peeling W, Mantell B, Shepard B: Postoperative irradiation in the treatment of renal cell carcinoma. *Br J Urol* 41:23, 1969.

5. Middleton R: Surgery for metastatic renal cell carcinoma. *J Urol* 97:973, 1967.

6. deKernion J, Ramming K, Smith R: The natural history of metastatic renal cell carcinoma: a computer analysis. *J Urol* 120:148, 1978.

7. Tykkä H: Active specific immunotherapy in the treatment of advanced renal cell carcinoma: a controlled clinical study. In Klippel KF, Gardilcic S (eds): *Immunotherapy in Urology*. München, Zuckschwerdt-Verlag, 1984, vol 9, p 49.

8. Middleton A: Indications for and results of nephrectomy for metastatic renal cell carcinoma. *Urol Clin North Am* 7:711, 1980.

9. Skinner D, deKernion J, Brower P, Ramming K, Pilch Y: Advanced renal cell carcinoma: treatment with xenogenic immune ribonucleic acid and appropriate surgical resection. *J Urol* 115:246, 1976.

10. O'Dea M, Zuncke H, Utz D, Bernatz P: Treatment of renal cell carcinoma with solitary metastases. *J Urol* 120:540, 1978.

11. Tolia B, Whitmore W: Solitary metastasis from renal cell carcinoma. *J Urol* 114:836, 1975.

12. Klippel KF, Altwein JE: Palliative Therapiemöglichkeiten beim metastasierten Hypernephrom. *Dtsch Med Wochenschr* 104:128, 1979.

13. Freed S: Nephrectomy for renal cell carcinoma with metastases. *Urology* 9:613, 1977.

14. Klugo R, Detmers M, Stiles R, Talley R, Cerny J. Aggressive versus conservative management of stage IV renal cell carcinoma. *J Urol* 118:244, 1977.

15. deKernion J: Hypernephroma—natural history and the influence of immunotherapy. *Proc Inst Med Chicago* 31:231, 1977.

16. Robson CJ, Churchill BM, Anderson W: The results of radical nephrectomy for renal cell carcinoma. *J Urol* 101:297, 1969.

17. Neidhart JA, Murphy GG, Hennick LA, Inise JA: Active specific immunotherapy of stage IV renal carcinoma with aggregated tumor antigen adjuvant. *Cancer* 46:1128, 1980.

18. Tykkä H, Oravisto KJ, Lehtonen T: Active specific immunotherapy of advanced renal cell carcinoma. *Eur Urol* 4:250, 1978.

19. Shapira DV, McCline CS, Henskaw EC: Treatment of advanced renal cell carcinoma with specific immunotherapy consisting of autologous tumor cells and *C. parvum*. *Proc Am Soc Clin Oncol* 20:348, 1979.

20. Schärfe T, Becht E, Klippel KF, Jacobi GH, Hohenfellner R: Active immunotherapy of stage IV renal cell cancer using autologous tumor cell. In Klippel KF, Gardilcic S (eds): *Immunotherapy in Urology*. München, Zuckschwerdt-Verlag, 1984, vol 9, p 59.

21. Tunn UW, Stieglitz J, Wierich W, Falkenberg FW, Binder A: Optimierung der spezifischen Immuntherapie durch exakte Zellklassifizierung. In Klippel KF, Gardilcic S (eds): *Immunotherapy in Urology*. München, Zuckschwerdt-Verlag, 1984, vol 9, p 47.

22. Nakano E, Tada Y, Idikawa Y, Fujoka H, Ishipasi M, Matsuda M, Takaha M, Sònoda T: Cytotoxic activity of peripheral blood lymphocytes grown with interleukin 2 against autologous tumor cells in patients with renal cell carcinoma. *J Urol* 134:24, 1985.

23. Droller MJ: Immunotherapy in genito-urinary neoplasia. *J Urol* 133:1, 1985.

24. McCune CS, Skapila DV, Henshaw EC: Specific immunotherapy of advanced renal carcinoma: evidence for the polyclonality of metastases. *Cancer* 47:1984, 1981.

25. Morales AD, Eidniger T: BCG treatment of adenocarcinoma of the kidney. *J Urol* 115:377, 1976.

26. Tallberg T, Tykkä H, Mahlberg K, Halttunen D, Lehtonen T, Kalima T, Sarna S: Active specific immunotherapy with supportive measures in the treatment of palliatively nephrectomized renal adenocarcinoma patients: a thirteen year follow up study. *Eur Urol* 11:233, 1985.

4
Section

Uncommon Renal Tumors

19

Mesenchymal and Capsular Tumors of the Kidney

Urs E. Studer, M.D.
Jean B. deKernion, M.D.

BENIGN MESENCHYMAL AND CAPSULAR TUMORS (TABLE 19.1)

Fibromas

Fibromas in the midzone of the renal medulla are found in as many as 40% of unselected autopsy populations (1). Those measuring 2 to 4 mm are firm, gray, and resemble fibroblasts; they are believed to be of interstitial medullary origin and have a characteristic lipid content (2). Lerman et al (3) therefore called them renomedullary interstitial cell tumors, rather then fibromas. Moreover, Xipell (1), in a systematic study on benign renal nodules, suggested that some of the fibrous nodules might be caused by tubular leakage or focal fibrosis occurring in relation to tubular damage, rather than true neoplasms. Further evidence that they cannot be considered fibromas in the usual sense is Prezyna et al's finding of high prostaglandin content, and its possible clinical implications are not yet clear (1, 4). Another kind is obviously the large fibroma, corresponding more closely to what is considered a typical fibroma. It is rarely found in the renal medulla. Glover and Buck (5) recently reviewed the literature and found eight reported cases of intramedullary fibroma. These can be partially calcified, they can produce a distortion of the caliceal system with pelviocaliectasis (6), and on renal arteriography, abnormal, tortuous vessels of varying caliber are apparent. This can make it difficult to discern intramedullary fibroma from renal cell carcinomas based on x-ray findings only. However, arteriovenous shunting and venous puddling of contrast medium do not usually occur (7).

While fibromas of the capsula are also rare, this is the site with the highest incidence in the kidney. A distinctive sign of difference, when compared to the intramedullary fibromas, is (as in other forms of

Table 19.1
Classification of Kidney Tumors

	Benign	Malignant
Tumors of renal parenchyma and capsule		
1. Epithelial tumors	Adenoma	Adenocarcinoma
	Papillary (cyst-)	Papillary (cyst-)
	Tubular	Clear cell
	Alveolar	Granular cell
		Mixed
		Spindle cell
	Oncocytoma	Alveolar cell
2. Mesenchymal/capsular tumors	Fibroma	Fibrosarcoma
		Fibroxanthosarcoma
	Hemangioma	Hemangioendothelioma
		Hemangiosarcoma
	Juxtaglomerular cell tumor	Hemangiopericytoma
	Lymphangioma	Lymphangiosarcoma
	Leiomyoma	Leiomyosarcoma
	Rhabdomyoma	Rhabdomyosarcoma
	Lipoma	Liposarcoma
	Chondroma/ossification	Osteogenic sarcoma
	Angiomyolipoma-hamartoma	
3. Neurogenic tumors	Neurofibroma	Neuroblastoma
		Symphathicoblastoma
		Schwannoma
4. Tumors of immature renal tissue	Mesoblastic nephroma	Nephroblastoma (Wilms' tumor)
		Embryonic carcinoma
5. Various tumors of different origin	Dermoid	Hemoblastoses
	Adrenal rests	Hodgkin's disease
	Endometriosis	Lymphomas
	Carcinoid tumor	Myelomas
	Granulomas	Leukemia
	Cysts	Metastases from other primaries
Tumors of the renal pelvis		
1. Epithelial tumors	Benign papilloma	Papillary tumor
		Transitional cell carcinoma
	Leukoplakia	Squamous cell carcinoma
	Glandular metaplasia	Adenocarcinoma
2. Mesenchymal tumors	Fibroma	Fibrosarcoma
	Hemangioma	Hemangiosarcoma
	Leiomyoma	Leiomyo(-myxo)sarcoma

capsular neoplasias) the fact that the blood supply derives typically from enlarged capsular vessels. Fibromas of the capsule can also compress, distort, or displace the kidney; however, as in other neoplasias of the capsula that do not invade the renal parenchyma, an intact kidney within the large mass of the neoplasm is seen during the nephrogram phase of angiography (7).

Hemangiomas

In 1971, Peterson and Thompson (8) summarized the literature on hemangiomas, including 150 reported cases since Virchow's original report in 1867. They discovered no preponderance of cases in males or females and an even distribution of occurrences in the right and left kidneys. The kidney is second to the liver among internal organs hosting these vascular tumors (9). Approximately 12% of hemangiomas are multiple (10), but less than 1% are bilateral (8). Most of the lesions are of the cavernous rather than the capillary type and are located in the medullary part of the kidney. Although they usually measure less than 2 cm, Samellas et al (11) reported one that measured 3 cm in diameter. Larger hemangiomas are rare and predominantly found in the subcapsular region (12).

Hematuria, which can be massive (13), does not always occur in hemangiomas, and many are incidental findings at autopsy only (14). Macroscopically, according to their content of blood, they are red or dark blue, soft, and poorly encapsulated.

Since pure hemangiomas tend to be small, at most a deformity of one calix on the intravenous pyelogram (IVP) can be expected. This may account in part for the difficulty of detecting them radiographically (13). Another reason is that some do not opacify at all, this helps to explain the numerous reports of preoperative angiograms that failed to demonstrate renal hemangiomas which were later detected by histologic examination. Feczko (13) estimated the proportion of false negative angiograms to be around 50%. This is supported by findings of Jonsson (15), who demonstrated angiographically only four of eight hemangiomas or arteriovenous malformations that were later found at surgery. Lesions that can be visualized on arteriography usually show rapid filling of a coil of blood vessels, well demarcated, and consisting of numerous, densely arranged, tortuous vessels. Emptying is delayed, and contrast medium may still be present when it has disappeared from other renal vessels of the same caliber showing marked intensity of the contrast in the capillary phase (16). Surgical excision is recommended only for patients who suffer repeated severe bleeding. The correct preoperative diagnosis of a benign renal hemangioma can lead to the preservation of normal renal tissue by doing a partial nephrectomy only. However, since radiologic findings in a benign angioma can resemble those found in a renal cell carcinoma, the latter should always be considered in the differential diagnosis.

Juxtaglomerular Cell Tumors of the Kidney

This tumor, originating from a particular part of the vascular structure (the pericytes of afferent arterioles in the juxtaglomerular apparatus) is extremely rare. Squires et al (17) recently reviewed the literature and found 15 published cases in the English literature (17). Nevertheless, interest in this tumor is 2-fold: because it is benign it is important to separate it from the better known, malignant hemangiopericytoma, which will be discussed later. Second, it usually causes severe hypertension by secreting renin. The mean age at the time of diagnosis is 24 years, with the oldest 57 (17).

The tumors so far published were all well circumscribed, encapsulated, and located in the cortical area. They are usually small. Three were less than 1 cm in diameter, but one measured 4.5 cm (17). The pathogno-monic findings at the electron microscopic examination are character-istic rhomboidal granules with a crystalline matrix, apparently repre-senting the immature, "protogranule" of renin, such as described by Biava and West (18) in human juxtaglomerular cells. The tumor cells are occasionally surrounded by nonmyelinated nerve fibers, such as those seen in a normal juxtaglomerular apparatus (17, 19, 20).

According to Squires et al (17), no correlation is found between tumor size and severity of hypertension, the leading symptom that enables diagnosis and treatment. The mean of the highest reported systolic and diastolic blood pressures was found to be 216/141 mm Hg. In addition, most of the patients with a juxtaglomerular cell tumor show attendant hyperaldosteronism and hypokalemia; the mean of the lowest observed values is 2.9 mEq/liter.

In 9 of 10 published cases the preoperative renal vein renin values indicated correctly the lateralization of the tumor, and this examination can certainly be of great importance when evaluating the patient. Moreover, it seems reasonable to attempt selective blood samplings from different renal veins, such as those performed by Bonnin et al (21), in case a tumor cannot be demonstrated on a preliminary ultrasound and/or axial computed tomography (CT) examination. This might enable the surgeon to cure the patient by means of a partial nephrectomy with preservation of the normal portion of the kidney, since in none of the reported cases has a recurrence or metastasis developed. All patients for whom data were available had significantly decreased or normalized postoperative blood pressure. Treatment success seems to be time re-lated, with partial blood pressure response only in patients who had hypertension for several years and who evidenced consecutively non-necrotizing hypertensive arterial damage in the nontumorous portion of the kidney (17).

Lymphangiomas

Joost et al (22) reviewed the literature in 1977 and found 20 cases of benign renal lymphangioma reported. At the time of diagnosis, the patients' average age was 33 years. Flank mass was the leading symptom in half of the patients; 30% had hematuria and/or pain, i.e., the classical triad for renal cell carcinoma. Moreover, since lymphangiomas are tumors of variable density because the ectasis of lymph vessels ranges from millimeters to centimeters (cavernous type), and since arteriog-raphy usually shows a poorly vascularized area with some small, irreg-ularly shaped vessels, the definitive diagnosis of a benign vascular tumor tends to be made only after a radical nephrectomy for suspected renal cell carcinoma has been performed.

Myomas

Leiomyomas, predominantly found in the renal cortex, are the second commonest mesenchymal tumors in the kidney, after the more frequent, mainly intramedullary fibromas (discussed above). Leiomyomas are the most frequent benign tumors of mesenchymal origin in the renal cortex, followed by the mixed mesenchymal nodules and the lipomas. Xipell (1) found an incidence of 5% in postmortem serial sections with a thickness measuring 2 to 3 mm in 500 different kidneys. However, leiomyomas are not the most common benign tumors of the cortex: according to the same author, benign epithelial tumors (adenomas), occur more frequently, with an incidence of 22% (see Chapter 20).

As in renal fibromas, small lesions, measuring just a few millimeters, are the rule; larger lesions measuring several centimeters are very rare. Foster (23) reviewed the literature in 1956 and found 22 cases of clinically significant leiomyomas. Unless they are not very big, such as reported by Clinton-Thomas (24), the diagnosis is likely to be an incidental finding or a misinterpretation of radiographic findings on IVP or renal angiogram, suggesting falsely malignant lesions because of atypical (however few) vessels within the mass (25–27). Furthermore, possible calcifications of leiomyomas, such as in the uterus, have been noted repeatedly and may also mislead to a diagnosis of renal cell carcinoma (27–29). A preoperative diagnosis of a benign leiomyoma thus seems rarely possible. Even in case of a cytologic interpretation of material aspirated through a fine needle, the benignity of the myomatous tumor could not be assessed reliably, since interpretation of malignant potential—as in all mesenchymal neoplasias—can be difficult even after histologic review of numerous sections of a leiomyoma.

Even rarer than large leiomyomas are the *rhabdomyomas*, which can grow to large size. Ney and Friedenberg (16) presented a case in which the aorta, the vena cava, and a ureter were displaced. The mass was hypovascular and angiography showed no major vessels suggesting malignancy; however, capillary vessels branched abnormally.

Lipomas

Pure intrarenal lipomas have an even lower incidence than leiomyomas. Xipell (1) found them in 0.8% of thoroughly examined kidneys, coinciding with the 1% incidental findings at autopsies reported by Robertson and Hand (30) in 1941. These authors suggested that lipomas could originate other than by possible rests of embryonal fat or fatty metaplasia of perivascular or mesenchymal interstitial tissue. They hypothesized that peripelvic embryonal fatty tissue can be carried into the cortex of the kidney by the collecting tubules which extend up toward the capsule to unite with the convoluted tubules. Whatever their origin, they must certainly be distinguished from so-called fibrolipomatosis, a secondary process usually associated with parenchymal destruction. Radiographically, lipomas appear as well defined, radiolucent masses which, once again, are hypovascular or even avascular on angiographic study (7). CT is the examination of choice, since the Hounsfield unit of fatty tissue varies significantly from those of a renal cell carcinoma or other benign mesenchymal tumors. Diagnosis becomes difficult as soon as other mesenchymal components are part of the mass, such as in a lipofibroma.

A special form of lipoma, although extremely rare, is the *myelolipoma*, consisting of mature adipose tissue with several islands of hematopoietic cells. It occurs more frequently in the adrenals than elsewhere in the retroperitoneal space. The presence of myeloid tissue is not well understood; is it a lipoma with ectopic hematopoietic islands, or does the whole tumor derive from ectopic bone marrow (which has a high amount of lipid-containing cells)? This question was raised earlier (31) but has not yet been answered. No correlation with blood dyscrasia seems to exist in myelolipomas of the adrenals (32).

Mixed Mesenchymal Nodules

This term can be interpreted in two ways. It expresses the combination of two of the above mentioned benign tumors, e.g., a fibrolipoma or a myolipoma, or, if the neoplasm contains myxoid structures, a fibromyxoma or a myxolipoma. Mixed mesenchymal nodules can also include combinations of the above mentioned tumors with angiomatous parts, the so-called angiomyolipomas or hamartomas (see Chapter 21).

MALIGNANT MESENCHYMAL AND CAPSULAR TUMORS (TABLE 19.1)

Sarcomas of the kidney are rare. Farrow et al (33) found 26 cases of primary renal sarcoma in 2386 examined renal malignancies at the Mayo Clinic, and Saitoh and colleagues (34) found 19 sarcomas in 2651 kidney tumors, an incidence of approximately 1%. These proportions may vary according to time and some subjective preferences of the pathologists. During the last century, sarcoma was the predominant diagnosis for most kidney tumors. Even today with more sophisticated diagnostic equipment, it is not always easy to establish the line of separation between an anaplastic carcinoma which may have areas with sarcoma-like structures and "true" sarcomas, or within the different groups of sarcomas, since all variations in these neoplasias occur. Furthermore, it is not always clear whether a mesenchymal tumor can still be considered benign or potentially invasive. Thirteen of 30 cases classified as benign angiolipoma by Price and Mostofi (35) were previously considered malignant by the referring pathologists. These inevitable differences in individual evaluations when attributing a given tumor to one or another diagnostic group are most likely the main reasons for seemingly important differences in reported survival or cure rates for certain rare sarcomas.

Leiomyosarcomas are the most common histologic subgroup, comprising 50 to 60% of the sarcomas. Nevertheless, their absolute number is still small. Niceta et al (36) reviewed the literature in 1974 and noted 66 cases published worldwide. The highest incidence was found in women in the fourth to sixth decades of life. Leiomyomas are followed by the liposarcomas, rhabdomyosarcomas, fibrosarcomas, and hemangiopericytomas, each accounting for 5 to 20% of all sarcomas according to the various reported series (33, 34, 37–42). They occur predominantly at the same age as the leiomyosarcomas. Even rarer are reported cases of osteogenic sarcoma (37), malignant schwannoma (33), or primary malignant histiocytoma/fibroxanthoma (38, 43).

The origin of many, if not most of the sarcomas, probably except for some deriving from vascular structures, must be attributed to the renal capsule, the perirenal or peripelvic tissue (44). Half of the leiomyomas and hemangiopericytomas as well as all five liposarcomas reported by Farrow and colleagues (33) were intimately attached to the renal capsule with compression but no invasion of the renal parenchyma.

Symptoms of renal sarcomas, as in the benign mesenchymal tumors, are the same as observed in renal cell carcinoma: flank mass, pain, hematuria, together with nonspecific signs of fatigue, malaise, and weight loss (33, 39). Hemangiopericytomas (the malignant form of juxtaglomerular cell tumors) rarely maintain their potential for secreting renin. One case was reported by Robertson et al (45). Two patients presented with hypoglycemia that was relieved after removing the hemangiopericytoma, but in one case, it reappeared after development of a local recurrence (33, 46). This was also observed in extrarenal hemangiopericytomas (47), and in one woman additional signs of masculinization disappeared after removal of the retroperitoneal pelvic mass (48).

Radiologic studies do not provide sufficient discernible characteristics between sarcomas and other renal tumors. Frequently large, the masses may displace the kidney and can cause hydronephrosis on the IVP; sometimes they present with calcifications (especially the leiomyosarcoma and osteogenic sarcoma). In contrast to the renal cell carcinoma, angiography chiefly reveals sparse, stretched tumor vessels supplied by capsular arteries. Zones of avascularity are frequent owing to necrosis and hemorrhage in the sarcomas (7). Arteriovenous shunting, pooling, and tumor staining are rare (41). Because of their dense, irregularly branching, capillary-like vessels, hemangiopericytomas usually show increased vascularity. According to Angervall and co-workers (49), who studied the angiographic findings in hemangiopericytomas mainly of the limb, many irregular tumor vessels of varying caliber are found. The tumor vessels can be so abundant that a diffuse opacification of the tumor area takes place, making it impossible to distinguish one capillary from another. However, despite the high vascularity, early filling of veins (pointing to arteriovenous shunting) was not observed.

Surgery has been the treatment of choice, despite the poor prognosis. Beside local recurrences, early metastases are found in lymph nodes, liver, and lung (33, 34, 44). Adjuvant conventional radiation therapy alone was not reported to improve the results of surgery. This seems to be valid also for better vascularized tumors, such as the hemangiopericytomas (47). However, adjuvant chemotherapy may be beneficial; Beccia et al (50) reported one, and Helmbrecht and Cosgrove (51) reported two patients (combined with radiation therapy) successfully treated with surgery and chemotherapy. A patient of deKernion's (52) with poorly differentiated and unresectable sarcoma received intra-arterial doxorubicin and radiation therapy. The residual fibrous mass was subsequently excised, and the patient was free of disease 2 years after surgery. Although these few cases of adjuvant chemotherapy have not yet proven that this procedure is of definitive value in renal sarcomas, and since the number of sarcomas is limited, a controlled study to answer this question is unlikely to be performed. Nevertheless, the limited experiences reported suggest that surgery with adjuvant chemotherapy, eventually combined with radiation, may be a reasonable curative approach.

REFERENCES

1. Xipell JM: The incidence of benign renal nodules (a clinicopathological study). *J Urol* 106:503, 1971.
2. Coulson WF: *Surgical Pathology.* Philadelphia, JB Lippincott, 1978, vol 1, p 493.
3. Lerman RJ, Pitcock JA, Stephenson P, Murihead EE: Renomedullary interstitial cell tumor (formerly fibroma of renal medulla). *Hum Pathol* 3:559–568, 1972.
4. Prezyna A: The renomedullar body. A newly recognized structure of renomedullary interstitial cell origin associated with high prostaglandin content. *Prostaglandins* 3:669–678, 1973.
5. Glover SD, Buck AC: Renal medullary fibroma. A case report. *J Urol* 127:758, 1982.
6. Polga JP: Renal medullary fibroma presenting as a calcified mass with neovascularity. *J Urol* 116:105, 1976.
7. Elkin M: *Radiology of the Urinary System.* Boston, Little, Brown, and Co, 1980, pp 337–338.
8. Peterson NE, Thompson HT: Renal hemangioma. *J Urol* 105:27, 1971.
9. White EW, Braunstein LE: Cavernous hemangioma: a renal vascular tumor requiring nephrectomy, an unusual entity. *J Urol* 56:183, 1946.
10. Hamm FC: Angioma of the kidney. *J Urol* 55:143, 1946.
11. Samellas W, Morphis LG, Bakopoulos CV: Hemangioma of the kidney. *J Urol* 116:653, 1976.
12. Rives HF, Pool TL: Hemangioma of the kidney. *JAMA* 125:1187, 1944.
13. Feczko PJ: Renal hemangioma: a cause of massive hematuria. *Urology* 13:447, 1979.
14. Edward HE, DeWeerd JH, Woolner LB: Renal hemangiomas. *Mayo Clin Proc* 37:545, 1962.
15. Jonsson K: Renal angiography in patients with hematuria. *AJR* 116:758, 1972.
16. Ney C, Friedenberg RM: *Radiographic Atlas of the Genitourinary System,* ed 2. Philadelphia, JB Lippincott, 1981, p 595.
17. Squires JP, Ulbright TM, deSchryver-Kecskemeti K, Engleman W: Juxtaglomerular cell tumor of the kidney. *Cancer* 53:516, 1984.
18. Biava CG, West M: Fine structure of normal human juxtaglomerular cells: specific and nonspecific cytoplasmic granules. *Pathology* 49:955, 1966.
19. Barajas L, Bennet CM, Connor G, Lindstrom RR: Structure of a juxtaglomerular cell tumor: the presence of a neural component. A light and electron microscopic study. *Lab Invest* 37:357, 1977.
20. Barajas L: The innervation of the juxtaglomerular apparatus. An electron microscopic study of the innervation of the glomerular arterioles. *Lab Invest* 13:916, 1964.
21. Bonnin JM, Cain MD, Jose JS, Mukherjee TM, Perret LV, Scroop GC, Seymour AE: Hypertension due to a renin-secreting tumour localized by segmental renal vein sampling. *Aust NZ J Med* 7:630, 1977.
22. Joost J, Schaefer R, Altwein JE: Renal lymphangioma. *J Urol* 118:22, 1977.
23. Foster DG: Large benign renal tumors: a review of the literature and report of a case in childhood. *J Urol* 76:231, 1956.
24. Clinton-Thomas CL: A giant leiomyoma of kidney. *Br J Surg* 43:497, 1956.
25. Palmer FJ, Tynan AP: Leiomyoma of the kidney. *J Urol* 112:22, 1974.
26. Summers JL: Leiomyoma in an atrophic kidney. *J. Urol* 125:414, 1981.
27. Fishbone G, Davidson AJ: Leiomyoma of the renal capsule. *Radiology* 92:1006, 1969.
28. Crabtree EG: Leiomyoma of the kidney associated with hemorrhagic cyst. *J Urol* 52:480, 1944.
29. Petkovick S: Myomatous tumours of kidney. *Urol Cutan Rev* 55:730, 1951.
30. Robertson TD, Hand JR: Primary intrarenal lipoma of surgical significance. *J Urol* 46:458, 1941.
31. Dodge OG, Evans DMD: Haemopoiesis in a presacral fatty tumor (myelolipoma). *J Pathol Bacteriol* 72:313, 1956.

32. Plaut A: Myelolipoma in the adrenal cortex (myeloadipose structures). *Am J Pathol* 34:487, 1958.
33. Farrow GW, Harrison EG Jr, Utz DG, ReMine WH: Sarcomas and sarcomatoid and mixed malignant tumors of the kidney in adults, parts 1–3. *Cancer* 22:545, 1968.
34. Saitoh H, Shimbo T, Wakabayashi T, Takeda M, Ogishima K: Metastases of renal sarcoma. *Tokai J Exp Clin Med* 7:356, 1982.
35. Price EB Jr, Mostofi FK: Symptomatic angiomyolipoma of the kidney. *Cancer* 18:761, 1965.
36. Niceta T, Lavengood RW Jr, Fernandez M, Tozzo PJ: Leiomyosarcoma of the kidney: review of the literature. *Urology* 3:270, 1974.
37. Biggers R, Stewart J: Primary renal osteosarcoma. *Urology* 13:674, 1979.
38. Chen KTK: Fibroxanthosarcoma of the kidney. *Urology* 13:439, 1979.
39. Busuttil A, More IAR: Two malignant soft tissue tumors of the kidney: an ultrastructural appraisal. *J Urol* 112:24, 1974.
40. Cano JY, d'Altorio RA: Renal liposarcoma: case report. *J Urol* 11:747, 1976.
41. Grammayeh M, Wallace S, Barrett AF: Sarcoma of the kidney; angiographic features. *AJR* 129:107, 1977.
42. Ordonez NG, Bracken RB, Stroehlein KB: Hemangioperizytoma of kidney. *Urology* 20:191, 1982.
43. Klugo RC, Farah RN, Cerny JC: Renal malignant histiocytoma. *J Urol* 112:727, 1974.
44. Gupta OP, Dube MK: Rare primary renal sarcoma. *Br J Urol* 43:546, 1971.
45. Robertson PW, Klidjian A, Harding LK, Walters G: Hypertension due to a renin secreting renal tumor. *Am J Med* 43:963, 1967.
46. Simon R, Green RC: Perirenal hemangioperiocytoma. A case associated with hypoglycemia. *JAMA* 189:181, 1984.
47. Backwinkel KD, Diddams JA: Hemangiopericytoma. Report of a case and comprehensive review of the literature. *Cancer* 25:896, 1970.
48. Howard JW, Davis PL: Retroperitoneal hemangiopericytoma associated with hypoglycemia and masculinisation. *Del State Med J* 31:29, 1959.
49. Angervall L, Kindblom LG, Nielsen JM, Stener B, Svendsen P: Hemangiopericytoma. A clinicopathologic, angiographic and microangiographic study. *Cancer* 42:2412, 1978.
50. Beccia DJ, Elkurt RJ, Rane RJ: Adjuvant chemotherapy in renal leiomyosarcoma. *Urology* 13:652, 1979.
51. Helmbracht LJ, Cosgrove MD: Triple therapy for leiomyosarcoma of the kidney. *J Urol* 112:581, 1974.
52. deKernion JB: Renal tumors. In Walsh PC, Gittes RF, Perlmutter AD, Stamey TA (eds): *Campbell's Urology*, ed 5. Philadelphia, WB Saunders, 1986, p 1294.

20

Renal Oncocytoma

Michael M. Lieber, M.D.
Taiji Tsukamoto, M.D.

INTRODUCTION

The identification of a new or previously overlooked clinicopathologic diagnosis such as "renal oncocytoma" is an exciting occurrence in any medical specialty. The very idea that there is a relatively common diagnostic entity (contained in essentially all medium or large series of tumors previously classified as renal cell carcinoma) overlooked by generations of urologists and pathologists is intriguing from all sorts of viewpoints. Moreover, the seminal, key observation and start of the renal oncocytoma era can be exactly dated to the publication of Klein and Valensi in 1976 (1). The extent of the semirevolutionary change in understanding of this diagnosis since then is simply attested by the numbers: Prior to 1975 there had only been six individual case reports of renal oncocytoma (2–6). Now there are well over 200 individual cases already published and, of course, hundreds of other recognized cases not published. Indeed, if there are approximately 14,000 new cases of renal cell carcinoma in the United States each year and slightly more than 3% of these are "really" renal oncocytomas, then one can estimate that approximately 500 new cases of renal oncocytoma may be discovered annually in the United States. So this is not such a rare "beastie." Rather, oncocytoma is just an unusual renal neoplasm which most urologists, uroradiologists, and pathologists will come upon from time to time. Consequently, a review of the published experience with this tumor seems timely and appropriate.

HISTOPATHOLOGY

"Oncocytes" by definition are large neoplastic cells with an intensely eosinophilic granular cytoplasm. "Oncocytomas" by definition are tumors composed strictly of oncocytes. Oncocytomas are not uncommon and have been identified previously in the salivary glands (7–12), thyroid (13–16), parathyroid (17–19), adrenal, and other organs and anatomic sites (20–22). Histochemical and ultrastructural studies have demonstrated that the eosinophilic granularity of oncocytes results from the packing of the cytoplasm of the oncocyte with mitochondria. The exact cell type or tissue origin that gives rise to an oncocytoma in the kidney or in these other organs is unknown (23).

Many renal cell carcinomas which behave as aggressive cancers contain eosinophilic granular cells either alone or in combination with "clear cell" neoplastic cell elements. Eosinophilic granularity of such cancer cells is also due to packing of their cytoplasm with numerous mitochondria. Renal cell carcinomas made up of granular cells are not oncocytomas. Rather, the term "renal oncocytoma" has come, by general usage, to apply to a renal neoplasm made up only of a pure population of the very best differentiated eosinophilic granular cells or oncocytes (1, 24). Since renal tumors which are composed strictly of well differentiated oncocytes behave in a benign fashion, this nosologic differentiation appears to be a useful point. But malignant-behaving renal neoplasms can have "oncocytic features," and this subtle distinction is quite important for the pathologist and urologist to bear in mind. The typical microscopic appearance of renal oncocytoma is illustrated in Figure 20.1.

GROSS MORPHOLOGY

Oncocytomas occurring in the kidney often have a typical macroscopic appearance which differs markedly from the typical gross appearance of most renal cell carcinomas (1, 24) (Fig. 20.2). Renal oncocytomas are generally well encapsulated with a well defined fibrous capsule, and the tumor tissue rarely penetrates the renal capsule or invades other local structures. The renal pelvis, the intrarenal collecting

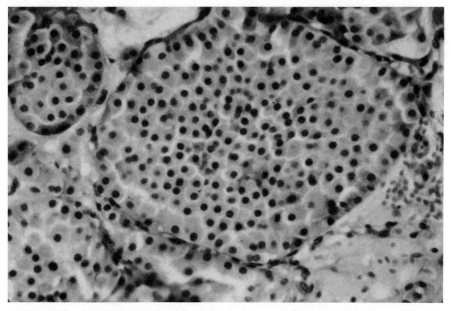

Figure 20.1. Typical histology of renal oncocytoma. The tumor is made up of a pure population of very well differentiated cells with an intensely eosinophilic granular cytoplasm.

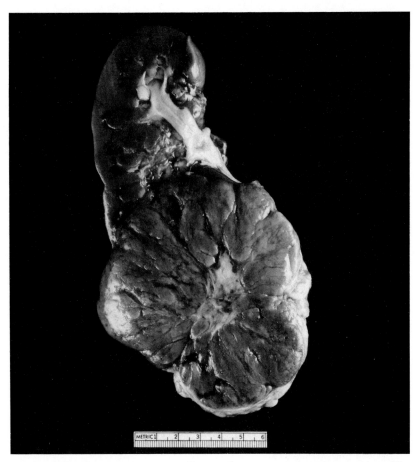

Figure 20.2. Gross appearance of a renal oncocytoma on cut section. The large central stellate scar is obvious. The lobular tumor tissue shows no evidence of hemorrhage or necrosis, and the cut surface of the tumor is brown in color.

system, and perinephric fat generally are not invaded. Even when such tumors grow fairly large, the adjacent normal renal parenchyma can be quite intact. On cut section, small renal oncocytomas generally have a homogeneous appearance with no hemorrhage or necrosis within the tumor. The cut surface of the tumor is usually dark brown or mahogany in color; this contrasts sharply with the gross appearance on cut section of a typical renal cell carcinoma, which often shows yellowish tumor tissue with hemorrhage and necrosis. Large oncocytomas commonly show a prominent stellate central scar which gives them an almost pathognomonic gross appearance. The central scar in a large renal oncocytoma is often obvious as well by computed tomographic (CT) examination of such a tumor or on ultrasound exam and can serve further to suggest the diagnosis preoperatively.

INCIDENCE OF RENAL ONCOCYTOMA

Through mid-1984, there have been 11 separate reports in which renal cell carcinoma specimens, solid renal tumor specimens, or radical nephrectomy specimens in a given institution have been reviewed to search for cases typical of renal oncocytoma (1, 24–33). These series are presented in Table 20.1. Of a total of 4304 renal tumor samples reviewed in these collected series, 149 instances of typical renal oncocytoma were identified. This suggests an incidence of approximately 3.4% for renal oncocytoma among tumors previously classified generally as renal cell carcinomas, but sometimes as renal adenomas. If the Mayo Clinic series is excluded (5), the frequency of renal oncocytoma is 87 in 1597 (5.4%).

To date, a total of 210 patients have been reported in the English literature with typical renal oncocytoma (1, 24–66) (Table 20.2). Only patients with the best differentiated renal tumors that generally fit the diagnosis of renal oncocytoma as described in the publication of Klein and Valensi have been counted here. Among these 210 patients, 196 patients were identified in clinical series and 14 patients have been identified from autopsy studies. In this total group of 210, there have been 142 male patients and 65 female patients (for 3 patients the sex was not given), for a male to female ratio of 2.2:1.

The ages of patients with renal oncocytoma vary considerably (Table 20.3). In clinical series, patients have ranged from 15 to 94 years of age; in autopsy series, patients have ranged from 57 to 93 years of age. The

Table 20.1
Series of Renal Oncocytoma Reported in the English Language[a]

Authors	No. of Renal Oncocytomas	No. of Renal Neoplasms Reviewed	Incidence of Oncocytoma (%)
Klein and Valensi (1976)	13	185[b]	6.6
Akhtar and Kott (1979)	2	49[b]	3.9
Sarkar et al (1979)	11	189[c]	5.5
Yu et al (1980)	5	102[b]	4.7
Lieber et al (1981)	62	2707[b]	2.3
Mitchell and Shilkin (1982)	6	36[c]	14.3
Merino and LiVolsi (1982)	14	249[b]	5.3
Barnes et al (1983)	7	247[b]	2.4
Choi et al (1983)	7	89[c]	7.2
Fairchild et al (1983)	11	208[d]	5.0
Maatman et al (1984)	11	243[b]	4.3
Total	149	4304	3.4

[a] Only Grade 1 tumors considered.
[b] Renal cell carcinomas.
[c] Renal adenomas and carcinomas.
[d] Radical nephrectomy specimens.

Table 20.2
Total Number of Renal Oncocytoma Patients Reported

210 Patients
$\begin{bmatrix}$ Clinical series = 196 Patients
Autopsy series = 14 Patients $\end{bmatrix}$

Male = 142 Patients
Female = 65 Patients
Unknown = 3 Patients

(Male to female ratio = 2.2:1)

Table 20.3
Age and Sex Distribution of Patients with Renal Oncocytoma

Age (Years)	Male	Female	Total
15–19	1	0	1
20–29	2	0	2
30–39	7	8	15
40–49	11	3	14
50–59	28	9	37
60–69	32	13	45
70–79	25	9	34
80–89	6	4	10
90–99	2	0	2
Total	114[a]	46[b]	160

[a] Including 5 patients with renal oncocytoma found incidentally at autopsy.
[b] Including 2 patients with renal oncocytoma found incidentally at autopsy.

median age for male patients has been 63 years, and the median age for female patients has been 62 years. These figures are slightly older than the median age for patients with typical renal cell carcinoma, which in most large series is around 55 years. Table 20.3 presents the age and sex distribution for patients with renal oncocytoma for whom this information could be recovered from the literature.

CLINICAL PRESENTATION

As pointed out originally by Klein and Valensi and subsequently confirmed by the other authors writing about renal oncocytomas, these tumors generally are not symptomatic. The majority have been discovered incidentally during the course of evaluation for some unrelated symptom or at postmortem examination. In every series reported, the majority of tumors were discovered incidentally, and in an occasional series, none of the patients with oncocytomas had any symptoms (Table 20.4). For 182 patients in the collected clinical series for which details are available, only 57 patients (31%) were symptomatic at the time of diagnosis. One hundred twenty-five of 182 patients (69%) had oncocytomas found incidentally. For 177 patients in the clinical series, the following signs and symptoms were reported (Table 20.5): gross hematuria, 12%; abdominal or flank pain, 17%; abdominal or flank mass, 19%; microscopic hematuria, 23%. The low incidence of signs and symptoms mirrors the benign local growth behavior of renal oncocytomas and the fact that these tumors do not metastasize. Since the tumors rarely invade the collecting system or renal pelvis, gross hematuria is unusual. Therefore, the most common presenting sign/symptom, an abdominal or flank mass, reflects the large size which many renal oncocytomas attain before being detected.

Techniques for radiologically imaging the kidneys and the retroperitoneum have improved dramatically in the past decade. The widespread availability of high quality excretory urography with nephrotomography and the frequent application of CT scanning of the abdomen now frequently turn up previously asymptomatic renal mass lesions. Because of these improved scanning techniques, it seems likely that many more

Table 20.4
Patient's Status at Presentation: Oncocytoma Symptomatic or Incidentally Found (182 Patients in Clinical Series[a])

Patient's Status	No. of Patients
Symptomatic	57 (31%)
Tumor incidentally found	125 (69%)
Total	182[a] (100%)

[a] Fourteen patients without details are excluded.

Table 20.5
Major Symptoms and Signs Related to Renal Oncocytoma (177 Patients in Clinical Series)

Symptoms and Signs	No. of Patients
Gross hematuria	21 (12%)
Abdominal or flank pain	30 (17%)
Abdominal or flank mass	33 (19%)
Microscopic hematuria	40 (23%)

Table 20.6
Laterality of Renal Oncocytoma

Laterality	No. of Patients	
Unilateral	185	(94%)
Right	83	
Left	79	
Not stated	23	
Bilateral	11	(6%)
Total	196	(100%)

oncocytomas will be discovered in the future and at a smaller size than has occurred previously.

MULTIFOCAL OCCURRENCE AND BILATERALITY

There is no evidence to suggest a preference for side (right or left) or site within the kidney for renal oncocytomas. For 196 cases reported, 185 (94%) of the tumors were unilateral (Table 20.6). Of this unilateral group, 83 were present in the right kidney, 79 were in the left kidney, and in 23 cases the side was not identified. Eleven of 196 (6% of the patients) had bilateral tumors. Both bilateral renal oncocytomas (synchronous or asynchronous) and bilateral tumors with a renal oncocytoma on one side and typical renal cell carcinoma on the other side also have been reported.

Multifocal renal oncocytomas occurring in multiple locations within one kidney also have been described. The term "oncocytomatosis" has been applied to this entity (59). Multiple oncocytomas in one kidney have been reported in 10 patients (28, 30, 32, 33, 53, 54, 56, 64, 65). In 11 patients with bilateral renal oncocytoma, 5 patients had a solitary oncocytoma in each kidney, 3 patients had a solitary oncocytoma on one side and multiple oncocytomas on the other, and 3 patients had multiple oncocytomas in both kidneys (Table 20.7). Thus, although

Table 20.7
Number of Tumors in Renal Oncocytoma Patients

Oncocytomas	No. of Patients
Unilateral renal oncocytomas	182
Solitary oncocytoma	172 (90%)
Multiple oncocytomas	10 (5%)
Bilateral renal oncocytoma	11
Solitary oncocytoma in both kidneys	5 (3%)
Solitary oncocytoma in one kidney and multiple in other	3 (1%)
Multiple oncocytomas in both kidneys	3 (1%)
Total	193

Table 20.8
Size of Renal Oncocytomas in Clinical and Autopsy Series

Size[a] (cm)	Clinical Series	Autopsy Series	Total
<1	3		3
1	6	5	11
2	10	2	12
3	18	1	19
4	17	1	18
5	20	1	21
6	22	1	23
7	14	1	15
8	12		12
9	8		8
10	10	1	11
11	5		5
12	2		2
13	3		3
14	4		4
15	4		4
16	2		2
20	1		1
23	1		1
	162 tumors in 146 patients	13 tumors in 9 patients	175 tumors in 155 patients

[a] In patients with numerous oncocytomas (oncocytomatosis), the size of largest tumor is selected.

solitary unilateral renal oncocytomas make up 90% of reported cases, multiple and bilateral tumors occur in various combinations, so that this possibility, which could markedly influence treatment options, should always be borne in mind when approaching an individual case from the clinical or pathologic point of view.

TUMOR SIZE

The size of renal oncocytomas in clinical and autopsy series is reported in Table 20.8. Tumors found in autopsy series have been fairly small. For 13 tumors identified in 9 patients, the median size was 2 cm. But for 162 tumors reported in 146 clinical patients, the median size was 6 cm. Thus, as can be seen from reviewing the table, half the tumors were larger than 6 cm in size and a number were larger than 10 cm in diameter. So oncocytomas are not generally inconsequential renal masses.

RADIOLOGIC FINDINGS

The majority of renal oncocytomas have been discovered because an excretory urogram or CT scan of the abdomen was performed for some unrelated reason. On excretory urography, ultrasound examination, and CT scanning, most oncocytomas simply have the typical appearance of a solid renal mass lesion. Sometimes for larger tumors, the prominent central stellate scar region is imaged and can suggest the diagnosis of a large oncocytoma. However, a similar, nonhomogeneous internal appearance can result from central hemorrhage or necrosis in a renal cell carcinoma. To date, angiography has been the test which has traditionally suggested the presence of renal oncocytoma preoperatively. Ambos and colleagues (38) presented the most extensive angiographic study of renal oncocytomas published to date. They described four typical angiographic signs that suggested the presence of a renal oncocytoma: (a) the "lucent rim sign," (b) a homogeneous capillary nephrogram phase, (c) the absence of clearly wild neoplastic vessels, and (d) the spoke-wheeled appearance of the feeding arteries.

The authors collected 42 cases from the literature in which details of angiographic findings were reported (Table 20.9). In this collected group of 42 cases, 31 (74%) of the patients showed a sharp and smooth margin, often with a lucent rim sign, 21 (50%) showed the spoke-wheel vascular pattern, and 13 (31%) showed the homogeneous nephrogram. Atypical angiographic features included an avascular or hypovascular pattern seen in 7 patients (17%), microaneurysms in 3 patients (7%), and marked arteriovenous shunting in 1 patient (66). In 14 cases of oncocytoma seen at the Mayo Clinic in which angiography was performed, CM Johnson (Department of Diagnostic Radiology) reviewed the angiograms. He thought that one-half of the tumors had a typical appearance, suggesting the possibility of an oncocytoma. The other seven tumors had either a hypovascular appearance or had an angiographic pattern that could not be reliably differentiated from a standard renal cell carcinoma.

Table 20.9
Typical or Atypical Major Angiographic Features (for 42 Cases with Details of Angiography)

Findings	No. of Patients
Typical features	
"Spoke-wheel" vascular pattern	21 (50%)
Homogeneous nephrogram	13 (31%)
Sharp and smooth margin (often with "lucent" rim)	31 (74%)
Atypical features	
Avascular or hypovascular pattern	7 (17%)
Microaneurysms	3 (7%)
Arteriovenous shunting	1 (2%)

Thus, at present, there is no preoperative radiologic imaging test which can be used "to make" the preoperative diagnosis of a renal oncocytoma. Attempts to find a radiopharmaceutical agent which would be selectively taken up into oncocytes have been made and are still being pursued (53), but none has been proven as yet. This creates quite a dilemma for the urologic practitioner, since among 100 cases of solid mass lesions identified by ultrasound or CT scanning, 3 to 5 probably will be renal oncocytomas.

TREATMENT

Until the present, nearly all renal oncocytomas were considered to be renal cell carcinomas preoperatively and most patients were treated by radical nephrectomy (Table 20.10). Thus, in the experience reported in the literature, for 162 patients with unilateral renal oncocytoma described, 151 were treated by nephrectomy. Only 2 patients are described who were treated by a partial or heminephrectomy, and 3 patients were treated by "tumor excision." On first review, it is difficult to take issue with the radical nephrectomy approach since renal oncocytomas behave as benign neoplasms (vide infra) and total surgical excision by total nephrectomy has been and is almost certain to be curative.

Nevertheless, with improving diagnostic tools, such as CT scanning, many renal oncocytomas are now being discovered at a small size in a renal location such as in the upper or lower pole or far laterally, where a substantial fraction of the kidney could be saved, even if the renal oncocytoma were totally excised with a margin of normal renal parenchyma. This presents a new and challenging problem for urologists since most likely, in good conscience, one can no longer simply remove every kidney with a solid mass lesion in it. This issue is discussed below under "Diagnostic and Therapeutic Strategy."

The treatment for bilateral renal oncocytoma is more of a surgical challenge, and a number of different approaches have been used. Four

Table 20.10
Treatment for 171 Patients with Renal Oncocytoma

Treatment	No. of Patients
Treatment for unilateral renal oncocytoma	162
Radical or simple nephrectomy	151
Partial or heminephrectomy	2
Tumor excision	3
"Surgical removal"	5
None	1
Treatments for bilateral renal oncocytoma	9
Radical nephrectomy—bench excision of tumor— autotransplantation; tumor excision (in situ)	1
Radical nephrectomy—bench excision of tumor— autotransplantation; radical nephrectomy— bench excision of tumor—autotransplantation	1
Nephrectomy; partial nephrectomy	3
None	4
Total	171

patients with bilateral renal oncocytoma have received no treatment at all other than biopsy and follow-up. Three patients have been treated by nephrectomy on one side and partial nephrectomy on the other, and other patients have been treated by nephrectomy on one side, and bench excision of tumor and autotransplantation on the other side. A number of patients with multifocal oncocytomas in a solitary kidney have had these tumors simply enucleated (67).

PROGNOSIS

For 196 clinical patients with renal oncocytoma who are reported in the literature, 133 (68%) are alive without tumor recurrence (Table 20.11). Twenty-eight patients (14%) have died of causes unrelated to the oncocytoma, 3 patients have been lost to follow-up, and in 32 cases, details of the clinical course of patients were not included in the report. To the authors' knowledge, there have been no instances reported in which metastases, local or distant, have been associated with a typical, well differentiated, "grade 1" renal oncocytoma in the now numerous series reviewed herein. Also to the authors' knowledge, there have been no cancer-related deaths associated with a typical renal oncocytoma. Indeed, for the 62 patients with typical renal oncocytomas (grade 1 tumors) in the Mayo Clinic series, the actuarial survival curve for the tumor-bearing patients was slightly better than for an age- and sex-matched control group (24). Thus, by their local behavior within the kidney, by their local invasiveness into other organs (which does not occur), by the absence of nodal metastases or spread to distant organs, and by the fact that they are not a cause of death, typical renal oncocytomas behave like benign rather than malignant tumors.

Once again, it is important to emphasize that other "oncocytic" renal tumors do occur in the kidney and that such higher grade oncocytic (or granular cell) renal tumors or oncocytic tumors which are mixed with clear cell elements or spindle cell elements do behave as malignant neoplasms, do metastasize, and do cause cancer deaths (24, 30). Not every granular cell renal neoplasm is a renal oncocytoma. This term should be reserved exclusively for the best differentiated members of this class.

Since no deaths or metastatic behavior have been reported in the world's literature for patients with "grade 1" renal oncocytomas, it certainly does appear reasonable to separate renal oncocytomas from

Table 20.11
Clinical Courses of Patients with Renal Oncocytoma

Clinical Course	No. of Patients
Patients alive without recurrence	133 (68%)
Patients dead of unrelated causes	28[a] (14%)
Patients lost to follow-up	3 (2%)
Patients without details of clinical courses in reports	32 (16%)
Total	196 (100%)

[a] Including one patient with unknown cause of death.

the diagnostic category of renal cell carcinomas since oncocytomas do not behave like carcinomas. The terms "oxyphilic adenoma" or "proximal tubular adenoma with oncocytic features" have been suggested (1) as more appropriate than renal oncocytoma. But it seems unlikely that the commonly used and traditional term oncocytoma will be displaced at this late date.

And, as commented upon before, if 3 to 5% of cases previously classified as renal cell carcinoma are really oncocytomas, we are doing less well in treating true renal cancer than had been thought.

DIAGNOSTIC AND THERAPEUTIC STRATEGY

Large renal mass lesions which are diagnosed in the presence of an anatomically and functionally normal contralateral kidney should not present much of a diagnostic or therapeutic dilemma. Renal oncocytomas are new growths and probably will continue to grow unless they are surgically excised. If such a surgical excision cannot be safely performed with the salvage of a significant renal fraction, then removal of the tumor and the kidney is obviously a straightforward approach. For this reason, the diagnosis of a 6- or 8-cm solid renal mass lesion occurring in the hilum of the kidney with a normal kidney on the other side, with typical features of an oncocytoma by CT scan or angiographic appearance, should not provoke extensive head scratching.

But a more difficult diagnostic and therapeutic situation is occasioned by the more common setting in which a small—for example, 3- or 4-cm—renal mass lesion is found incidentally on either the upper or lower pole of the kidney when CT scanning is performed for some other unrelated problem. A substantial fraction of such small, incidentally discovered tumors will be oncocytomas that could be simply treated by total surgical excision. Such a tumor could probably be well treated by straightforward guillotine type partial nephrectomy. An additional approach for a tumor which appeared likely to be a resectable oncocytoma would be to perform intraoperative frozen section biopsies. Tumors examined by biopsy which proved to be typical, very well differentiated oncocytomas could be treated by enucleation just outside the tumor capsule or by quite limited partial nephrectomy. For a solid renal mass lesion discovered by excretory urography, ultrasound, or CT scanning in a very poor risk or elderly patient, fine needle aspiration could be performed with the fairly confident assumption that a skillful cytologist could identify typical oncocytes so that the poor risk patient might be spared surgical exploration.

All of this throws a real monkey wrench into the previously straightforward algorithms for treating patients with solid renal mass lesions by a technically straightforward radical nephrectomy. But there is no reason to think that a young patient, with or without a normal contralateral kidney, should need a radical nephrectomy as proper treatment for a 2-, 3-, or 4-cm suitably located renal oncocytoma. Until the day arrives when new diagnostic methods will allow the confident preoperative diagnosis of an oncocytoma and its clear differentiation from renal cell carcinoma, urologic surgeons will have to struggle with these difficult and unsettled and unsettling issues.

Nevertheless, even though their existence makes a urologist's professional life more difficult, renal oncocytomas do exist, they do not behave as carcinomas, and, therefore, they require a change in the previous ways of thinking and acting about solid renal mass lesions.

REFERENCES

1. Klein MJ, Valensi QJ: Proximal tubular adenomas of kidney with so-called oncocytic features: a clinicopathological study of 13 cases of a rarely reported neoplasm. *Cancer* 38:906–914, 1976.
2. Zippel L: Zur kenntnis der onkocyten. *Virchows Arch* 308:360–382, 1942.
3. Poroshin KK, Galyl-Ogly GA: Oncocytic adenomas. *Arkh Pathol* 27:43–49, 1965.
4. Wasilkowski A, Dabrowski H: Eosinophilic adenoma of the kidney (oncocytoma). *Pol Przegl Chir* 43:1051–1054, 1971.
5. Berger G, Clermont A, Pinet F, Loire R: Pluricentric oncocytoma of the kidney (microangiographic study). *Arch Anat Pathol (Paris)* 21:287–292, 1973.
6. Blessing MA, Wienert G: Onkozytom der Niere. *Zentrabl Allg Pathol Anat* 117:227–234, 1973.
7. Jaffe RH: Adenolymphoma (onkocytoma) of parotid gland. *Am J Cancer* 16:1415–1432, 1932.
8. Batsakis JG, Martz DG: Oxyphil cell tumor of submaxillary gland. *US Armed Forces Med J* 14:1383–1386, 1960.
9. Bazaz-Malik G, Gupta DN: Metastasizing (malignant) oncocytoma of the parotid gland. *Z Krebsforsch* 70:193–197, 1968.
10. Blank C, Eneroter C, Jakobssin P: Oncocytoma of the parotid gland: neoplasm or nodular hyperplasia. *Cancer* 25:919–925, 1970.
11. Sun CN, White HJ, Thompson BW: Oncocytoma (mitochondria) of the parotid gland: an electron microscopic study. *Arch Pathol* 99:208–214, 1975.
12. Gray SR, Cornog JL, Seo IS: Oncocytic neoplasms of salivary glands: a report of fifteen cases including two malignant oncocytomas. *Cancer* 38:1306–1317, 1976.
13. Chesky VE, Dreese WC, Helwig CA: Hurthle cell tumors of the thyroid gland: report of 25 cases. *J Clin Endocrinol* 11:1535–1548, 1951.
14. Frazel EL, Duffy BJ Jr: Hurthle-cell cancer of the thyroid. *Cancer* 4:952–956, 1951.
15. Horn RC: Hurthle cell tumors of the thyroid. *Cancer* 7:234–244, 1954.
16. Thompson NW, Dunn EL, Batsakis JG, Nishiyama RH: Hurthle cell lesions of the thyroid gland. *Surg Gynecol Obstet* 139:555–560, 1974.
17. Roth SI, Olen E, Hausen LS: The eosinophilic cells of the parathyroid (oxyphil cells), salivary (oncocytes), and thyroid (Hurthle cells) gland: light and electron microscopic observations. *Lab Invest* 11:933–941, 1962.
18. Tandler B, Hutter RVP, Erlandson RA: Ultrastructure of oncocytoma of the parathyroid gland. *Lab Invest* 23:567–568, 1970.
19. Arnold BM, Kovacs K, Horvath E, Murray TM, Higgins HP: Functioning oxyphil cell adenoma of the parathyroid gland: evidence for secretory activity of oxyphil cells. *J Clin Endocrinol Metab* 38:458–462, 1974.
20. Hamperl H: Oncocytomas of different organs. *Acta Union Int Cancer* 20:854, 1964.
21. Briggs J, Evans JNG: Malignant oxyphilic granular-cell tumor (oncocytoma) of the palate. *Oral Surg* 23:796–802, 1967.
22. Black WC III: Pulmonary oncocytoma. *Cancer* 23:1347–1357, 1969.
23. Tremblay G: The oncocytes. In Baqusz E, Jasmin G (eds): *Methods and Achievements in Experimental Pathology.* Basel, Karger, 1969, vol 4, pp 121–140.
24. Lieber MM, Tomera KM, Farrow GM: Renal oncocytoma. *J Urol* 125:481–485, 1981.
25. Aktar M, Kott E: Oncocytoma of kidney. *Urology* 14:397–400, 1979.
26. Sarkar K, Ejeckman GC, McCaughey WTE, Tolnai G: Oncocytic tumors of the kidney (so called "renal oncocytomas"). Abstracts, IAP Annual Meeting. *Lab Invest* 40:282, 1979.

27. Yu GSM, Rendler S, Herskowitz A, Molnar JJ: Renal oncocytoma: report of five cases and review of literature. *Cancer* 45:1010–1018, 1980.
28. Mitchell KM, Shilkin KB: Renal oncocytoma. *Pathology* 14:75–80, 1982.
29. Merino MJ, LiVolsi VA: Oncocytomas of the kidney. *Cancer* 50:1852–1856, 1982.
30. Barnes CA, Beckman EN: Renal oncocytoma and its congeners. *Am J Clin Pathol* 79:312–318, 1983.
31. Choi H, Almagro UA, McManus JT, Norback DH, Jacobs SC: Renal oncocytoma: a clinicopathological study. *Cancer* 51:1887–1896, 1983.
32. Fairchild TN, Dail DH, Brannen GE: Renal oncocytoma: bilateral, multifocal. *Urology* 22:355–359, 1983.
33. Maatman TJ, Novick AC, Tancino BF, Vesoulis Z, Levin HS, Montie JE, Montague DK: Renal oncocytoma: diagnostic and therapeutic dilemma. *J Urol* 132:878–881, 1984.
34. Sos TA, Gray G Jr, Baltaxe HA: The angiographic appearance of benign renal oxyphilic adenoma. *AJR* 127:717–722, 1976.
35. Tessler AN, Kurusu S, Klein MJ, Valensi QJ: Proximal tubular adenoma of kidney. *Urology* 10:203–206, 1977.
36. Milstoc M: Renal oncocytoma: a rare case of renal adenoma. *J Urol* 118:856–857, 1977.
37. Weiner SN, Bernstein RG: Renal oncocytoma: angiographic features of two cases. *Radiology* 125:633–635, 1977.
38. Ambos MA, Bosniak MA, Valensi QJ, Madayag MA, Lefleur SS: Angiographic patterns in renal oncocytomas. *Radiology* 129:615–622, 1978.
39. Pearse HD, Houghton DC: Renal oncocytoma. *Urology* 13:74–77, 1979.
40. Johnson JR, Thurman AE, Metter JB, Bannayan GA: Oncocytoma of kidney. *Urology* 14:181–185, 1979.
41. Ejeckman GC, Tolnai G, Sarkar K, McCaughey WTE: Renal oncocytoma: study of eight cases. *Urology* 14:186–189, 1979.
42. Chaudhry AP, Slotkin E, Satchidanand SK, Shenoy S, Gaeta JF, Nickerson PA: Light and ultrastructural studies of renal oncocytic adenoma. *Urology* 14:392–396, 1979.
43. Weedon D, Splatt AJ, Moore WE: Proximal tubular adenoma of the kidney. *Aust NZ J Surg* 49:250–252, 1979.
44. Wojtowicz J, Karwowski A, Konkiewicz J, Lukaszewski B: Case report: renal oncocytoma. *J Comput Assist Tomogr* 3:124–125, 1979.
45. Barth KH, Menon M: Renal oncocytoma: further diagnostic observations. *Diag Imag* 49:259–265, 1980.
46. Bono AV, Caresano A, Roggia A, Gianneo E: A case of renal oncocytoma. *Eur Urol* 6:247–248, 1980.
47. Kay S, Armstrong KS: Oncocytic tubular adenoma of the kidney: report of three cases with 28-year follow-up on one. In Fienoglio CM, Wolff M (eds): *Progress in Surgical Pathology*. New York, Masson Publishing, 1980, vol 2, pp 259–268.
48. Morales A, Wasan S, Bryniak S: Renal oncocytomas: clinical, radiological, and histological features. *J Urol* 123:261–264, 1980.
49. Kendall AR, Pollack HM, Petersen RO, Stein BS: Incidentally found renal mass. *J Urol* 124:269–273, 1980.
50. Bokinsky GB: Renal oncocytoma. *Urology* 17:364–366, 1981.
51. Bonavita JA, Pollack HM, Banner MP: Renal oncocytoma: further observations and literature review. *Urol Radiol* 2:229–234, 1981.
52. Harrison RH, Baird JM, Kowierschke SW: Renal oncocytoma: ten-year follow-up. *Urology* 17:596–599, 1981.
53. Lautin EM, Gordon PM, Friedman AC, McCormick JF, Fromowitz FB, Goldman MJ, Sugarman LA: Radionuclide imaging and computed tomography in renal oncocytoma. *Radiology* 138:185–190, 1981.
54. Rodriguez CA, Buskop A, Johnson J, Fromowitz F, Loss LG: Renal oncocytoma: preoperative diagnosis by aspiration biopsy. *Acta Cytol* 24:355–359, 1980.
55. Susman BR, Levin FA, Barland P, Fromowitz F: Vasculitis associated with renal oncocytoma. *NY State J Med* 81:1501–1503, 1981.
56. Woodward BH, Tannenbaum SI, Mossler JA: Multicentric renal oncocytoma. *J Urol* 126:247–248, 1981.

57. Moshman SE, Fromowitz FB, Lautin EM, Gendelman HE: Renal oncocytoma. *NY State J Med* 82:1471–1473, 1982.
58. Moura ACF, Nascimento AG: Renal oncocytoma: report of a case with unusual presentation. *J Urol* 127:311–313, 1982.
59. Warfel KA, Eble JN: Renal oncocytomatosis. *J Urol* 127:1179–1180, 1982.
60. Slasky BS, Bron KM: Aneurysms in renal oncocytoma. *Urology* 20:552–554, 1982.
61. Hara M, Yoshida K, Tomita M, Akimoto M, Kawai M, Fukuda Y: A case of bilateral renal oncocytoma. *J Urol* 128:576–578, 1982.
62. Shah I, Parekh N, Nakah PK, Taher S: Renal oncocytoma associated with diffuse lymphoma. *Urology* 22:314–317, 1983.
63. Hunt HA, Tudball CF, Sutherland RC, Westmore DD: Bilateral renal oncocytomas: a case report. *J Urol* 129:1220–1221, 1983.
64. Chen KTK: Multiple renal oncocytoma. *J Urol* 130:546–547, 1983.
65. van der Walt JD, Reid HAS, Risdon A, Shaw JHF: Renal oncocytoma: a review of the literature and report of an unusual multicentric case. *Virchows Arch* 398:291–304, 1983.
66. Raspa RW, Fernandes M, Ward JN: Bilateral renal oncocytoma: report of 2 cases and review of literature. *J Urol* 133:458–461, 1985.
67. Lieber MM: Renal oncocytoma. In Javadopour N (ed): *Cancer of the Kidney*. New York, Theime Stratton, 1984, pp 154–165.

21

Angiomyolipoma

Grant Williams, M.S., F.R.C.S.

The fact that angiomyolipoma is composed of mature components (blood vessels, muscle, and fat) in an abnormal pattern has led to various semantic arguments. It is usually regarded as a hamartoma, and, because it presents as abnormal swellings in the kidney or other tissues, its histogenic nature qualifies it to be regarded as a mesenchymal tumor. No true cases of metastases have been recorded.

It is surprising that, although this condition was described by Bourneville (1) over 100 years ago, episodic publications concerning it regularly appear. By 1965, Vasco et al (2) had collected 150 such cases, and 3 years later Farrow et al (3) had added a further 32 cases from the records of the Mayo Clinic.

INCIDENCE

Autopsy studies have implied its rarity. Small asymptomatic nodules were found to be angiomyolipoma in 0.07% of 4309 autopsies by Apitz (4), and these chance findings are occasionally seen in related living donors of a kidney for transplantation (G Williams, personal observation).

The association of angiomyolipoma with the tuberous sclerosis complex is well known; it is estimated to occur in up to 80% of cases of tuberous sclerosis. Moolten's (5) classical description has not been bettered, and it confirmed the earlier neurologic literature (6). The heredofamilial nature of angiomyolipoma in tuberous sclerosis is probably a manifestation of that same genetic defect, in that patients usually have other hamartomata, and even other renal hamartomata. However, the patient presenting only with a single angiomyolipoma and no other hamartomata does not appear to share the same genetic defect.

It has been stated that angiomyolipoma did not appear in colored races (7). However, it was more likely that cases of angiomyolipoma had simply not been noticed in colored races, and Udekwu (8) reported two cases in colored patients. Recently, Takashi et al (9) reported on 194 cases in the Japanese literature; whether this included the 147 cases reported the previous year by Noguchi et al (10) is not clear, but there is probably no particular racial preponderance.

Nothing is known about the age range at presentation nor about the rate of growth of the tumor. As the condition is a hamartoma, it is not surprising that it occurs in childhood (11).

ASSOCIATED CONDITIONS

The association with tuberous sclerosis (5) has been recorded in multiple publications. Moolten also pointed out the occasional association of angiomyolipoma with von Recklinghausen's neurofibromatosis and with von Hippel-Lindau disease. Systemic angiomatosis of the von Hippel-Lindau type is known to be associated with renal adenoma or renal adenocarcinoma, so this presumably explains the occasional report of angiomyolipoma with renal adenocarcinoma. Takeyama et al (12) could find only four previous reports of coincident renal cell carcinoma and angiomyolipoma and added a further case, occurring without the tuberous sclerosis complex, but there have been further reports of this association (13, 14). While this occasional association contributes little to the epidemiology of either condition, it is cause for caution when conservative therapy of angiomyolipoma is considered.

A further association with Potter type III polycystic kidneys has been noted (15), where of course Lindau's disease, with its higher incidence of renal carcinoma may also be associated (16). Fibromuscular dysplasia and the Sturge-Weber syndrome have also been reported as associated conditions (17). While there are occasional reports of polycystic kidneys with associated renal adenocarcinoma or even urothelial carcinoma, that association is probably fortuitous.

The genetic defects in adult polycystic kidney disease are caused by inheritance of an autosomal dominant gene, but this is different from the autosomal dominant gene with incomplete penetrance in Lindau's disease (18). This has been included in the general term "phakomatoses" (19), which includes tuberous sclerosis, which is also caused by a rare autosomal dominant gene with at least two modifying genes that affect phenotype expression (20). These genetic defects with their interfaces cause a high degree of suspicion of angiomyolipoma, either symptomatic or asymptomatic, in those conditions mentioned, but they do nothing to explain the etiology of angiomyolipoma when it occurs outside these conditions.

CLINICAL PRESENTATION

Classically this lesion presents as a symptom-free mass in the loin or as abdominal pain with hematuria. Of 30 patients discussed by Price and Mostofi (21), the predominant symptom was pain in the loin. This pain may be so severe that intra-abdominal hemorrhage is suspected. This may be associated with intraperitoneal hemorrhage (22), retroperitoneal hemorrhage (23), or intrarenal hemorrhage (24). Obviously the presenting symptoms vary from hypovolemic shock to hematuria, though only 8 of Price and Mostofi's 30 patients presented with hematuria.

There has been a recent report of angiomyolipoma proceeding to renal failure (25), but the European Dialysis and Transplant Association has no such situation recorded among 150,000 cases of renal failure (26). However, it is probable that many patients with tuberous sclerosis are not considered for kidney, transplantation or dialysis.

From this it may be seen that there are many erroneous views of this condition, the first being that they are rare. There were 80 publications 3 from 1982 to 1984 concerning this condition, describing at least 135 cases, with an additional 194 cases from the Japanese literature alone. The second misconception (27) is that angiomyolipoma presents with three varieties, namely (*a*) asymptomatic angiomyolipoma of the kidney associated with tuberous sclerosis, (*b*) tumors discovered incidentally at autopsy, and (*c*) symptomatic tumors not associated with tuberous sclerosis. Actually there are (*a*) asymptomatic masses, (*b*) incidental findings at autopsy, pyelography, sonography, or nephrectomy, and (*c*) symptomatic lesions which occur with or without association with tuberous sclerosis. The third error is to regard them as neoplastic. This last view is based on the observations that occasionally there may be lymph node involvement, vascular invasion, and extrarenal involvement.

Lymph Node Involvement

Lymph node involvement has been noted from early reports. Busch et al (28) pointed out that this is an example of multicentricity and that it is not metastatic. Long term survival with such lymph node involvement is commonplace, and no patient has yet been reported as dying from these "metastases." Nevertheless, this controversy continues (29). There has to date been no documented case of systemic dissemination following well documented lymph node involvement (30) where the nodes are entirely hamartomatous histologically. The previously discussed association with renal adenocarcinoma can lead to cases of nodal involvement with adenocarcinoma, as described by Schujman and associates (31). However, that does not mean that radiation therapy should be used in angiomyolipoma, as it was in 1 of Allen and Risk's (32) patients and in 3 of 30 cases reported by Price and Mostofi (21).

Vascular Invasion

This is frequently observed histologically, and the papers of Burkitt (33) and Berg (34) are usually quoted as evidence of vascular invasion. However, Burkitt reported his case as a liposarcoma with hepatic involvement, but both primary and "secondaries" contained mature elements of fat and smooth muscle in a milieu of blood vessels. Berg's patient showed "involvement" of the renal vein, but in fact died of bronchogenic carcinoma. There is no doubt that these mature elements are intimately involved with the abnormal vessels, but as with "nodal involvement," there has been no documented case of death from vascular invasion. Patients with extensive fatal renal angiomyolipoma die from hemorrhage, renal failure, or surgery, but they do not die from metastases. Reports of caval extension (35) are therefore of only academic interest unless there is a circulatory risk of "tumor" embolism.

Extrarenal Lesions

Early reports of this condition frequently used the phenomenon of extrarenal lesions as an indication of malignancy. However, if angiomyolipoma is accepted as a mixed mesenchymal lesion, then there is no particular reason why the lesions should not be noted elsewehere in the body. In addition to Burkitt's patient with liver involvement, there continue to be further reports. Goodman and Ishak (36) recorded angiomyolipoma in the liver, and Katz and associates (37) noted it in the fallopian tube. These extrarenal lesions tend to present as an abdominal mass, where pain in the mass is associated with intratumoral bleeding, but certainly they can occur without any renal involvement (38). Chen and Bauer (39) reported such an extrarenal lesion in the anterior abdominal wall and reviewed other extrarenal cases, including a lesion in the soft palate.

In the same way that nodal involvement is frequently noted, other organs, such as the spleen, can be involved (40). Apart from the previous observations on multicentricity, metastasis to the spleen is the most excessive rarity in any malignancy.

INVESTIGATION

Pyelography

A patient presenting with a large abdominal mass, pain, and bleeding, with or without hematuria, will usually be investigated by intravenous urography, which classically shows a space-occupying lesion with calyceal distortion (Fig. 21.1). It is vital to inspect the pyelographic findings on the other side because more than one lesion on the ipsilateral kidney and bilateral lesions are commonplace, especially in the phakoma complex. This also applies to patients with polycystic kidneys, Lindau's disease, and neurofibromatosis (12, 15), which may not be classical cases of tuberous sclerosis. It should be borne in mind that while multiple lesions are well documented, they may be entirely hamartoma or polycystic or adenocarcinoma, or all three. In addition to the space-occupying lesion, the films during and before pyelography may show a radiolucency due to the fat content of the hamartoma (41), although the significance of the radiolucency of fat had been earlier noted in a case of retroperitoneal lipoma (42). It cannot be assumed that this radiographic finding is always present, and Becker and associates (43) could only find this sign in 9% of their cases. However, Baron et al (44) found this valuable sign in five of six cases, especially when pyelography was combined with nephrotomography.

Sonography

Sonography of abdominal masses is now commonplace and is mandatory to document space-occupying lesions in the kidney. Pitts and

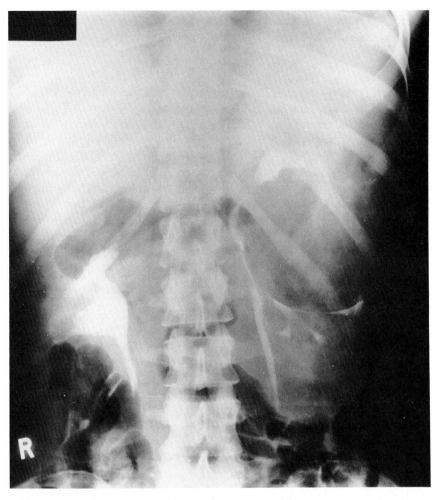

Figure 21.1. Intravenous pyelogram in a patient with tuberous sclerosis. There are space-occupying lesions in both kidneys. Radiolucency is seen in the left kidney.

associates (45) reported an 85% accuracy in diagnosing renal and extrarenal masses, although they did not include hamartomata. They later (46) extended their sonographic experience and pointed out that angiomyolipomata were the most echogenic lesions in over 300 consecutive renal studies. Sonography can therefore only be diagnostic of angiomyolipoma if the hamartoma is predominantly composed of fat, and there is now considerable doubt about whether there is a typical echographic pattern which allows sonography and nephrotomography always to diagnose these lesions (47).

Computerized Axial Tomography (CT)

This facility is not available in every hospital, but its diagnostic value in angiomyolipoma usually augments sonography and may dispense with angiography. There is little dispute that CT is usually diagnostic because of its sensitivity in detecting fat (48), which is not present in renal carcinoma (49). However, the patient presenting with an acute abdomen may be admitted to an institution where CT scanning is not performed or is not available. Despite the continuing claims (usually of radiologists) that angiomyolipoma should be diagnosed accurately pre-operatively, that is seldom the clinical situation. The didactic claims of Pitts et al (46) should be tempered by the clinical fact that this lesion, when it presents with pain, usually has intratumoral bleeding, which may confuse the sonographic or CT findings. This problem is considered by Perry et al (24), who found that the combination of pyelography, sonography, and CT scanning enabled a preoperative diagnosis to be made.

Angiography

This was the standard investigation following pyelography for many years. Love and Frank (50) noted the angiographic findings which were similar to those findings in renal adenocarcinoma. Silbiger and Peterson (51) felt that the multiple arterial aneurysms, well organized early arteriolar network, and late whorled appearances differentiated angio-myolipomata from renal carcinoma with its multiple arteriovenous fistulae (Fig. 21.2). However, they did note that the angiomatous mal-formation in angiomyolipoma was similar to renal carcinoma, in that neither disease demonstrates vasoconstriction from intra-arterial epi-nephrine, and most investigators now believe that the two lesions cannot be differentiated angiographically.

The demonstration of bilateral lesions (Fig. 21.3) raises doubts about a diagnosis of renal carcinoma where a synchronous presentation is a most rare finding, whereas it is common in angiomyolipoma. However, angiography should not be dismissed because therapeutic embolization may be a necessary therapeutic procedure to preserve renal tissue.

MANAGEMENT

The patient with an incidental finding of symptom-free angiomyoli-poma or the patient with asymptomatic tuberous sclerosis should be followed up by ultrasound. The natural history of small lesions is completely unknown.

However, the patient presenting with an abdominal mass, usually localized to one or both kidneys, should be investigated by pyelography, sonography, and, if possible, CT scanning. If these investigations infer a minimal residual renal tissue, then selective angiography and thera-peutic embolization should be considered.

However, if the patient has a large and sometimes expanding intra-renal lesion, then surgical removal is necessary. This surgical removal is usually a radical nephrectomy based on the mistaken diagnosis of renal carcinoma. However, although the lesions should be completely re-moved because of their well known local recurrence after incomplete removal, in fact conservative surgery should be considered (52). Ob-

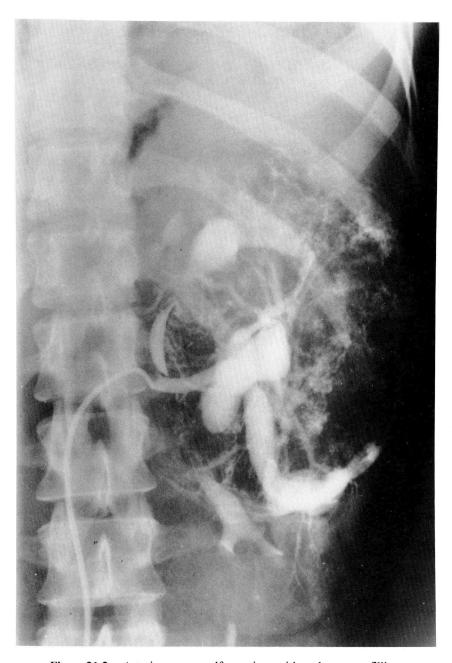

Figure 21.2. Arteriovenous malformations with early venous filling.

viously such a conservative policy must be based on accurate preoperative diagnosis. Attempts to do this by aspiration cytology (53) have been made, and intraoperative biopsy may be necessary before conservative surgery can be recommended (54). As Kaneti and colleagues (54) observed, nearly all cases of symptomatic angiomyolipoma have been treated by nephrectomy. It hardly needs to be emphasized that the use of radiotherapy or chemotherapy is misguided.

326   TUMORS OF THE KIDNEY

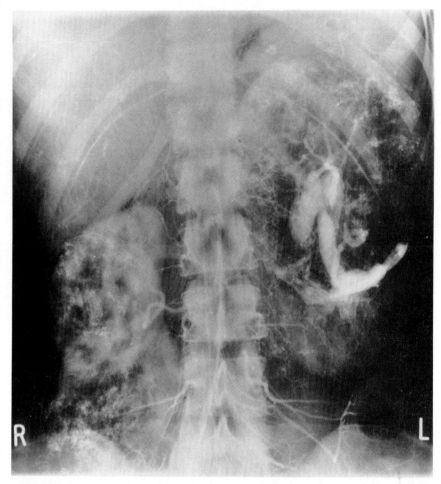

Figure 21.3. Aortogram showing bilateral tumors with considerable replacement of renal parenchyma.

CONCLUSIONS

1. Angiomyolipoma is a hamartoma, usually in the kidney but with occasional extrarenal manifestations.
2. It is said to occur in up to 80% of the phakomas (tuberous sclerosis, etc) but also occurs in other genetically determined conditions.
3. It can occur without these associated conditions.
4. The condition may be an incidental finding or may be symptomatic.
5. The commonest symptomatic presentations are a painful abdominal mass and/or hypovolemic shock and occasionally hematuria.
6. Although there are pyelographic, sonographic, and CT characteristics (55), they are seldom appreciated preoperatively. The angiographic findings are seldom conclusive.
7. The lesions are not neoplastic but are hamartomatous, and no death from metastasis has been recorded.
8. If death occurs from this condition, it is from hemorrhage, renal failure, or the complications of surgery.

9. While radical surgery is frequently performed for symptomatic lesions, conservative surgery or even therapeutic angioinfarction may be considered.
10. Asymptomatic lesions found at the time of donor nephrectomy should be locally excised. Other lesions, if small, may be followed up ultrasonically.

Acknowledgment. Thanks are due to Dr James McIvor, Consultant Radiologist, Charing Cross Hospital London, for the illustrations.

REFERENCES

1. Bourneville DM: Contribution a l'etude de l'idiotie. *Arch Neurol (Chicago)* 1:69–91, 1980.
2. Vasco JS, Brockman SK, Bomar RL: Renal angiomyolipoma—a rare case of spontaneous retroperitoneal hemorrhage. *Ann Surg* 161:577–581, 1965.
3. Farrow GM, Harrison EG, Utz DC, Jones DR: Renal angiomyolipoma. *Cancer* 22:564–570, 1968.
4. Apitz K: Die Geschwulste und Gewebsmiss bildungen der Nierenrinde III. *Virchows Arch* 311:328–359, 1943.
5. Moolton SE: Hamartial nature of tuberous sclerosis complex and its bearing on tumor problems. *Arch Intern Med* 69:589–623, 1942.
6. Critchley M, Earl CJC: Tuberous sclerosis and allied conditions. *Brain* 55:311–346, 1932.
7. Wilson, SAK: *Neurology*, ed 2. Stoneham, MA, Butterworth, 1954, vol 2, p 1031.
8. Udekwu FAO: Renal angiomyolipoma. *Int Surg* 46: 205–214, 1966.
9. Takashi M, Murase T, Yamamoto M, Sobajima T, Miyake K, Mitsuya H, Soma T, Ogisu B, Watanabe J, Ootake H: Angiomyolipoma of the kidney. Report of three cases and a statistical study of 194 cases in Japan. *Hinoyokika Kiyo* 30:65–75, 1984.
10. Noguchi K, Kawakami A, Yoshimura S: Angiomyolipoma—a case report and a statistical study of 147 cases in Japanese literature. *Hinoyokika Kiyo* 29:325–331, 1983.
11. Williams DI, Martin J: In Williams DI, Johnston JH (eds): *Pediatric Urology*, ed 2. Stoneham, MA. Butterworth, 1982, chap 32, p 397.
12. Takeyama M, Arima M, Sagawa S, Sonoda T: Pre-operative diagnosis of coincident renal cell carcinoma and renal angiomyolipoma in non-tuberous sclerosis. *J Urol* 128:579–581, 1982.
13. Silpananta P, Michael RP, Oliver JA: Simultaneous occurrence of angiomyolipoma and renal cell carcinoma. Clinical and pathological (including ultrastructural) features. *Urology* 23:200–204, 1984.
14. Graves N, Barnes WF: Renal cell carcinoma and angiomyolipoma in tuberous sclerosis: case report. *J Urol* 135:122–123, 1986.
15. Lynne CM, Carrion HM, Bakshandeh K, Nadji M, Russel E, Politano VA: Renal angiomyolipoma: polycystic kidney and renal cell carcinoma in a patient with tuberous sclerosis. *Urology* 14:174, 1979.
16. Frimodt Muller PC, Nissen HM, Dryebourg V: Polycystic kidneys as the renal lesion in Lindau's syndrome. *J Urol* 125:868–870, 1981.
17. Olsen S: *Tumours of the Kidney and Urinary Tract.* Copenhagen, Munksgaard, 1984, p 62.
18. Melmon KL, Rosen SW: Lindau's disease. Review of the literature and study of a large kindred. *Am J Med* 36:595, 1964.
19. Van der Hoeve J: Eye symptoms in phakomatoses. *Trans Ophthalmol Soc UK* 52:380, 1932.
20. Gunther M, Penrose LS: The genetics of epiloia. *J Genet* 31:413–430, 1935.
21. Price EB, Mostofi FB: Symptomatic angiomyolipoma. *Cancer* 18:761–774, 1965.
22. MacDougal JA: Renal hamartoma causing intraperitoneal haemorrhage. *Br J Urol* 32:280–281, 1960.
23. Canellas Anoz J, Molino-Trinidad C: Retroperitoneal haemorrhage secondary to a renal angiomyolipoma. *Rev Clin Esp* 172:239–240, 1984.

24. Perry NM, Webb JA, White FE, Whitfield HN: Hemorrhagic angiomyolipoma of the kidney. *J Urol* 132:749–751, 1984.

25. Imai H, Nakamoto Y, Miki K, Miyakuni T, Akihama T, Miura I, Miura A, Tsuburaya T, Harada M: Autopsy case of tuberous sclerosis accompanied by renal failure and systemic angiomyolipoma. *Nippon Naika Gakkai Zasshi* 72:778–783, 1983.

26. Wing AJ, Broyer M, Brunner FP, Brynger H, Challah S, Donkerwolcke RA, Gretz N, Jacobs C, Kramer P, Selwood NH: Combined report on regular dialysis and transplantation in Europe XIII 1982. *Proc Eur Dialy Transplant Assoc* 20:2–75, 1984.

27. Rao PN, Osborn DE, Barnard RJ, Beot JJK: Symptomatic renal angiomyolipoma. *Br J Urol* 53:212–215, 1981.

28. Busch FM, Bark CC, Clyde HR: Benign renal angiomyolipoma with regional lymph node involvement. *J Urol* 116:715–717, 1976.

29. Fernandez Larranga A, Nacariino Corbacho L, Uson-Calvo A: Renal angiomyolipoma and simultaneous involvement of regional lymph nodes—multicentric origin or metastases? *Acta Urol Esp* 8:155–156, 1984.

30. Bloom DA, Scardino PT, Ehrlich RM, Waisman J: The significance of lymph nodal involvement in renal angiomyolipoma. *J Urol* 128:1292–1295, 1982.

31. Schujman E, Meiraz D, Liban E, Servadio C: Mixed reno-medullary tumour: renal cell carcinoma associated with angiomyolipoma. *Urology* 17:375, 1981.

32. Allen TD, Risk W: Renal angiomyolipoma. *J Urol* 94:203, 1965.

33. Burkitt R: Fatal haemorrhage into perirenal liposarcoma. *Br J Surg* 36:439, 1949.

34. Berg JW: Angiolipomyosarcoma of the kidney. *Cancer* 8:759–763, 1955.

35. Kutcher R, Rosenblatt R, Mibudo SM, Goldman M, Kogan S: Renal angiomyolipoma with sonographic demonstration of extension into the inferior vena cava. *Radiology* 143:755–756, 1982.

36. Goodman ZD, Ishak, KG: Angiomyolipoma of the liver. *Am J Surg Pathol* 8:745–750, 1984.

37. Katz DA, Thom D, Bogard P, Dermer MS: Angiomyolipoma of the fallopian tube. *Am J Obstet Gynecol* 148:341–343, 1984.

38. Friis J, Hjorstrup A: Extra-renal angiomyolipoma. Diagnosis and management. *J Urol* 127:528–529, 1982.

39. Chen KTK, Bauer V: Extra-renal angiomyolipoma. *J Surg Oncol* 25:89–91, 1984.

40. Hulbert JC, Graf R: Involvement of the spleen by renal angiomyolipoma: metastasis or multicentricity? *J Urol* 130:328–329, 1983.

41. Crosett AD: Roentgenographic findings in the renal lesion of tuberous sclerosis. *AJR* 98:739, 1966.

42. Windholz F: Roentgen diagnosis of retroperitoneal lipoma. *AJR* 56:594, 1946.

43. Becker JA, Kinghabwalla M, Pollack H, Bosniak M: Angiomyolipoma (Hamartoma) of the kidney. An angiographic review. *Acta Radiol Diagn* 14:561, 1973.

44. Baron M, Leiter E, Brendler H: Preoperative diagnosis of renal angiomyolipoma. *J Urol* 117:701–703, 1977.

45. Pitts WR, Kazam E, Gershowitz M, Muecke E: A review of 100 renal and perinephric sonograms with anatomical diagnosis. *J Urol* 114:21–26, 1975.

46. Pitts WR, Kazam E, Gray G, Vaughan ED: Ultrasonography, computerised transaxial tomography and pathology of angiomyolipoma. Solution to a diagnostic dilemma. *J Urol* 124:907–909, 1980.

47. Volterrani L, Cappaccioli L, Ferrari F: Renal angiomyolipoma: is there a typical echographic aspect? *Radiol Med (Torino)* 68:123–125, 1982.

48. Bosniak MA: Angiomyolipoma (hamartoma) of the kidney: a pre-operative diagnosis is possible in virtually every case. *Urol Radiol* 3:135, 1981.

49. Sagel SS, Stanley RJ, Levitt RG, Geisse G: Computed tomography of the kidney. *Radiology* 124:359, 1977.

50. Love L, Frank SJ: Angiographic features of angiomyolipoma of the kidney. *AJR* 95:406–408, 1965.

51. Sibiger M, Peterson CC: Renal angiomyolipoma. Its distinctive angiographic characteristics. *J Urol* 106:363–365, 1971.

52. McQueeny AJ, Dahlen GA, Gebhart WF: Cystic hamartoma (angiomyolipoma) of kidney simulating renal carcinoma. *J Urol* 92:98, 1964.

53. Gleuthoj A, Partoft S: Ultrasounded percutaneous aspiration of renal angiomyoli-

poma. Report of two cases diagnosed by cytology. *Acta Cytol (Baltimore)* 28:265–268, 1984.
54. Kaneti J, Kruguak K, Hirsh M, Glickman L: Rupture of renal angiomyolipoma: conservative surgery. *J Urol* 129:810–811, 1983.
55. Bush WH, Freemy PC, Orme BM: Angiomyolipoma: characteristic images by ultrasound and computerised tomography. *Urology* 14:531, 1979.

Index

Page numbers in *italics* denote figures; those followed by "t" denote tables.

Insulin, 52, 62–63
INT vital stain, 263, 268
Interferon, 278
α-Interferon, 276
　activity in subrenal capsule assay, 248*t*
　DNA precursor assay results, 250*t*
Interleukin-2, 276, 278
Intracranial pressure, elevated secondary to cerebral
　　metastases, 52
Intravenous pyelography
　of adenocarcinoma, *159, 161*
　of enucleative surgery for pseudocapsule, *167*
　of hemangiomas, 299
　of solitary kidney with RCC, *129*
　of synchronous bilateral renal cell carcinoma, *151*
　postoperative, *134, 135*
　preoperative, 113–114
Intravenous urography, 15*t*
Iron, metabolic disorders of, 64
Isoantigens, blood group, prognostic value in RCC, 34

Juxtaglomerular cell tumors
　benign, 298*t*, 299–300
　malignant form (hemangiopericytomas), 298*t*, 302, 303

Kidney(s)
　left
　　carcinoma, control of inferior vena cava and, 103
　　lymphadenectomy procedure for tumors, 83–84
　　normal lymphatic drainage, 77, *78*
　　regional lymphatic drainage, 92–93
　lymphatic drainage, normal, 75–77, *78*
　　regional, 90–93
　right
　　lymphadenectomy procedure for tumors, *83*
　　normal lymphatic drainage, 76–77
　　regional lymphatic drainage, 91–92
　space-occupying lesions of (*see* Mass lesions)
　vascular supply, *117*
　venous drainage, collateral, 114–*115*
Kocher maneuver, 116

Lactate dehydrogenase-isoenzyme, 229
Langenbeck maneuver, 117, *118, 119, 120*
Laterality, of oncocytoma, 311–312*t*
Leiomyomas, 300, 302, 303
Leiomyosarcomas, 302
Ligaments, anatomic relationship to vena cava, *118, 119*
Lipomas, 301–302
Lipomatosis, sinusal, 4
Liposarcomas, 302, 303
Liver
　anatomic relationship to vena cava, 118, *119*
　function tests, 114
　metastases, surgical excision, 197
　nonmetastatic dysfunction, 54–55
Lung metastases, surgical excision, 196
Lymph nodes
　assessment by CT, 8–9
　drainage, of kidney, *78*
　involvement of (*see* Metastases, lymph node)
　regional, for renal cell carcinoma, 82
Lymphadenectomy
　extensive, 87
　　long-term survival, 80–81*t*
　　occurrence of metastases following, 79–80*t*
　for adenocarcinoma, 75–85

for renal cell carcinoma, 87–*95*
　recommendations, 95
　recommended approach, 82–*84*
morbidity and mortality, 81–82
regional, 87
　extent of, 93–*95*
　long-term survival, 80–81*t*
　survival rates and, 89–90
transperitoneal with subcostal xyphoumbilical flap,
　　82–*84*
with radical nephrectomy, 75
Lymphangiomas, 300
Lymphatic drainage
　of kidneys, normal, 75–76
　left, 77
　right, 76–77
Lymphatic metastases, 84–85
Lymphocytes, thymus-derived, 230
Lymphokines, 276

Magnetic resonance imaging, 12
　of venous dissemination, 101–102
Mainz University clinical trial
　patients and methodology, 283*t*
　preparation of vaccine, 283
　results, 285–*286*
　treatment protocol, 283–*284*
Mass lesions, 310, 316
　asymptomatic
　　assessment approach, current, 11–22
　　assessment, cost-effective approach, 22, 24–32*t*
　　confidence level of diagnosis, 12, 15–22
　　diagnostic assessment pathway for lesions discovered
　　　by CT, 13*t*
　　diagnostic assessment pathway for lesions discovered
　　　by IVU, 14*t*
　　etiologic composition, 15*t*
　　incidence, 25*t*
　　number diagnosed as benign by various techniques,
　　　26*t*
　　with cystic characteristics, 12, 13*t*
　　with solid tumor characteristics, 12, 13*t*
　benign tumors, diagnosis of, 17–18, 26*t*
　determination between cystic and solid, by intravenous
　　urography, 4
　inflammatory, number diagnosed after discovery by CT
　　and IVU, 26*t*
　vascular, diagnosis of, 20–21
Mayo Clinic, Urology Research Laboratory
　investigations in Urology Research Laboratory, 258
　soft agar colony forming assay studies, 259–260
Medroxyprogesterone acetate (MPA)
　adjuvant treatment, 218–219
　clinical experience, 214
　experimental data, 209
　inhibition of receptor binding, 213
　for metastatic disease, 190, 191
　therapeutic dosage, 215
　therapeutic trials, 198*t*
Megestrol acetate, therapy for advanced RCC, 214*t*
Mesenchymal nodules, mixed, 302
Mesenchymal tumors
　benign, 298*t*
　　fibromas, 297–298*t*
　leiomyomas, 300–301
　malignant, 298*t*, 302–304